THE
T-FACTOR
2000
DIET

THE
T-FACTOR
2000
DIET

MARTIN KATAHN, PH.D.

WITH JAMIE POPE, M.S., R.D.

W. W. NORTON & COMPANY

NEW YORK / LONDON

For information about permission to reproduce selections from this book, write to Permissions, W. W. Norton & Company, Inc., 500 Fifth Avenue, New York, NY 10110

The text of this book is composed in ITC Garamond Light
with the display set in Futura Light
Composition by Allentown Digital Services Division of R.R. Donnelley & Sons Company
Manufacturing by Haddon Craftsmen, Inc.
Book design by JAM Design

Library of Congress Cataloging-in-Publication Data

Katahn, Martin.
The T-factor 2000 diet / Martin Katahn, with Jamie Pope.
p.   cm.
First ed. published under title: The T-factor diet. New York :
Norton, 1989.
Includes bibliographical references and index.
ISBN 0-393-04724-5
1. Low-fat diet. 2. Reducing diets. I. Pope, Jamie.
II. Katahn, Martin. The T-factor diet. III. Title.
RM237.7.K38   1999
613.2'5—dc21 99-13380
CIP

W. W. Norton & Company, Inc., 500 Fifth Avenue, New York, N.Y. 10100
www.wwnorton.com

W. W. Norton & Company Ltd., 10 Coptic Street, London WC1A 1PU

1 2 3 4 5 6 7 8 9 0

To Gordon Kaplan, Ph.D., who, after losing 100 pounds,
recruited me to chair his dissertation committee
and designed the research study that led to the creation
of the Vanderbilt Weight Management Program.

Contents

Acknowledgments

Many people, including colleagues, friends, and formerly overweight individuals, have made significant contributions to this book. I would like to express my appreciation to:

Jamie Pope, M.S., R.D., for writing the chapter on childhood nutrition, taking major responsibility for developing the Fat Gram Counter, reading that part of the manuscript for which I had primary responsibility and suggesting ways in which I might make complex concepts more understandable to nonprofessional readers, inviting me as guest lecturer to the ongoing Vanderbilt Weight Management classes where we could introduce and discuss these new ideas and help participants put them into practice, designing the basic menus, developing many of the recipes, and analyzing nutrient values for all of them.

James O. Hill, Ph.D., professor of pediatrics and medicine at the University of Colorado Health Sciences Center, for checking my understanding of the complex biochemical and physiological processes that led to the formation of the Second Law of Energy Balance (any errors that remain in my explanation and illustrations are, of course, my responsibility) and arranging my interviews with successful participants in the National Weight Control Registry.

Enid Katahn for undying love and forbearance when my eyes glaze over as my mind becomes preoccupied with planning my day's work and she has to say "Hello? Hello?" to try to get me back on line, and for the many hours she spent devising, testing, and retesting nearly 100 recipes during the months I was writing this book.

Dikkie Schoggen for three of the recipes in this book that I consider to be among the best.

ESHA Research for the Food Processor for Windows, Nutrition Analysis and Fitness Software, which supplies the program we use to analyze our menus and recipes and especially to the technical staff at ESHA Research who have always been so helpful whenever we had a question during the dozen or so years we have used the program.

The participants in the National Weight Control Registry and the Vanderbilt Weight Management Program (their names have been changed to protect their privacy) for their insights and inspiration that they shared with me in the hope of helping others become as successful in managing their weight as they have been.

Starling Lawrence, editor in chief at W. W. Norton, with whom I have worked closely for eighteen years and twelve books going on thirteen, for making it his business to know as much about the field I work in as possible, which in turn has enabled him to hound me until I find ways to explain difficult scientific concepts so that persons outside the field will be able to understand them more easily.

Artie and Richard Pine, my literary agents for the past eighteen years, for believing in me and taking me on as one of their authors when I wrote to them in 1981 after having had my first book turned down by all six publishers to whom I had sent it on my own, but even more for the warm friendship and enthusiasm for my work that has developed over these years.

All of my other friends and helpers at W. W. Norton: associate editor Patricia Chui, managing editor Nancy Palmquist, copy editor Janet Byrne, director of manufacturing Andrew Marasia, corporate art director Debra Morton Hoyt, and publicist Holly Watson.

Dona Haywood, close friend from the first days of my arrival in Nashville thirty-seven years ago, to whom I have always turned to put everything else in her life on hold in order to transcribe, proofread, or do any other editing task that needed doing on a moment's notice.

Ed Porter and the entire technical staff of Info Computer, Joel Cipriano, Jonathan Eby, Richard McClellan, Kollins Bull, and Jeffery Kodsyz, for the design and maintenance of my home and office computing needs, especially at this time to Jeffery, who came to my rescue immediately when the power supply to the computer I was using to write the last page of this book went down and the monitor developed a glitch at the same time.

Again, thank you all very much.

THE
T-FACTOR
2000
DIET

Introduction

If you are an overweight person who has picked up this book to see if *The T-Factor 2000 Diet* can help you lose weight and keep it off, I imagine this may not be the first time you have tried to do this. I suspect that you already know one thing from your past experience:

Losing weight is hard enough, but keeping it off is a **very** hard thing to do!

If you haven't found the way to permanent weight management, you are one of a vast majority. Every year between 80 and 100 million people in the United States, about two-thirds of them women, go on a weight-loss diet. About 95 percent of them ultimately fail to reach and maintain their goal or, in fact, come anywhere near it. Sooner or later, they end up right back where they started or even fatter.

No other change in personal habits has this high a failure rate—not quitting smoking, nor defeating a drug or alcohol addiction. If you look at all the other things that you've accomplished in your lifetime, I think you will admit that losing weight and *keeping it off* has been one of the most difficult and frustrating things you have ever tried to do. And when you look at that failure rate, it seems that you have to be a hero to succeed!

But it doesn't have to be that way. Look at the flip side of that statistic. **Five percent of the people who try to lose weight and keep it off *do succeed!***

My goal in *The T-Factor 2000 Diet* is to show you what these successful people are doing, because, as extensive research over many years with more than 3000 persons *who have been successful* proves:

> *one way or another, successful people have discovered and continue to follow the weight-management principles that were introduced in the original T-Factor Diet ten years ago.**

While successful people demonstrate that you can *lose* weight on any reduced-calorie diet, when it comes to keeping it off, *permanent weight management requires that you make a permanent reduction in the fat content of your diet.*

According to their reports, successful people have, on the average, reduced fat to just under 25 percent of total calories. This is precisely the reduction that our subjects made in the original research in the Vanderbilt Weight Management Program back in 1987 and 1988, and which led to the publication of *The T-Factor Diet* in 1989. While virtually all successful people either cut out or severely limit certain high-fat foods or methods of preparation that use a great deal of fat (for example fried foods) about one-third of them, even years after losing weight, continue to count fat grams! Counting fat grams, the strategy popularized in *The T-Factor Diet,* is the simplest and most effective way to lose real fat weight, not water, and to make sure you don't outeat your energy needs and begin to slide back into your old fat eating habits when you reach your goal. Of course, I hope that once you find the low-fat foods you like you won't need to continue counting. But the fact that so many successful people continue to use that strategy certainly proves its utility.

SO WHY DO WE NEED A NEW T-FACTOR DIET?

In the original *T-Factor Diet* I explained the biochemical basis of obesity as it was known at that time. The research on which it was based had not yet been translated into the practical treatment of obe-

---

*In order not to interrupt the narrative, I review in considerable depth the research studies on which my conclusions are based in Appendix A. Interested readers will also find an extensive bibliography at the end of Appendix A. In the present instance I am referring to the findings of the National Weight Control Registry, an ongoing project at the Universities of Colorado and Pittsburgh.

sity. This research disclosed that the calories in protein, carbohydrate, and fat are not equally accessible to the human body for use and storage. Before the energy from these different sources ends up as fuel to power your basal metabolic functions and physical activity, it is processed and stored in different ways.

Today we know a great deal more about how the differences between nutrients can critically affect your weight. This new knowledge clearly indicates the kind of diet and physical activity that can lead to permanent weight management. I want to show you what you need to do to put this new knowledge to work for you. Here are a few of the key points that I will discuss later in this book.

PROTEIN, CARBOHYDRATE, AND FAT HAVE DIFFERENT EFFECTS ON YOUR APPETITE

We now know that all of the nutrients that supply energy to your body—carbohydrate, protein, and fat—differ in the strength of the physiological signals they produce, which in turn stimulate or "turn on" your appetite when you are eating. They also differ in the strength of their opposing physiological signals that stop further food consumption when you have had enough to eat. These are the signals that prevent you from going into positive energy balance— that is, gaining weight. If, looking at your diet in general, the physiological signals from the foods you eat that "turn on" your appetite remain stronger at energy balance than the signals generated by the foods that "turn off" your appetite, you will take in more calories than you can burn, which means, of course, that you will gain weight. You need to construct a diet where the turn-off signals become greater than the turn-on signals when you have reached energy balance. Most biochemists and physiologists studying obesity now believe that this is the dietary key to success in permanent weight management.

THERE'S A NEW LAW OF ENERGY BALANCE

We now know that, for your weight to become stabilized at a given level where you are neither gaining nor losing, there is more to consider than the familiar First Law of Energy Balance, which is expressed in mathematical form as:

$$\text{Energy in} = \text{Energy out}$$

New discoveries indicate stabilized weight requires that your intake of protein, carbohydrate, and fat each considered separately must be in balance with the amount of each that you burn. It's called the Second Law of Energy Balance. Weight stability requires that:

$$\text{Protein in} = \text{Protein out}$$
$$\text{Carbohydrate in} = \text{Carbohydrate out}$$
$$\text{Fat in} = \text{Fat out}$$

Now, what does this mean for you?

However many calories in protein or carbohydrate you eat each day, the body finds a way to burn them all up!

That is, the body quickly and automatically begins to adjust the protein-out and carbohydrate-out sides of the first two equations so that however much you eat of carbohydrate and protein, you adjust your fuel mixture and burn up virtually all the carbohydrate and protein calories. So, however many calories you consume of carbohydrate and protein, you burn all you eat.

This is not true for fat. Fat is handled in a different way.

The way the body adjusts the fat-out side of the equation to the fat-in side to arrive at a stable weight is not by quickly adjusting how much it burns in its fuel mixture, as it does with protein and carbohydrate. Instead, it simply puts fat calories into storage if you eat too many of them—or takes them out of storage if you aren't eating enough fat to maintain the present size of your fat stores. Whereas carbohydrate and protein burning go up and down according to how much carbohydrate and protein you eat, it's your body fat *and not fat burning* that goes up and down according to how much fat you eat. This is extremely important for you to understand. To paraphrase Jean Pierre Flatt, a scientist in the Department of Biochemistry and Molecular Biology at the University of Massachusetts Medical Center and one of the pioneers in the field of obesity research,

within the boundaries set by your heredity and certain lifestyle factors such as the amount of physical activity in your daily life, *the fat content of your body is adjusted to the fat content of your diet.*

As fantastic as this may sound, here's an example of how it can work. If at some point in your life you gradually gained about 22 pounds of body fat, it was the result of eating an average of about 20 grams of fat more each day than you were able to burn in your fuel mixture. On average, it takes about 22 pounds of body fat to promote the burning of 20 grams of fat in the body's fuel mixture! Want to peel off those 22 pounds? Hold your protein and carbohydrate consumption constant and just cut the fat in your diet by about 20 grams a day! Just as you gained weight gradually over time, you will now lose it gradually over time.

Now, before going on, let's be clear on one point. It's not the conversion to fat of the carbohydrate you eat that makes you fat (as some diet writers who have not kept up with the latest research in biochemistry continue to claim). When it comes to carbohydrate, what you eat is what you burn. Except under certain extreme conditions not likely to be seen in everyday life (such as when research subjects consume a surplus of 1500 carbohydrate calories every day for several days over and above their energy needs), carbohydrate *is not* converted to fat for storage.

Carbohydrate counts, though, in an important, if indirect, way.

By eating excessive amounts of carbohydrate you can actually stop your body's ability to burn fat *dead in its tracks!* It will simply stop using the fat from the other foods you eat (meat, dairy products, etc.) for fuel! Research shows, however, that this is unlikely to happen as long as you stick with unprocessed, naturally occurring carbohydrate foods such as fruits, vegetables, and whole grains (including minimally processed whole-grain breads and cereals). These are "good carbohydrates." With good carbohydrates (you'll find an extensive list in Chapter 4) you can eat all you want because these foods generate turn-off signals to your appetite before you have eaten so much that they can suppress your body's ability to burn fat.

But there is a new villain in town.

It's those "imitation," highly processed *fat-free* desserts, pastries, snack foods, and candies!

Yes, modern *junk*-food science has found a way to outwit Mother Nature by creating new kinds of foods with a taste and texture that mimic the original full-fat versions. In the past, it has been virtually impossible to consume too much carbohydrate in unrefined natural form—fresh fruits, vegetables, and grains—because, as I just said, unrefined natural carbohydrates generate physiological signals in which "turn off is greater than turn on" when you reach energy balance. In the past, you could only consume too much carbohydrate by adding fat to carbohydrate foods.

Now, for the first time in human history, it has become easy to outeat your caloric needs with new kinds of carbohydrate foods: the artificially created, refined carbohydrate foods made to taste *as if they contain fat*. These imitations are really fake foods because they have very little nutritional value except for calories. They are marketed by an industry that claims they are healthful and good for you because they are fat-free. I believe that no harm was originally intended in their creation, because just about everyone, including most nutrition experts, thought they would prove to be a boon to persons who wanted to reduce the fat in their diets. It just hasn't worked out that way!

Imitation fat-free foods are "energy dense," which means that they contain far more calories per unit of weight or volume than unrefined natural carbohydrates. In fact, along with the taste and texture of fat, they often contain just as many calories as the high-fat foods they were designed to replace. The calories come from sugar and refined flours, artfully blended with various gums and forms of lipid that do not, by law, have to be counted as fat, although they do contain fatty acids.

Because these foods simulate the taste and texture of fat, they can turn on your appetite just like the real thing. You can outeat your needs for carbohydrate with these imitation foods because they do not generate turn-off signals when you have reached energy balance. Perhaps an example will make this even more clear. A medium-size (5-ounce) apple contains about 80 calories; 5 ounces of a fat-free apple streusel or crumb cake will contain 300 or more calories. Obviously, you are much more likely to take in excess calories consuming fat-free apple streusel than you are by eating fresh apples.

Remember that the body quickly adjusts to burn the carbohydrate you eat each day. When you eat too much of it, it may suppress fat burning so that the fat in other foods goes into your fat cells. When you eat a low-fat diet, there is no danger of this happening from "good carbohydrates." With a healthful low-fat diet, you simply can't eat enough fruits, vegetables, and whole grains unless you add fat to them. This is not so with the energy-dense, "bad" carbohydrates I am referring to. There's a similar if not greater problem with *reduced*-fat foods in the dessert, pastry, and snack categories. Because they can do an even better job than the fat-free products of approaching the taste and texture of the original foods they were designed to replace, they may encourage you to overeat to an even greater extent.

I'll explain what you need to do if you wish to include any of these foods in your diet in Chapter 4. In essence, you need to think of them as though they actually contain the fat that has been re-placed with sugar and other artificial ingredients that simulate the taste of fat. Better yet, read the opinions that successful people have about these fat-free foods and what they have done about them in their quest for success in Chapters 2 and 11. You may just want to eliminate them from your diet altogether!

YOU HAVE A FAT-CONSUMPTION THRESHOLD

We now know that there is a certain threshold for fat consumption, determined in part by your heredity and in part by your lifestyle. When you go above that threshold in your fat consumption, you gain weight. Go below it, you lose weight.

The fat-consumption threshold is influenced to a large extent by the amount of physical activity in your daily life as well as by the ratio of carbohydrate to fat in your diet. As I just explained, exces-sive consumption of carbohydrate can suppress your body's ability to burn fat in its fuel mixture. Research on people who have lost a significant amount of weight and have been able to maintain their losses for many years indicates that the average fat-consumption threshold is around 25 percent of total calories. But their success also involves a significant increase in physical activity. As you will see, the amount of fat that you can consume and not gain weight is di-rectly related to the level of physical activity in your daily life.

Remember my illustration of how 22 pounds of fat weight may be gained by beginning to eat an average of 20 grams of fat more than you burn each day? Walking around at a moderate pace for be-tween forty minutes and an hour burns about 20 grams of fat (the exact amount of time will depend to a great extent on your weight and how fast you walk). That's why one expert pointed out that you have a choice. On the one hand, out of the total fat you eat each day, about 20 grams will be burned as a result of having stored an extra 22 pounds of fat on your body. On the other hand, you can take a walk for forty to sixty minutes every day, burn 20 grams of fat in that activity, and in time end up weighing about 22 pounds less.

And there is one thing more that you must understand about your fat-consumption threshold that is not appreciated by many health professionals. Weight gain is not always achieved (nor is obesity maintained) by eating too much fat spread evenly over time in your daily diet. In fact, recent research suggests that *eating too much fat in just one or two meals each week may be the culprit.* That one festive meal, that one visit to the Sunday brunch buffet, where people often eat 80 to 120 grams of fat in one meal without realizing it, can do it. Whether you are just 10 pounds overweight or 50, you may be maintaining that extra fat weight with just one or two such meals a week!

Every extra fat gram that you eat and don't burn off in your fuel mixture is going to stay put in your fat cells. Your body does not make an automatic adjustment and compensate for the extra fat when you have a high-fat meal. You must make a conscious effort to compensate—by cutting back on fat in future meals, increasing your physical activity, or both. As you will see in Chapter 11, people who have lost significant amounts of weight have learned the truth of this statement. Most successful people do deviate from their basic low-fat diets on occasion. They do not deny themselves a delicious high-fat dessert or a complete festive meal, but they take corrective action before it can put their success in danger.

HEREDITY PLAYS AN IMPORTANT ROLE IN THE DEVELOPMENT OF OBESITY

We now know that there are at least a dozen hereditary factors that can influence your predisposition to obesity. However, *except in the tiny fraction of cases in which severe endocrine abnormalities exist,* the hereditary factors are much less important than environmental conditions and the personal behaviors that are a response to these environmental conditions. From a dietary standpoint, the obesity genes can take over when a person is surrounded every day, day in and day out, with a great variety of easily available, highly palatable foods. Under these conditions, the unfortunate obesity-prone individual must find ways to constantly restrain his appetite. He will always need to exercise restraint as long as he is faced with foods in which the turn-on signals to eat and continue to keep on eating remain stronger than the turn-off signals at the point when consumption has already equaled energy needs.

LET'S GET THE ROLE OF INSULIN AND OBESITY STRAIGHT

Many fad diet writers are dispensing inaccurate information about the role of insulin in obesity and suggesting high-protein/high-fat diets that in the long run may prove dangerous. It's not an overactive insulin response to carbohydrate that makes most people fat. It's the other way around. *Eating more fat than your body can burn each day and lack of physical activity make people fat.* Although hereditary factors are sometimes involved and some people are hyperinsulinemic without being fat, in the case of overweight persons, it's obesity that leads to hyperinsulinemia (overproduction of insulin) and insulin resistance. The final outcome can be noninsulin-dependent diabetes mellitus (NIDDM). And it's a fact that between 80 to 90 percent of the people who do end up with NIDDM (sometimes called Type II or adult-onset diabetes) as a result of obesity can normalize their insulin and glycemic responses to carbohydrate by simply *losing weight and increasing daily physical activity.*

If you suffer from NIDDM and if treatment already requires medication, the T-Factor 2000 Diet is likely to help you reduce your need for that medication, if not dispense with it altogether. Of course, since diabetic diets must be individually designed to suit differing needs, you must show *The T-Factor 2000 Diet* to your doctor before you make any changes. Point out the special section for diabetics on the role of high-fiber carbohydrates and an increase in monounsaturated fatty acids in the regulation of glucose, insulin, and lipid levels in Appendix C, and see if he doesn't agree!

But for now, here is some serious advice:

If you have a single close relative with diabetes, there is an increased likelihood that you, too, may have inherited a familial disposition to diabetes. the T-Factor 2000 Diet is an effective diabetes prevention program. You need to be on such a program right now!

THE BIGGEST, FATTEST LIE OF THE 1990s

Before you continue with what you can expect to find in *The T-Factor 2000 Diet,* I need to correct a serious misconception about fat consumption in the United States.

Many authors of high-protein/high-fat weight-loss diets have disputed the fact that too much fat in the American diet is the major cause of obesity in this country. They point to recent data from the National Health and Nutrition Examination Survey (NHANES III, 1993) indicating that the percent of calories from fat in the American diet has gone down since a decade or two ago. According to the report, it has gone down from 37 percent of total calories to only 34 percent. But we as a nation are getting fatter! How can the population be getting fatter while, as these writers put it, "fat consumption is going down" if too much fat in the diet is the nutrient primarily responsible for obesity?

Well, it's true, unfortunately, that Americans are fatter today than ever before. Except for a few islands in the Pacific, we are the fattest nation in the world. Fifty-four percent of the population is overweight, and 33 percent of us are downright obese, up from only 25 percent a decade ago. Those figures don't lie! The people who participated in the study were weighed in person on extremely accurate scales.

But it is not true that we are eating less fat.

WE ARE EATING MORE FAT THAN EVER BEFORE!

I can understand how journalists may often lack the time to investigate the original research, and I can understand how the news media only quote what appear to be the highlights of an expert's statements about the study. What I don't understand is how any professionally trained person can make the statement that fat consumption has gone down in the United States. It hasn't, but it can be made to look that way.

All you have to do is take a look at the figures, and you will see that the conclusion depends on which statistic you choose to focus your attention on. In an absolute sense, weight in grams each day, the data in NHANES III indicate that we are, in fact, *eating more fat.*

But we also report eating many more calories. Comparing the 1970s with 1993, per-day consumption of fat by women went up, from 62.5 grams to 69 grams (562.5 calories to 621 calories), while total calories increased, from 1531 to 1831.

$$562.5/1531 = .37 \text{ or } 37 \text{ percent}$$
$$621/1831 = .34 \text{ or } 34 \text{ percent}$$

Similarly, for men, comparing the 1970s with 1993, the reported per-day consumption of fat went from 101.5 to 105.4 grams (913.5 calories to 948.6 calories), while total calories increased, from 2457 to 2751.

$$913.5/2457 = .37 \text{ or } 37 \text{ percent}$$
$$948.6/2751 = .34 \text{ or } 34 \text{ percent}$$

So, while we report eating more fat, because we report eating so many more calories than were reported in previous National Health and Nutrition Examination Surveys, *the proportion of fat, relative to the total, has gone down.*

What's even worse than the misrepresentation of data is that what people report they eat has little to do with what they really eat. The data are faulty to begin with!

Numerous articles have appeared in the scientific literature in an effort to correct the misinterpretation of government dietary surveys that are presented to the public in the media and by fad diet writers. These and many other studies have also pointed out that people seriously underreport both total calories and fat intake on all surveys. The underreporting of calories runs an average of only about 10 percent among persons who are not overweight, but it runs an astonishing 30 percent to 55 percent among the overweight. Most of the underreporting of calories is due to underreporting fat in the diet, **and over half the population of the United States is overweight. With over half the population overweight, and with this half underreporting their food consumption by 30 percent or more, think of what this does to the data.** Indeed, the underreporting is so great that in many surveys of eating habits a large percentage of the respondents would not be able to sustain basal metabolic processes and obtain the energy required in sedentary activities if they actually ate what they claim to eat!*

---

*Fortunately, average caloric needs for a given height and weight can be calculated scientifically, and persons with such extreme deviations from what would be necessary to keep them alive and engaging in sedentary activity are usually eliminated from the research.

If someone attempts to convince you that overconsumption of fat is not the most dangerous feature of the American diet because of its relationship to obesity, heart disease, certain cancers, plus a host of other ills, and if that same person makes dietary recommendations that fail to include a reduction of your fat intake, then he or she is doing you a serious disservice.

MAKE THE "T" IN T-FACTOR YOUR "THIN" FACTOR

The "T" was chosen as part of the title of the original T-Factor Diet because it stands for two processes involved in your metabolism: *thermogenesis,* and the *thermic* effects of food and exercise. Both words are of Greek origin, *therme* meaning heat, and *gignesthai* meaning to be born (the Greek word became *genesis* in Latin). As applied in fields such as nutrition, physiology, and biochemistry, thermogenesis refers to the heat created as a byproduct as your body carries out all of the metabolic processes necessary to stay alive (for example, circulation of blood, digestion, breathing) and physical activity. Just like an automobile engine, which heats up as it generates the energy to turn the wheels on a car, so the body heats up as it does its work. Thermogenesis accounts for the burning of about 75 percent of the energy contained in the food you eat each day. Only 25 percent is put directly to use in basal metabolic processes and physical activity. In engineering terms, the human body is only 25 percent efficient. In terms of weight management, this suggests that (unlike what you want in your car's motor) the more heat you generate, the easier it is to manage your weight. *The T-Factor 2000 Diet* shows you how to increase thermogenesis, which means simply how to burn extra calories and prevent them from ending up in your fat cells.

The *thermic effect of food* refers specifically to the energy it takes to eat and digest your food, and to get its nutrients circulating in your bloodstream to their specific target areas. Typically, it takes the energy equivalent of about 10 percent of the calories in each meal to do this work. Many overweight people experience a deficit in the thermic effect of food. They may spend as little as 4 percent of calories getting this work done (about 30 calories less than normal after a 500-calorie meal). This, in turn, means that these calories are left over for other functions, including storage in your fat depots. In a single day, a deficit in the thermic effect of food can add up to over 100 surplus calories. The thermic effect of food is greater in active people, and the thermic effect of a high-carbohydrate diet is greater than that of a high-fat diet, especially after weight loss. By magnifying the thermic effect of food via a high-carbohydrate diet, you may be able to consume over 100 calories more each day without having it relegated to your fat depots, as it may have been in the past.

The *thermic effect of exercise* refers to both the additional energy used during exercise in comparison with the resting state and the additional energy that is used in the hours following exercise as the body repairs and regenerates tissue. The thermic effect of exercise can equal hundreds of calories during and following an hour's worth of physical activity each day. The activity does not have to be done all at once. Benefits are obtained even if the activity is done five to ten minutes at a time. All kinds of activity that are equivalent to a brisk walk confer a number of other benefits in addition to burning calories. These include better control over blood glucose, glycogen storage, insulin secretion, and blood lipids, which I'll discuss in Chapter 9. Every research study on weight management shows that the thermic effects and other benefits of exercise can play an important role in magnifying your success in losing weight and a *key* role in preventing the pounds from creeping back afterwards.

There is one other thermic effect that becomes important under certain circumstances: *adaptive thermogenesis*. This refers to the body's ability to either waste or conserve energy. You probably already know that metabolism slows during periods of starvation in the interests of prolonging life. It can also speed up to burn surplus calories in the case of drastic overconsumption, as you will see in one of the studies quoted later in this book.

The T-Factor 2000 Diet will show you how to put these important thermic effects to work for you. But there is much more to the T-Factor 2000 Diet program than its valuable impact on thermogenesis and the thermic effects of exercise. It's a complete enabling program that shows you, as you greet the millennium, how to deal successfully with every factor that has so far kept you out of the ranks of those who win the struggle with obesity.

HERE IS WHAT TO EXPECT

The scientific background. I want you to understand the scientific background of the T-Factor 2000 Diet. Knowledge is power. Once you understand the scientific background, and see that successful people, in spite of all the many predisposing genetic factors, and sometimes without even knowing it, are following T-Factor principles, you will be committed and motivated enough to succeed. I will summarize the scientific background in the next two chapters. A full discussion of the research, with references, will be found in Appendix A.

Successful weight management requires more than just going on a diet. The day-to-day directions for how to put the T-Factor 2000 Diet into practice follow in the next several chapters. I'll start with the important preparations you must make *before* you embark on a weight-loss campaign. As successful people have discovered, there is much more to becoming a successful loser than going on a diet. If you have ever had the feeling that the world conspires to keep you fat, you're right! At least here in America, we live in an environment that has resulted in over half the population becoming overweight! If you are going to beat the odds, there are interpersonal, economic, emotional, psychological, and time-management issues that must be resolved.

There is a lot to learn from the success of others. Based on personal interviews and research studies, I will show you what formerly overweight people are doing to keep it off. Of course they changed their eating habits. You'll see how they discovered the dangers of imitation fat-free and reduced-fat foods and how they plan a healthful diet that maintains their losses. You'll also see why they place such a high priority on physical activity and how they go about fitting it in to their daily lives. But, what's even more important, because they could not have made these behavior changes without having done it, I'll show you how they surmounted the emotional, psychological, and social barriers encountered when overweight people try to change the things in their lives that have been keeping them fat. Their inspiration, commitment, and continuing motivation flows from a new philosophy of life. Many of these successful people went through a kind of "born again" experience that resulted in a change of values and priorities. They found a new vision of the kind of person they wanted to be, and this vision gave them the power to take control of their appetites, change those aspects of the environment that formerly led to failure, and respond differently to environmental influences that cannot be changed. I think their successful experiences will be an inspiration to you and show you how to sustain your own commitment and motivation.

I am very happy to say that I am one of those successful persons myself. I lost 75 pounds thirty-five years ago, as of this writing. If you have that amount of weight to lose, I'll show you how I did it with a modern, up-to-date version of my own, wonderfully effective, quick Rotation Diet. If you have a great deal of weight to lose, as I did, it's an excellent, frustration-free way to go about it. On the new T-Factor 2000 Rotation Plan you can lose up to 10 pounds or more on each rotation and never be burned out or hit plateaus while dieting. The most important benefit associated with using the new T-Factor 2000 Rotation Plan is that while losing weight quickly you will also be following the basic T-Factor 2000 dietary principles that will enable you to keep it off, just as I have done for the past thirty-five years!

Think about this for a moment. If you have ever dieted before, lost weight, and then regained it, what was missing in the dietary plan that you followed? Why didn't it prepare you for permanent weight management? With the T-Factor 2000 Diet you will not be faced with coming off a weight-loss diet and then having to design a new way of eating to prevent your regaining weight.

But as I said earlier, there is a great deal more to successful weight management than just going on a diet. If you are serious about changing your eating and activity behavior, it will have an impact on your relationship with other people and almost everything else that goes on in your life. Unless you learn how to change your own eating environment, or how to restrain yourself if you remain surrounded by highly palatable foods, you are sure to fall victim once again to temptation and make poor food choices. The same family responsibilities and work schedule may still interfere with becoming and remaining an active person. So I'll show you, from interviews and research, how successful people in a variety of different circumstances have found ways to deal with these matters. And since both Jamie and I, each of us with a strong hereditary predisposition to obesity and a history of being overweight, have learned how to deal with these same issues ourselves (Jamie is also the working mother of a three-year-old daughter), we'll go into detail with our personal experience in managing our daily lives because we think it may be of help to you.

Menus and recipes. We have worked hard to develop menus and recipes to satisfy every taste preference. In addition to recommendations for persons who prefer the complete range of foods found in the typical American diet, which includes meat, poultry, and fish, we have devised a vegetarian version and menus for "part-time" vegetarians, which is, by the way, where I fit. More and more people are cutting back on their meat consumption in order to reduce their risk of heart disease and certain cancers. But did you know that people who have been successful in managing their weight report, right at the top of the list of changes they have made in their diets, a significant cutback in their meat consumption? This is not surprising, since meat is one of the primary sources of fat in the American diet. However, if you prefer to include meat in your diet, we have some delicious recipes for low-fat cuts of beef and pork that will cut your animal fat intake by 50 to 80 percent.

My *number-one* consideration in the development of the recipes in this book has been taste!

No matter how important it may be to lose weight, if the menus and recipes that we suggest don't appeal to you and satisfy your taste preferences, there is little likelihood that you will continue to use them.

As a former fat man, having inherited the preferences for all the qualities in foods and their preparation that can result in obesity—remember that I was once 75 pounds overweight!—I have always enjoyed the pleasures of good eating, and I still do. The taste and enjoyment of food remain my primary concern in every recipe, and I will show you that you do not have to give up palatable foods to lose weight. My wife, Enid, Jamie, and I created most of the recipes in this book. A few were contributed by participants in the Vanderbilt Weight Management Program and friends. We include many styles of food preparation from different culinary traditions, and every recipe was tested by Jamie or me. We feel certain that you will find many dishes that suit your personal tastes and that you will want to make them a part of your menus from now on.

While the majority of recipes in *The T-Factor 2000 Diet* are new, I have included some all-time-favorites, chosen on the basis of the many fan letters I have received in the years I have been developing low-fat recipes.

Of course, cost and convenience are also important when you attempt to make permanent changes in your diet. Our personal experience shows that healthful eating for weight management does not have to be any more expensive than the typical American diet. And except for some special-occasion recipes, most of our recipes can be prepared in twenty minutes or less, once you get familiar with them. But food preparation must not become a bore or a burden. So, in the recipe chapter you will also find some suggestions that can double your pleasure and efficiency in food preparation.

Physical activity. With my appetite and genetic predisposition for obesity, I don't think I would ever have been able to maintain a weight loss of 70 pounds for the past thirty-five years without becoming an active person. I'm not alone, however. *Every single research study of which I am aware shows that an increase in physical activity may be the key to long-term weight management after a significant loss of weight.* On average, successful people report an increase in physical activity that amounts to an energy expenditure of about 2800 calories a week. That's equivalent to about 80 minutes of walking every day. But think about it for a moment—if, as I explained earlier in this Introduction, about 40 minutes of walking will burn 20 grams of fat, 80 minutes ought to take care of 40 grams. Think about the freedom this can give you to include some high-fat foods in your diet without danger of gaining weight! Without physical activity, those fat grams would end up right back in your fat cells once again.

I know from personal experience, however, that physical activity doesn't feel very good when you are overweight and you are first getting started. Nevertheless, speaking again from personal experience as well as on the basis of research studies, one of the most important benefits of becoming an active person is the change it can make psychologically and emotionally in your life. Getting active will do even more than losing weight to increase your self-esteem, satisfaction with your body, and emotional well-being. For this reason, it is very important to me that I show you how to experience the pleasure and terrific satisfaction that can go with becoming a more active person.

From a physiological and biochemical perspective, there have been a number of new discoveries showing how physical activity can play a part in weight management and your physical health. Although all kinds of physical activity can be helpful in managing your weight, I will explain why the so-called fat-burning, low-to-moderate aerobic exercise (such as walking at a moderate pace) that experts have been recommending for the past decade may not all by itself be the most effective way to help you lose weight and maintain the loss. The best exercise involves a balanced program in which activity burns both fat and carbohydrate in your fuel mix, and which builds fitness and endurance, increases your metabolic rate, regulates blood sugar and triglycerides, and prevents the development of insulin resistance and hyperinsulinemia (or cures them if these disorders already exist). This is the program I will describe for you in Chapter 9.

How to help the children in your family handle the weight issue. In Chapter 10 Jamie will give you some suggestions for how to help your children learn to manage their weight *without dieting*. We are facing two major kinds of weight problems with our children. On the one hand, we have an obesity epidemic, with more children overweight than ever before. These children often learn all the wrong ways to manage their weight, such as going on a very low-calorie diet, or engaging in unhealthy kinds of food restrictions, only to return to eating the typical American high-fat diet that will make them grow up to be fat adults. They tend to spend many more hours in front of the TV set than in any kind of physical activity. On the other hand, we have some teenagers, most often girls, who are compulsively trying to reach an unhealthy state of thinness as a result of the unrealistic images they view on magazine covers and TV. Jamie will show you how family attitudes and behaviors can help remedy these problems.

Now let's begin.

I am eager to show you how you, too, can become a member of that select group of people who have gone beyond dieting and achieved final victory over fat.

CHAPTER 1

Why Am I Fat?

GENETIC FACTORS MAY PREDISPOSE TO OBESITY

Heredity plays an important role in predisposing a person to obesity. Adopted children are much more like their biological parents in weight than they are their adoptive parents, and studies show that the weights of identical twins are much more alike than those of same-sex fraternal twins. In studies comparing fraternal and identical twins, the variability in the weight of fraternal twins is about twice as large as that of identical twins.

The chances of a child becoming obese are fifty-fifty if one parent is obese, and four to one if both parents are obese. You are quite likely to see the genetic influence on your own weight by comparing your body build with that of your parents and siblings. Just take a look at where you store your body fat. You will most likely find that it's in the same places as one of your parents, but, if not a parent, one of your siblings. I take after my mother. Slim hands, narrow feet and legs, but plenty of fat around the hips. In fact, when I was an overweight child I felt my mother had started out to make a girl and changed her mind halfway. At my largest, I was 59 inches around the most substantial part of my buttocks—I still keep a pair of the made-to-order pants I had tailored in 1952, when I was twenty-four years old, as a memento.

Research has uncovered a rather depressing long list of genetic factors that, acting alone or in various combinations, can increase a person's likelihood of becoming obese. But you should understand that they only *predispose* you to a weight problem; they don't constitute an imperative. The predisposition only shows itself in a particular environment, one in which a great variety of highly palatable foods is easily available and which encourages a sedentary lifestyle.

One of the best examples of this genetic/environmental interaction can be seen in the Pima Indians. The original home of the Pima Indians is in Mexico, but a group of them migrated long ago to Arizona and now live on a reservation. The Pima Indians living in Arizona eat a high-fat diet and are sedentary. They are obese and many of them suffer from diabetes. The group that remained in Mexico eats a traditional low-fat diet and their lifestyle calls for a great deal of physical exertion. They remain thin and diabetes is rare.

We all know people, perhaps only a few, who seem to be able to eat a high-fat diet, remain sedentary, and, while they may add an inch or two around the waist as they grow older, never get fat. They obviously do not possess genetic factors that could interact with the environment and result in obesity. If you are overweight, you do! You cannot eat and act as persons without a predisposition to obesity and expect to be as thin. I say this because you are going to have to find a way to work with your body. By making changes in your eating and activity level, you can reverse the environmental influences that allow your predisposition to be expressed. *You can beat your genes!* That is one of the most important messages of this book. Just read the stories in Chapter 11. They will show you how people who were once as much as 100 pounds or more overweight have fought the good fight and won. You can do it, too.

PROTEIN, CARBOHYDRATE, AND FAT IN THE PROBLEM OF OBESITY

To understand why the T-Factor 2000 Diet can solve your weight problem, you need to know how the body deals with the energy contained in the food you eat. Does overeating on protein, carbohydrate, and fat act in the same way and contribute equally to a weight problem?

Protein

Overeating on protein does not contribute directly to a weight problem. On any given day, if you are eating a mixed diet and double up on your protein intake—for example, by eating a steak at lunch *and* dinner instead of your usual habit of just one at dinner—your body has several ways of dealing with the extra protein calories without turning them into fat for storage. Although the way it does this is not yet fully understood, it seems to work in the following way:

To begin with, the liver and other protein tissues can expand a little in size by taking in a small amount of the extra amino acids that are broken down from the extra protein you have eaten.* Other amino acids are broken down and converted to glucose (the form of carbohydrate the body burns as fuel), while still others are broken down to ketones (which share some chemical characteristics of both fat and glucose and can also be burned). Then, both the glucose and ketones to which the extra protein was converted are burned in the body's fuel mixture. In addition, the body seems to speed up the recycling of amino acids among its own tissues. Normally, the body breaks down and recycles between one-half and one pound of its own protein tissue each day, and recombines the amino acids for use by other body cells throughout the body. At the same time, it eliminates 50 or 60 grams of its own tissue amino acids and replaces them with new amino acids from your diet. This whole process may speed up, burning off the energy contained in the extra amount of protein in your diet.

The end result of all these processes is that *within the range that a person consuming a mixed diet might vary his intake, the extra protein has little or no effect on body fat stores.* The body has a way of adjusting the amount of protein burned in its fuel mixture to the amount in the diet. In other words, *when it comes to protein, we burn what we eat.*

---

*Proteins are combinations of various amino acids. To use them, the body breaks down the protein we eat into individual amino acids and then recombines them in various ways for use in our structural tissues, and to make hormones, enzymes, and antibodies to fight disease. In order to carry out all of the functions performed by amino acids in our bodies, the system creates 30,000 different combinations from the 20 different amino acids we obtain from the foods we eat!

Carbohydrate

Because carbohydrates play such an important role in supplying energy for certain bodily functions and because overconsumption of carbohydrates—those "bad" junk-food carbohydrates—can play an important although indirect role in obesity, I want to spend considerable time describing how the body uses and stores carbohydrate.

Before they can be used by your body, the various forms of dietary carbohydrate (sugars and starches) must be broken down and converted to glucose, the simple sugar that the body uses for energy. Since each meal of a mixed diet usually contains enough carbohydrates to make several times the amount of glucose that can be burned immediately or even in the next couple of hours, most of the glucose is converted to glycogen for storage. Glycogen is the storage form of carbohydrate energy in which hundreds of glucose molecules are strung together in many branched chains, held in reserve, and then quickly broken down into individual glucose molecules as needed. The liver and muscle cells are the major storage sites for glycogen, and both can make the conversion, glucose to glycogen and back again.

Glucose has some unique functions as a provider of energy in the human body. At this very moment, billions of glucose molecules are splitting within your brain cells, providing the energy that fuels their function and enables you to understand what you have been reading. Glucose, almost exclusively, supplies the energy used by brain cells, and by the rest of the nervous system and other tissues, such as red blood cells. Except in highly active people, the brain and central nervous system use about two-thirds of the glucose that's burned each day. Because your brain cells and these other tissues do not store glycogen, they rely on a constant supply of glucose in the bloodstream. The liver keeps them supplied from its store of glycogen by continually sending enough glucose into the bloodstream to maintain stable concentrations between meals and during sleep.

Glucose is also the quick-start fuel for all muscular activity. When you get up from a chair, run up a flight of stairs, or start rearranging your furniture, glycogen that's stored in your muscles will be immediately broken down to glucose and will supply all the fuel that's needed in the first few moments of any physical activity. Within seconds, a portion of the glycogen stored in the liver is broken down to glucose and sent to the muscles to keep them going. As time progresses, in light to moderate activity, the muscles begin to switch from a predominance of glucose in their fuel mixture to a predominance of fat. All in all, under normal circumstances, glucose provides about half the energy used by your body each day, while fat supplies the other half (remember that protein is broken down to either glucose or ketones when making its energy available for metabolic functions).

Although the body may need 1000 or more calories a day from glucose, the liver and muscles have limited storage capacity. Together, the liver and muscles normally store only between 200 and 400 grams of glycogen (about one-third of it in the liver, and two-thirds of it spread throughout your musculature). In energy terms, this amounts to between 800 and 1600 calories, which is not much more than a day's supply.

There is an important physiological reason for this limitation in the amount of glycogen storage: in order to store glycogen it must be combined with water. It takes 3 parts water to put 1 part glycogen into solution for storage. Thus the storage of glycogen adds three times its weight in water plus the weight of the glycogen to the body. Storing just 110 grams of glycogen, which weighs about ¼ pound, adds ¾ pound of water to your liver and muscles. In contrast, fat is stored almost 4½ parts fat to only 1 part water. Since glycogen supplies 4 calories of energy per gram, while fat supplies 9, a pound of glycogen/water storage nets you only about 450 calories, while a pound of fat/water storage nets you about 3500 calories. It would take 8 pounds of glycogen storage to equal the energy contained in 1 pound of fat. So nature, in its wisdom, chose fat as the preferred vehicle for long-term storage of energy, and puts only about a one-day supply of glucose in its short-term store. (See box "The reason for rapid weight loss . . . " for how this relates to weight loss on high-protein/high-fat diets that eliminate most carbohydrates from the diet.)

THE REASON FOR RAPID WEIGHT LOSS
on a high-protein/high-fat/low-carbohydrate diet and its dangers.

Because the body stores glycogen in the ratio of 3 parts water to 1 part carbohydrate, a cutback of just 450 calories of carbohydrate in the diet leads to a loss of about 1 pound of water/glucose mixture. Then, even though the diet may contain a large amount of protein, it still contains fewer calories than the body needs to maintain its weight. This forces the body to convert some of its own amino acids to glucose to feed the brain and red blood cells, which causes the loss of a great deal of water, since muscle tissue is also about 70 to 80 percent water. In addition, the byproducts of breaking down protein for use as energy are toxic and must be eliminated from the body as quickly as possible. More water is lost as the kidneys work to flush them out of the system. So, converting and burning just 450 calories of protein also leads to about 1 pound of water loss and possibly a little more. People have been known to lose 7 pounds in two days when they eliminate virtually all the carbohydrate from their diets. But as much as 6½ pounds of it is water! The loss of body fat is not greater on diets of this kind than on any other diet that reduces energy intake to the same degree.

In the absence of carbohydrate in the diet and with glucose reserves depleted, remnants of the fat molecules that are being broken down to supply energy are combined to form ketone bodies. Ketones can be burned by some parts of the brain in place of glucose. However, some ketones are actually acids (keto acids). As their concentration in the blood rises, the pH of the blood declines (the blood becomes more acidic) and the kidneys work to restore acid balance. Again, more water is used to flush toxins from the system. When keto acids appear in the urine, it is a sign that the kidneys may not be able to maintain proper acid balance in the blood and that body chemistry is going awry. This can be especially dangerous for people with poor kidney and liver function, and serious cases of liver and kidney damage have been reported. Other risks include dehydration and hypotension (low blood pressure) resulting from sodium loss and water imbalance, promotion of atherosclerosis resulting from a high saturated-fat intake, and increased uric acid levels and risk for gout. Many people suffer from constipation, and nausea is an occasional side effect. It is difficult to build endurance and enjoy physical activity on such a diet because, with glycogen stores depleted, slight exertion brings on fatigue. The impact on the brain when it is forced to switch its source of fuel is not clear, but one recent study showed that people may lose some of their ability to perform certain kinds of mental tasks when their diets have insufficient carbohydrate and the brain is forced to run on ketones rather than glycogen.

The limited ability to store carbohydrate means that our body's storage depots must be replenished frequently if the concentration of glucose in the blood is to remain stable and the supply to both the brain and the musculature ensured. If carbohydrate is omitted from the diet, the body's entire supply would be exhausted in about a day. For these reasons, the body has developed strict mechanisms to adjust the amount of glucose that it burns in its fuel mixture to the amount in storage and the influx at mealtimes. Some examples will make this clear.

Think of the body's glycogen stores as residing in two related reservoirs, one in the liver, another spread throughout the musculature. Normally the body likes to keep this reservoir system at about half its maximum capacity, which is about a one-day supply. There is room to adapt to changing circumstances: the body can temporarily put some extra glycogen in liver storage after a large meal, and it can establish a higher baseline storage level should a person chronically overeat on carbohydrate relative to the demands he makes on the total reservoir system. In addition, the reservoir system can adapt to the demands of exercise when a sedentary person becomes more active. As it senses the chronic need for more glucose as a result of more daily exercise, the musculature expands its glycogen storage to a higher baseline level.

If the reservoir gets low for some reason—for example, a person skips a meal or engages in a long bout of intense activity—the body cuts back on glucose burning in favor of fat to preserve its precious supply of glycogen. If the reservoir becomes overloaded and is not regularly brought back to baseline, experts now believe that the increased amount of storage in the reservoir may exert pressure on the body to burn more glucose in its mixture. This will reduce the amount of fat that it burns. Obviously, anything that reduces your ability to burn fat can have important consequences for weight management. I'll discuss the implications of chronically overloaded glycogen stores in the next section, on fat, and in the next chapter, when I discuss the Second Law of Energy Balance. I'll discuss the importance of physical activity in preventing overloaded glycogen stores in Chapter 9.

The tightness with which the body adjusts the rate of carbohydrate burning to carbohydrate intake has been demonstrated in research subjects by examining the fuel mixture before and after meals. At rest several hours after a meal, the body relies primarily on fat in its fuel mix. A relatively small percentage of the fuel is glucose that is being converted from glycogen stores in order to maintain the blood glucose concentration essential for brain function and other dependent tissues. In the hours between meals or overnight, the glycogen reservoir may become depleted by 50 to 100 grams—that is, by several hundred calories—as a result of maintaining basic metabolic functions and any physical activity that has taken place. In terms of the analogy with a reservoir, it may be only one-quarter full.

Right after eating, as carbohydrate is being absorbed from the intestine, the body switches to a fuel mix comprised primarily of carbohydrate and places a high priority on bringing the glycogen reservoirs back up to half-full. During the first hour to two hours after a meal, fat makes up a relatively small portion of the body's fuel mixture. Over the next several hours, the mix is gradually reversed. The process is diagramed in Figure 1-1.

Studies like this show that when carbohydrate comes into the system, the body quickly switches to carbohydrate burning and puts some of the carbohydrate back into liver and muscle storage as glycogen to replace what was burned between meals.

But what happens if a person overeats on carbohydrate, and more is taken in than can be burned between meals or in a twenty-four-hour period?

Many people are under the mistaken impression that when they eat too much carbohydrate it gets turned to fat and ends up in their fat cells. This is simply not true except in highly unusual circumstances that hardly anyone will voluntarily endure. The body resists turning carbohydrate to fat for storage! Here are just two of the many studies that demonstrate this fact.

In one of the first ground-breaking studies, subjects were given a 2000-calorie test load of carbohydrate (500 grams). Measurements of any possible conversion of carbohydrate to fat for storage and whether the subjects experienced any gain or loss in total body fat were done at fourteen hours and twenty-four hours after the test load.

In order to create conditions that would be most likely to force the body to convert carbohydrate to fat, some of the subjects in this experiment had been previously made accustomed to a very high-carbohydrate diet in order to fill their glycogen reservoirs to the

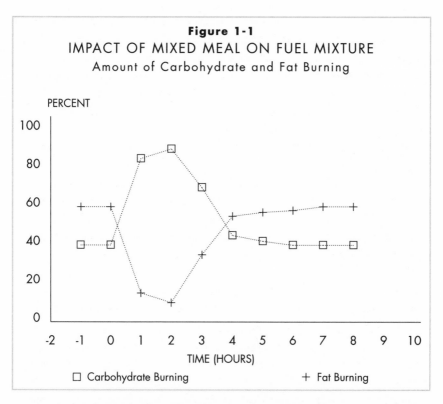

Figure 1-1
IMPACT OF MIXED MEAL ON FUEL MIXTURE
Amount of Carbohydrate and Fat Burning

□ Carbohydrate Burning   + Fat Burning

A meal is eaten at time 0. Carbohydrate burning increases quickly, while fat burning is depressed. The situation is reversed over the next several hours until fat again becomes the major part of the fuel mixture in the body at rest.

maximum. Thus there would be no place for carbohydrate to be stored—it would have to be burned or converted to fat for storage. Nevertheless, when measurements were taken at fourteen hours, only 81 calories (9 grams, or about 4 percent) were converted to fat for storage. **But even this small conversion to fat was temporary!** After twenty-four hours *all* subjects were in negative fat balance. Because the body still required a certain amount of fat in its fuel mix to meet the energy needs of the body in the final ten hours, they were in negative fat balance by an average of 35 grams of fat. That is, in spite of ingesting 2000 calories of carbohydrate, in the twenty-four hours that followed, they burned 315 calories in fat withdrawn from fat stores.

This study, as well as others that followed, proved that even after the consumption of an extremely large amount of carbohydrate—an amount equal to 125 teaspoons of sugar!—there is no net gain in body fat. So, even if you plan to eat more than 125 teaspoons of sugar at a sitting, which I think is hardly likely, there is no need to worry about your body converting carbohydrate to fat for storage.

So what does it take to force the body to convert carbohydrate to fat for storage, and how likely is this to happen?

It is possible to force the body to convert a portion of dietary carbohydrate to fat following sustained excesses of carbohydrate in the diet. However, before such conversion takes place it is necessary to maximize the body's ability to store glycogen and then saturate the glycogen reservoirs. In another ground-breaking study, researchers first completely saturated their subjects' liver and muscle storage sites and kept them saturated on a high-carbohydrate diet.

Then, each day, in order to maintain complete saturation of glycogen stores and, in addition, encourage the conversion of carbohydrate to fat, they fed their subjects 1500 more calories than they had burned on the previous day. Before any appreciable conversion of carbohydrate to fat took place, there was a massive increase in glycogen storage. While the maximum seen on a high-carbohydrate diet without such overfeeding is usually about 400 grams, by eating 1500 calories more than normally burned each day, glycogen stores reached an average of 810 grams. Then, because the body resists converting carbohydrate to fat for storage and speeds up its metabolic processes as it tries to burn off any excess, metabolic rate increased an average of 35 percent.*

Little by little, the body began to convert carbohydrate to fat, but in order to continue the conversion, by the seventh day of overfeeding, subjects had to eat 5000 calories a day, 4000 of it in carbohydrate! If the research subjects had continued to overeat beyond the seventh day, some 70 to 75 percent of the excess intake would have been converted to fat and retained in fat storage from that point on.

So, while it is possible to force the conversion of carbohydrate to fat for storage, to do so glycogen stores must first increase by about 500 grams over their normal level (about 2000 calories over normal). That is, just as the previously quoted study showed, the body can handle periodic loads of 2000 calories of carbohydrate without contributing to fat synthesis and storage. The energy obtained from

---

*Metabolic rate does not increase in this way to adjust to overconsumption of fat! The increase in metabolic rate on overconsumption of carbohydrate, which burns off a portion of the calories in the surplus, is one way the body protects itself from having to convert carbohydrate to fat.

overeating on carbohydrate goes first to glycogen storage, while at the same time the body attempts to defend itself against excess energy storage *when it comes in the form of carbohydrate* by increasing its metabolic rate dramatically. In order to continue conversion of carbohydrate to fat, massive amounts of carbohydrate over and above energy needs, such as were used in this study, would have to be ingested on a daily basis.

If carbohydrate is not converted to fat for storage, how, then, can excess carbohydrate in the diet affect your weight? Can you eat all the carbohydrate you want and never add a pound?

The answer is "yes" and "no."

It depends on the packaging!

On the one hand, you **can** eat as much carbohydrate as you want when it is packaged as fruits, vegetables, and whole grains (or minimally processed whole grains such as are found in whole-grain cereals and breads). In the case of fruits, vegetables, and whole grains, it's *only* the addition of fat that can increase their ability to "turn on" your appetite to the point where you will not stop when you reach energy balance. For example, it's the salad dressing that results in an intake of more calories than your body can burn and ends up in your fat cells, not the greens and other vegetables in the salad; and it's the meat sauce and cheese that does the same for pasta, not the wheat; and it's the fat in the crust and filling, not the apples, in the apple pie.

On the other hand, it's a big, fat "no!" if you are into those imitation, processed fat-free desserts, snacks, pastries, and confections that are designed to simulate the taste of fat. Their "turn on" can be just as great as the foods they are designed to replace, and their impact on your weight can be almost as disastrous. You will see exactly why after I discuss the role of fat in the diet and in your metabolism.

Fat

Fat, stored in our fat cells as triglycerides, constitutes our large long-term energy supply. This stored supply may be as much as 100 times larger than the glycogen reservoir in the average person. In terms of calories, it can add up to 150,000. In the seriously obese person it can be considerably greater than that.

The fat we eat contains the compounds that impart flavor, tenderness, and the mouth-watering quality that helps turn on our appetite. Fat is also responsible for the aromas created by a steak sizzling on the grill and onions in the frying pan. These are the qualities, unfortunately, that can seduce you into eating beyond your energy needs. The palatability of high-fat foods sends strong signals that stimulate your appetite. But, while eating, it generates very weak opposing physiological signals that you have had enough when you reach energy balance, and even these weak signals tend to arrive too late to turn you off before you have eaten too much.

During digestion, the fats in our food are broken down into their component fatty acids. Some of the fatty acids are released directly into the bloodstream and go to the liver, where they are used to make cholesterol and combined in various ways to suit the needs of different body cells. By far the largest proportion of fatty acids are recombined into triglycerides by cells in the intestinal wall and then sent to your fat cells for storage.* Almost none of the fat you eat is made available immediately upon absorption as fuel. Whether you consume 6 grams of fat or 40 grams of fat at a given meal, there is virtually no effect on the fuel mixture that your body burns right after you eat, or for the next several hours after that meal.

This is in direct contrast to carbohydrate.

As you may recall from the previous section, carbohydrate intake has a powerful effect in promoting carbohydrate burning. When you eat a meal that contains carbohydrate, the body quickly alters its fuel mixture to a predominance of carbohydrate and minimizes the contribution of fat. Carbohydrate burning is closely tied to carbohydrate intake. And, as I explained in the section on protein, protein burning is also adjusted to protein intake. These operate independently of the fat content of the diet. Adding as much as 300 or 400 calories of fat to a meal has no impact on the fuel mixture that your body burns. In fact, even when 700 or 800 calories in fat are added to a meal, there is only a small increase in fat burning.

What this means in practice is that we tend to burn in our fuel mix each day all the protein and carbohydrate that we obtain in our diets. The rest of our need for energy during that day will be made up by fat.

Let us see what this means in relation to a person's daily diet.

Assume you need 2000 calories a day to maintain a stable weight.

---

*I have left out a number of steps; the interested reader can consult a textbook, such as *Understanding Normal and Clinical Nutrition,* by E. N. Whitney, C. B. Cataldo, and S. R. Rolfes (Belmont, CA: West/Wadsworth, 1998).

If you eat 1300 calories combined in protein and carbohydrate, your body will burn those 1300 calories, and there is room in the diet for 700 fat calories. Eat more fat than that, it will go into storage and you gain weight. Eat less fat than that, and your body will take some out of storage to burn in its fuel mixture, and you lose weight. If you up your intake to 1400 calories combined in protein and carbohydrate, the body will also up the amount of protein and carbohydrate that gets burned in the fuel mix to equal what you have eaten. Now there will be room for only 600 fat calories in your diet without putting some into storage and gaining weight. In order to pull fat from fat storage to burn in your fuel mixture and lose weight, you would now have to eat less than 600 calories in fat.

In other words, fat fills the gap between your total energy needs and the amount of protein and carbohydrate you eat in your diet. With respect to protein and carbohydrate, you burn what you eat.

On the other hand, the amount of fat in your diet has no direct effect on the amount of protein and carbohydrate that gets burned. While the combined amount of protein and carbohydrate affects how much fat you burn, no matter how much fat you eat, it will have no impact on how much carbohydrate or protein you burn— you will still burn whatever carbohydrate and protein you have eaten. Even if you eat as much as 80 grams of fat at a single meal, it will have only a small impact on your fuel mixture.

This is a very important point. And I know it sounds confusing, but I think it's essential that you understand what it means for weight control. Let me show you how it works, with a real example from one of the first and most important research studies to demonstrate this relationship between the burning of carbohydrate, protein, and fat.

In this study the research subjects ate two breakfasts, on different days, that had exactly the same amount of protein and carbohydrate but varied in fat content.

On each of the two days, the diet had 120 calories in protein and 292 calories in carbohydrate.

On the low-fat day it had only 54 calories in fat.

On the high-fat day it contained 414 calories in fat.

Following each of the breakfasts, the researchers measured the amounts of protein, carbohydrate, and fat burned by these subjects in their fuel mixtures during the next nine hours.

On both days the total energy needs in the nine hours following breakfast were quite similar: The research subjects burned about 760 to 780 calories. On each of the days they burned almost exactly the same number of protein and carbohydrate calories as were contained in the breakfast—that is, about 120 protein calories and about 292 carbohydrate calories. *The difference in fat consumption had no effect on carbohydrate or protein burning.* This reflects the tight regulation that exists between protein and carbohydrate consumption and protein and carbohydrate burning. *You will burn what you eat, but only with respect to carbohydrate and protein.*

The situation is completely different with fat. *What you eat has no direct effect on fat burning.*

This is important for weight management because on both days the subjects needed to burn approximately 360 calories of fat in their fuel mixtures in order to meet basal metabolic requirements and the cost of physical activity.

Think about this: Regardless of the fat content of the breakfast—it didn't matter if it was high or low—the body still burned the same total calories and the same amount of fat.

On the low-fat day, when the diet contained only 54 calories in fat, the body took about 306 calories out of fat storage to meet its 360-calorie requirement.

On the high-fat day, when the diet contained 414 calories in fat, the body used the dietary fat to meet its needs for fat in the fuel mixture, which was about 360 calories, *and had about 54 calories left to be put in fat storage.*

The conclusion is obvious: **Cut the fat in your diet for permanent weight loss.**

As I mentioned in the Introduction, if you cut 20 grams of fat a day from your diet, the likely loss may run about 22 pounds. A number of other studies show that a 10 percent cut in fat consumption, for example from 40 percent of total calories to 30 percent, results in an average weight loss of 12 pounds. When you cut the fat, assuming carbohydrate and protein remain constant as in the above study, the fat that you burn in your fuel mixture will come out of your fat cells. The amount of fat in that mix will be gradually reduced as your fat stores are depleted. Weight loss, which under these circumstances is all fat loss, will stop when the body has completely adjusted the proportion of protein, carbohydrate, and fat in the fuel mixture to match the ratio of these nutrients in the diet.

Do you really know how much fat you eat each day? In the government nutrition study that I quoted in the Introduction, women reported consuming an average of about 70 grams of fat a day, and men about 105. However, when overweight people are asked to record their food intake, they underestimate calories (mostly fat calories) by 30 to 55 percent. Do you? Do you think you can estimate your intake more accurately than registered dietitians do? A couple of years ago at a convention, over 200 registered dietitians were asked to estimate the calories and fat content of five different restaurant dinners that were placed right before their eyes. On average, they underestimated the calories by 37 percent and the fat content by 49 percent.

Considering the degree of underreporting that's common, if you are an overweight woman, it is quite likely that you are in reality consuming an average of 100 grams of fat a day, or even more! If you are an overweight man, you may be consuming 130 to 150 grams of fat a day. In Chapter 3, before you start the T-Factor 2000 Diet, I am going to give you an easy little exercise to do that Jamie and I recently introduced in the Vanderbilt Weight Management Program. I am excited about the usefulness of this exercise because it never fails to surprise the participants while they are doing it, and it never fails to change the way they relate to food when they finish doing it. It takes just one day, and you don't have to count anything! Not calories or fat grams. But it will quickly show you whether or not you are aware of how much you are eating, and, of much greater consequence, it will help give you just the right amount of control you need over your appetite to achieve successful weight management. Be sure to do it!

But first, if you have already been trying to cut the fat in your diet and have been eating imitation fat-free or reduced-fat desserts, snacks, pastries, and candies, you better think again. You have not been doing yourself any favors. I think this will become clear from the following discussion of the First and Second Laws of Energy Balance and the impact of overeating carbohydrates on your *fat-consumption threshold*.

CHAPTER 2

Getting from Fat to Thin

THE FIRST AND SECOND LAWS OF ENERGY BALANCE

The First Law of Energy Balance, with which I'm quite sure you're familiar, states that stable weight requires:

Energy in = Energy out

In other words, figured over time, on average, you must burn the same number of calories each day as you eat to maintain a stable weight. Eat more calories than you burn, you gain weight. Eat fewer calories than you burn, you lose weight. This is a law of physics. There is no way you can get around it!

I've already mentioned, however, that calories contained in various food sources may not be equally available for use to the human body. It takes a bit more energy to transform the calories in carbohydrate and protein for use or storage than it does the calories in fat. In addition, the calories in the fiber portion of carbohydrate foods cannot be broken down for use to any appreciable extent. These calories are always included in the nutritional information labels on packaged foods, and in the calorie information on fruits, vegetables, and grains in calorie counters, but almost all fiber calories pass through your body unused.

So the First Law of Energy Balance obviously means *available* or *usable* "Energy in = Energy out" in weight-stable individuals.

As increasingly sensitive scientific instruments for examining how the body adjusts its fuel mixture to the dietary mixture became available in the last ten to fifteen years, scientists began to realize that the First Law of Energy Balance was not sufficient to describe the weight-stable human body. Recent research has shown that carbohydrate, protein, and fat are regulated separately, with virtually no conversion taking place between carbohydrate and fat, as I explained in the previous chapter. Each must be in balance or the entire system can be thrown out of kilter. This has led to the formulation of the Second Law of Energy Balance, which states that stabilized body weight requires:

Protein energy in = Protein energy out
Carbohydrate energy in = Carbohydrate energy out
Fat energy in = Fat energy out

In the last chapter I explained that within the range seen in persons consuming a mixed diet, the body has mechanisms to adjust the energy it derives from protein to the amount of protein in the diet. Thus an increase in the amount of protein in the diet results in the addition of little if any fat to storage.

I also explained that carbohydrate is tightly regulated by the human body. That is, increases or decreases in the amount of carbohydrate in the diet are quickly reflected in the body's fuel mixture. Right after a meal, even if it contains only a small amount of carbohydrate, the body increases carbohydrate burning, restores glycogen reserves in the liver and muscles, and decreases the amount of fat in its fuel mix. Then, over the next several hours, while a person is pursuing sedentary activities or is asleep, the ratio of carbohydrate to fat in the fuel mix is gradually reversed and fat becomes the predominant fuel.

In contrast with carbohydrate, the amount of fat in a meal has virtually no immediate effect on the body's fuel mixture. Whether you eat 6 grams of fat in a meal (54 calories) or 46 (414 calories), the burning of whatever carbohydrate and protein you have eaten has priority. Your fuel mix will be quickly adjusted to match the amount of protein and carbohydrate in your diet, but not the fat.

This is what you need to remember:

Under all but the most extreme conditions, the amount of protein and carbohydrate in your diet will be burned in your body's fuel mixture. The amount of fat that gets burned depends upon the gap between your total energy needs and the amount of protein and carbohydrate energy in your diet. If you take in more energy in the form of fat than the gap between your total energy expenditure and your combined protein and carbohydrate energy intake, it will go into your fat cells. If you take in less energy in the form of fat than the gap between your total energy expenditure and the amount of protein and carbohydrate energy in your diet, the body will withdraw fat from your fat cells and burn it in its fuel mix.

Thus, if over a certain period of time you eat more fat than you can burn in your fuel mix, it leads to an enlargement of your fat stores.* Larger fat stores promote the burning of more fat in the fuel mixture. When the amount of fat you burn in your fuel mix is equal to the amount of fat in your diet, weight gain stops. Within the boundaries set by your heredity and level of physical activity, the amount of fat on your body is adjusted to the amount of fat in your diet. Changes in the amount of fat stored in your body take place so that your body can equalize the amount of fat it burns in its fuel mix to the amount of fat in your diet.†

The main reason that an increase in physical activity promotes weight maintenance after a significant weight loss is that physical activity can take the place of an enlarged fat store. I repeat the illustration from the Introduction: On the one hand, it may take about 22 pounds of fat on your body to promote the burning of 20 grams of fat each day; on the other hand, it takes about forty minutes to an hour's worth of physical activity. (The time depends on your weight and the intensity of the activity.) Another way of looking at this is that physical activity can add several hundred calories to your

---

*An increase in the size of the body's fat storage is accompanied by the development of a form of insulin resistance that promotes higher levels of circulating free fatty acids. (Insulin is the hormone that facilitates the transport of glucose into your body cells for use as fuel. At the same time, it blocks the release of fat from your fat cells for use in the body's fuel mixture.) Insulin resistance, by causing an increase in circulating free fatty acids, increases fat burning relative to glucose burning, and helps to make fat burning equal to your dietary fat intake. The insulin resistance that develops as a result of obesity is a mechanism that the body uses to promote fat burning. Thus insulin resistance, in promoting fat burning, is the body's way of trying to defend itself against further fat weight gain. However, when insulin resistance develops, the body has difficulty handling carbohydrate in your diet. It is accompanied by hyperinsulinemia, high levels of sugar in the blood, and an increased risk of diabetes.

†When you begin to eat more fat than you can burn in your fuel mixture, your fat cells expand to accept the fat, and in some cases, more fat cells may be created. As a result of this expansion of fat stores, more fat begins to circulate in the system for use as fuel. When the expansion of existing fat cells or creation of new fat cells results in the circulation of enough fat for use as fuel to equal the amount of fat you are eating in your diet, weight gain due to the amount of fat in your diet will stop.

total energy needs each day, thus widening the gap between your total needs and your combined protein and carbohydrate intake each day. Those forty to sixty minutes of activity will burn 20 grams of fat.* Without those minutes of physical activity, 20 grams of fat (180 calories) would exceed the gap between your total needs and your combined protein and carbohydrate intake. Instead of being burned as fuel for activity, the excess fat would start getting deposited in your fat cells until, little by little, a fraction of an ounce at a time, you gained about 22 pounds. Is it any wonder that an increase in physical activity is so important for weight maintenance after a significant loss of weight?

CARBOHYDRATE AND WEIGHT MANAGEMENT

Right now I want to explain how overeating on carbohydrate can prevent you from losing weight and even make you gain weight. Because of the high priority given to the burning of carbohydrate in your diet, *overeating on carbohydrate can prevent your body from burning all the fat in your diet!* Since the carbohydrate must be burned, overeating on carbohydrate leaves less room for fat in the gap between your combined protein and carbohydrate intake and your total energy needs. And this is why energy-dense, imitation, fat-free foods and reduced-fat foods that have an increased amount of sugar can prove to be a curse rather than a blessing.

As you may recall from one of the studies I discussed in the previous chapter, the body does not convert carbohydrate to fat for storage unless a person takes in a tremendous amount of extra carbohydrate calories more than his energy expenditure, every day, on a continuing basis. In the study I described it took 1500 extra calories added to the diet each day, which in turn led to a 35 percent increase in the metabolic rate. This resulted in the need to eat over 5000 calories a day in order to obtain just several hundred calories of new fat to be placed in storage. Overeating to this extent causes a great deal of discomfort. People are not normally willing

---

*The activity will burn a good deal of the carbohydrate in your diet as well, which makes the gap even larger because, as you will see in a moment, by burning carbohydrate in activity you prevent excess carbohydrate in your diet from interfering with fat burning.

to do it, except for research purposes and then only for a limited time.

The real question for practical purposes is: How can consuming a few hundred extra calories in carbohydrate on a daily basis, over and above a person's total energy needs, interfere with weight management if they are not going to get converted to fat?

It does so indirectly by *lowering your fat-consumption threshold*.

An illustration may help clarify the issue.

Imagine a woman who consumes an average of 2000 calories a day, containing an average of 50 percent of calories in carbohydrate, 35 percent in fat, and 15 percent in protein. She has been weight stable for a long period of time, with just the usual fluctuations of a couple of pounds, up or down, around her steady weight.

In terms of calories for each nutrient, these percentages amount to:

1000 calories in carbohydrate
700 calories in fat
300 calories in protein

Now imagine that for one reason or another, she chooses to add about 300 calories a day in carbohydrate to her diet on a continuing basis. This is rather hard to do with naturally occurring carbohydrate foods like fresh fruit, vegetables, and whole grains unless you add fat to them in their preparation. For example, 300 calories would mean eating four good-size apples or four full cups of shredded wheat. Most people would find this hard to do—their appetite would be satisfied with just one apple or one cup of shredded wheat. But it's now very easy to do with fat-free desserts, snacks, pastries, and candies because these generally contain about four times the number of calories per unit of weight or volume compared with foods like fresh apples or shredded wheat. For example: a 5-ounce apple contains 80 calories; 5 ounces of a famous fast-food chain's fat-free apple bran muffin contains just over 300 calories.

As a result of the addition of 300 extra carbohydrate calories, her body will respond in two ways. It will increase the amount of carbohydrate in its fuel mixture, and it will increase the amount of glucose it converts to glycogen for storage. Her glycogen stores will remain higher than previously as long as she continues to eat the extra carbohydrate, and the heightened stores will put continual pressure on her body to burn more carbohydrate rather than fat.

Since her daily energy needs remain quite close to the original

2000, her body will replace the fat that it formerly burned in its fuel mixture with carbohydrate.

Whereas prior to adding the extra carbohydrate to her diet she was burning 700 calories of fat in her fuel mixture, the added carbohydrate will suppress fat burning by perhaps 75 percent of the amount of additional carbohydrate, give or take a few percentage points. That is, should she continue to consume 700 calories in fat, around 225 will be shunted to her fat cells for storage. The amount is not exactly equal to the total carbohydrate increase, because carbohydrate tends to produce a greater thermic effect than fat. That is, more energy is given off as heat in the metabolism of carbohydrate than of fat, and there are additional energy costs in the use and cycling of glucose to glycogen and back.

What the overconsumption of carbohydrate has done is to lower her *fat-consumption threshold* from 700 calories to about 475 calories. As long as she eats those 300 extra carbohydrate calories, she cannot eat more than 475 calories in fat without putting any of the overage in her fat cells for storage. While the exact amount that a person's fat-consumption threshold will be lowered as a result of increased carbohydrate consumption will vary from person to person, the following conclusion holds true for *everyone:*

IF YOU INCREASE THE AMOUNT OF CARBOHYDRATE ENERGY IN YOUR DIET, YOU MUST DECREASE THE FAT ENERGY IN THE DIET BY AN ALMOST EQUAL AMOUNT.

I'm quite sure you are asking at this point, "How can you be recommending a high-carbohydrate diet, and only picking on imitation, refined, energy-dense, fat-free carbohydrate foods as threats to weight management, and not all carbohydrates?"

There is a big difference between the body's response to unrefined, more natural foods, such as fruits, vegetables, and whole grains, and its response to high-fat foods and energy-dense fat-free foods that are designed to simulate the taste of fat. **Each of the nutrients—protein, carbohydrate, and fat—has a different impact on appetite and on energy balance.** In fact, most obesity researchers believe that *the difference in the impact that carbohydrate, protein, and fat have on stimulating your appetite and satisfying your appetite during and after eating may be as important as, if not of greater importance than,* the difference in the way their energy component is handled by the human body.

Here is why.

HOW PROTEIN, CARBOHYDRATE, AND FAT
AFFECT THE APPETITE

Carbohydrate, protein, and fat do not have identical effects on your appetite. At any given level of hunger, fat, via the compounds that impart flavor, tenderness, and palatability, along with the aromas that go with the cooking of so many different foods, generates strong signals that turn on your appetite to a much greater extent than either carbohydrate or protein. At the same time, while you are eating, the consumption of fat generates weak opposing physiological signals to stop eating as your intake approaches energy balance. Because the signals to continue eating high-fat foods remain stronger than the signals such foods generate to stop eating at the point of energy balance, high-fat foods tend to encourage unintended overeating (or what scientists are now calling "passive overconsumption").

The studies that I will discuss below show that, calorie for calorie, carbohydrate satisfies your appetite much more effectively than fat. Meals with a high carbohydrate-to-fat ratio suppress hunger more quickly than meals with a high fat-to-carbohydrate ratio. In other words, the more carbohydrate relative to fat in a meal, the quicker your hunger is satisfied and your appetite is turned off. The more fat, the more likely you are to take in more calories than you need. The difference in impact on weight is reflected in a host of studies that show that, *all over the world,* the greater the fat-to-carbohydrate ratio in the diet, the greater the prevalence of obesity.

Many research studies have shown that when people are given an opportunity to choose from a selection of high-carbohydrate foods or high-fat foods and can eat as much as they want, as at a buffet, they take in far more calories from the high-fat selection before they feel satisfied and stop eating than from the high-carbohydrate selection. This has been verified both in observational studies of people eating in restaurants "in the real world" and in studies where participants in the research are offered a selection of either high-fat foods or high-carbohydrate foods on different days. In other words, fat turns on appetite to a greater extent than carbohydrate.

Research has also shown that obese people as a group seem to prefer the flavor of fat more than thin people, and, as a group, obese individuals consume a diet that is higher in fat than the diet of lean people. A preference for fat appears to have a genetic basis.

Children of obese parents prefer, and consume, a diet with a larger fat content and lower carbohydrate energy percentage than children of lean parents. When diners are observed in restaurants that offer both a buffet, with a wide assortment of highly palatable foods, or the opportunity to order from a menu, more obese than lean patrons choose the buffet, while more lean than obese persons choose to order from the menu.

Many people have the mistaken notion that fat in a meal satisfies their hunger for a longer period of time than carbohydrate. This is not true!

Here are just two of the many studies that prove that notion is wrong.

In one study that examined the effect of fat and carbohydrate on hunger and subsequent eating behavior, subjects consumed 1) a basic breakfast of 440 calories; 2) the basic breakfast plus 362 additional calories in fat; or, 3) the basic breakfast with 362 additional calories in carbohydrate. The addition of fat did not suppress hunger or lead to a lower intake of food as snacks between meals than did the breakfast without the fat. In contrast, adding 363 calories in carbohydrate significantly suppressed the experience of hunger and the amount of food eaten as snacks in comparison with the amount eaten after the basic breakfast.

In another study, subjects were offered a buffet containing either a selection of high-fat foods or a selection of high-carbohydrate foods at dinnertime. The average caloric intake from the high-fat meal was 1336 calories, while from the high-carbohydrate meal it was 677 calories. In spite of this difference in caloric intake at dinner, there was hardly any difference in the amount of calories eaten in snacks later that evening, or in meals during the entire next day. In fact, the slight difference that was observed was in the opposite direction from what you might expect—the participants who had the high-carbohydrate meal the evening before ate somewhat less the next day. In other words, extra fat did not lead to a longer suppression of hunger or any reduction in caloric intake in the meals eaten the next day as compensation for having eaten so much at the evening meal.

These are just a couple of the studies among scores in the literature that show, simply put, that:

1. fat turns on appetite;
2. people eat more when exposed to a selection of high-fat foods;

3. additional fat does not suppress hunger for a longer period of time than a high-carbohydrate meal, and;

4. having eaten many more calories in a high-fat meal does not automatically reduce your appetite and result in a lower intake of calories at future meals.

Is it any wonder that, whenever the diets of different groups of people are compared, either across cultures or among groups in the same country, as the ratio of fat to carbohydrate in the diet goes up, obesity goes up?

What about the imitation, fat-free, energy-dense carbohydrates created to taste like high-fat foods and replace them in the diet?

Here I'm speaking primarily of fat-free desserts, snacks, pastries, and candy. There are several major problems with these foods.

• They are meant to simulate the taste and texture of fat. This means that they are likely to have the same impact on your appetite and on the control mechanisms that come into operation as when you eat high-fat foods. Just like the real things, the signals they send when you have eaten enough to reach energy balance are rather weak, and late in arriving. Fruits, vegetables, and whole-grain foods have a strong ability to turn off your appetite before you have overeaten, largely because of their bulk. They contain fiber and, in the case of fruit and vegetables, a high percentage of water per unit of weight or volume. Naturally occurring, unprocessed carbohydrates are foods of low energy density—that is, they have fewer calories per unit of weight or volume. The processed imitation foods are high in energy density—that is, they squeeze in many calories per unit of weight or volume. You get a much quicker and stronger sense of fullness before you have consumed more than your energy needs from natural foods of low energy density than from energy-dense imitation foods (the feeling of fullness is among the first appetite turn-off signals generated during eating). Remember my example: a 5-ounce apple contains about 80 calories; a 5-ounce portion of a fat-free apple streusel or a fat-free apple bran muffin may contain over 300 calories. That's about as many calories as would be found in a "real" strudel or cake, but in the case of the fat-free dessert, the major calories come from sugar and refined flour. *Energy-dense fat-free foods that simulate the taste and texture of fat can be just as ruinous to your weight-management efforts as the original high-fat versions.*

• The impression that "fat-free" is somehow healthy, or at least without danger to your weight-management efforts, is created by the hype in the marketing of fat-free foods, and it can have a serious psychological impact. It can reduce your guard against overeating. Whereas when you eat a high-fat food you are likely to attempt a certain amount of restraint if you are interested in weight management, you are likely to make less of an effort with a fat-free food. Many experts now believe that the substitution of fat-free desserts, snacks, pastries, and candies can lead, if you're not careful, to a significant increase in total calories. **A similar if not greater warning must be issued with respect to the reduced-fat and low-fat versions of foods in these categories, because, while reducing the fat, they make a significant increase in the carbohydrate content (mainly sugar). Since they taste even better than the fat-free versions, they are even more likely to encourage overconsumption.** Once again, in spite of the decrease in fat, the increase in carbohydrate intake resulting from consumption of reduced-fat foods can end up shunting a larger proportion of the other fat in your diet to storage than to burning in your fuel mix.

• One of the most dangerous results of the long-term inclusion of refined, fat-free, energy-dense items like desserts and snacks is a nutrient-poor diet. Fake foods often take the place of fruits, vegetables, and healthier grain foods. This means a lower intake of vitamins, minerals, and thousands of other health-promoting phytochemicals,* found only in plant foods, which are either completely lacking in the ingredients used in fat-free foods in the first place or refined out of them during processing.

If you insist on including these imitation foods in your diet, I'll show you how to protect yourself from their dangers in Chapter 4, when you begin the T-Factor 2000 Diet. However, after reading what successful participants in the Vanderbilt program have to say about these imitation fat-free foods, you may realize you'll lose weight faster and keep it off more easily if you completely rid your diet of these junk foods.

I want to emphasize once again that when I refer to imitation energy-dense fat-free foods I'm referring primarily to foods in the dessert, snack, pastry, cookie, and confection categories. *I think it is a good idea to use either fat-free or low-fat dairy products.* How-

---

*Phytochemicals (from the Greek word *phyto,* meaning plant) are now thought to play an important role in protecting against cancer and heart disease.

ever, while fat-free dairy products are not likely to overly stimulate your appetite, the same is not true of certain reduced-fat or low-fat products such as 2% cottage cheese and part-skim ricotta and mozzarella cheeses. You must still use discretion in the use of reduced-fat and low-fat versions of higher-fat foods.

FAT-FREE IMITATION FOODS? READ THESE REMARKS IF YOU INCLUDE THEM IN YOUR DIET AND ARE HAVING TROUBLE MANAGING YOUR WEIGHT.

Jamie directs the in-house weight-management program for faculty and staff at Vanderbilt University. She stays in touch with all participants via e-mail. Here are some of their responses to a question, asked in December 1998, about fat-free imitation foods.

I'm probably a real typical case. I came into the program BINGEING on fat-free foods like snack bars, cookies, and breakfast bars. I would check the fat content on the packages and think I was getting away with something. Since I've been in the class and done a couple of food diaries and listened to you, I have pretty much avoided them—and have lost weight and kept it off! I still do eat rice cakes and raisins for a snack—both of which are fat-free, but I don't think you mean these. —CH

If I keep it around then I just eat "fat-free" junk in huge volumes. It's fat-free, but it's junk food all the same. A poor substitute for healthy eating. Too much sugar (most of the fat-free stuff is still very high in calories) then becomes a vicious cycle for me. I have found that eating all the sugar makes me crave more sugar. . . . In effect once I get started on the stuff, I have a hard time stopping. Bottom line is that I was eating a lot of fat-free "junk" foods, but getting no exercise. When I cut down on the volume of junk, added more fruits and vegetables, made more careful selections when eating out, and (most importantly) added 30 minutes of stair-stepping every night, the weight finally started coming off. —RM

Previous to the class I did buy many more fat-free cookies and pastries, but after going thru the class last Jan.–May and logging in the fat grams AND calories, I learned to beware the "fat-free" items because of the false but implied assumption one gets that one can eat more freely (many more servings)! —PT

I think SnackWell's does a good job with fat-free cookies, but I think I'd rather have 2 regular Oreos vs. 4 fat-free cookies. I definitely steer away from the fat-free chips. . . . I've had friends who have had very bad experiences with the olean products! My brother-in-law didn't even make it to the bathroom after eating a bag of fat-free Doritos! Yikes!!!! —MFR

I never really had a problem with SnackWell's until the mint cremes came out. I can't have them in the house. My husband will eat a box of the chocolate chip SnackWell's in about five minutes. If I buy them for me, I either have to hide them or buy a sacrificial box for him. I do have to monitor myself with olean products. I've learned that the baked potato with catsup thing (as gross as I thought it sounded in class) is a better option for me than olean products. One little piece of real, dark, slightly bitter chocolate is much more satisfying than two boxes of SnackWell's. —LAK

I use no fat-free sweets for the same reason you gave in the class. I ate the whole box! —BF

Before I came into the program, I sometimes ate some SnackWell's cookies, but they were so sweet I stopped doing that. I have really tried to cut down on my sugar consumption and that pretty much cuts out the fat-free sweets—they seem overloaded with sugar! As far as sugar-free chips or crackers or stuff, I eat Matzo crackers or Wasa bread, which are both pretty much fat-free, sugar-free. —MC

Prior to entering the program, if I did buy something like the SnackWell's cookies I would typically overeat—most of the cookies in one sitting!

By the way, I was standing in the checkout line at a local convenience store the other day when I noticed a shelf stocked with "FAT-FREE" blueberry muffins. Out of curiosity I picked one up to see the nutrition label. The first thing that caught my eye was the serving size: ⅓ of the muffin!!! which contained almost 200 calories, but no fat, so eating the whole muffin (who would actually eat ⅓ of a muffin?) would give zero fat grams and a whopping 600 calories. No way to justify eating that sort of thing. —PG

ARTIFICIAL SWEETENERS

I have held from the time of their introduction that artificial sweeteners (sometimes referred to as high-intensity sweeteners) are of very little help in weight management. I believe they only keep your taste for sweetness alive and stand in the way of your cultivating a taste for other flavors, such as are found in herbs and spices. I think their use is counterproductive because the chemical composition of these sweeteners can alter your response to the natural sweetness found in fruits and vegetables. Whether it does or not may depend on the particular artificial sweetener that you use, and the degree to which your taste buds respond to various fruits.

Here is a little experiment for you to try.

If you drink any kind of diet soda, take a sip of that soda and then taste a piece of fruit. When I have done a taste test of this kind at lectures and press conferences, a majority of those who participate report that fruits such as apples, oranges, melons, strawberries, and other berries have an off-flavor—are even bitter.

The basic issue that must be resolved in the use of artificial sweeteners as a replacement for sugar in weight management is whether they lead to a reduction in your caloric intake or to compensation. That is, do they lead to an increase in the consumption of other carbohydrates, fat, or protein following a meal or snack in which they are consumed? The answer appears to be yes. Research shows that if artificial sweeteners are used in a breakfast cereal, then lunch and dinner meals tend to be larger. The compensation in caloric intake may come via an increase in fat! While it's true that some individuals may benefit by their use in the context of a broad program of weight management, after many years of debate, experts are now pretty much in agreement: people who use artificial sweeteners tend to eat more later to make up for the energy saved. In fact, comparing people who use sugar with those who use artificial sweeteners over a long period of time, there is much evidence that sugar users stay thinner than persons who use artificial sweeteners.

Take stock of your own situation. Do you use artificial sweeteners? Have you lost weight since you began to use them, or are you heavier? Perhaps you use them as a result of a fear, fostered by the industry and sometimes by misguided health professionals, that you would be in even worse shape without them. You may change your mind about using them as you read on and put the T-Factor 2000 Diet in action.

IT'S TIME TO SWITCH GEARS AND ACCENT THE POSITIVE

I've spent a good deal of time on the negative, pointing out the dangers of: 1) too much fat in the diet; 2) the inclusion of certain categories of fat-free or reduced-fat foods; and 3) the use of artificial sweeteners. While there is no way around the need for restraint, negativity is not the best approach to a weight-management regimen. You need to focus on the positive—not so much on what's coming out of your diet but on what's going in, and the great benefits to be gained thereby.

The T-Factor 2000 Diet includes all you want to eat of healthful, natural, unprocessed fruits and vegetables and whole grains (or minimally processed grains in whole-grain breads and cereals), with enough fat in their preparation to make sure you end up with a delicious diet. You'll find over 135 recipes in Chapter 8 to prove that eating healthy can taste great, too. But before we jump into the diet itself, let's look at the preparations you need to make in order to assure yourself that you are going to be 100 percent successful. As successful persons will tell you, *"There's much more to permanent weight management than just going on a diet."*

CHAPTER 3

There's More to Permanent Weight Management Than Just Going on a Diet

Are you *really* ready to lose weight and willing to do what it takes to keep it off?

If you have tried to lose weight before and found yourself regaining part or all of the weight you lost, I think you must agree that it would be wrong to pull punches and tell you that a miracle has occurred and it will suddenly be easy. You already know it can be hard work. In the end, it's going to boil down to a question of motivation.

But take it from a former fat man—there really is a lot to look forward to! I'll tell you my story later in this chapter. Losing 75 pounds back in 1963 changed my life in ways I had never imagined until it happened. You must keep your eyes on the goal and make a commitment to a plan that will get you there, day by day, step by step, and you *will* get there.

But if you have a great deal of weight to lose, you must control your impatience. You cannot leap from here to there. You must set interim objectives that you feel certain you can reach, and take pride each time you pass a mile marker along the way. And even if you have just 10 pounds to lose, which you may be able to do quickly on the new T-Factor 2000 Rotation Plan, you will still face the problem of keeping it off.

So let's take a look at some of the many obstacles you are likely to face, and see what kind of planning has been successful in surmounting them for me and for other successful people.

From day one, you will face the same environment that may have encouraged poor eating habits in the past—*unless you are willing to make some changes in that environment*. The best way to deal with this obstacle is to take command and change every aspect of that environment that's within your power to change so that you are not constantly tempted by the foods that keep you fat. We'll show you how to do this—and still stay friends with the people you live and work with!

What about exercise?

You simply *must* make physical activity a priority and an integral part of your daily life. At least 90 percent of the people who have been successful in losing weight and *keeping it off* point to an increase in physical activity as a key factor in weight maintenance no matter what diet they used to lose the weight they've lost. I am going to do everything I know how to do to inspire you to become an active person. Becoming an active person will do more for your ego and for your mental and emotional well-being than just losing weight by itself. I'll focus on physical activity in Chapter 9. In Chapter 11 I'll let some successful people tell you in their own words what physical activity means to them. But first, let's talk about your diet.

What about your taste preferences?

Don't kick yourself if you like a well-seasoned steak, or that delicious combination of sweetness with fat in desserts, pastries, and, of course, in chocolate. It's absolutely normal, part of the human genetic heritage, to respond with salivation, increased gastric secretions, even an anticipatory insulin response at the sight or smell of tasty foods. This is a built-in physiological reaction that's preparing your body to handle the food it expects to receive. Indeed, *it's abnormal* to try to limit your consumption of highly palatable foods if you live in an environment in which you have to face them, right in front of your nose, day in and day out whenever you must make an eating choice! It means you must fight Mother Nature.

I think it's obvious that the first step is to take command and construct a safe eating environment in your home if you eat most of your meals there. But you cannot always avoid foods that will tempt you to outeat your energy needs when you are invited to a friend's home or find yourself in a restaurant, celebrating some special occasion. This will require some restraint and the ability to make choices that will satisfy your appetite without threatening your ability to manage your weight.

In time almost everyone discovers that their taste preferences change and many of the high-fat foods they previously liked lose their attractiveness. We've got to find a way to stick with it, to make better choices, and to learn how to prepare different foods with different seasonings until that happens. Many successful people have told me that after avoiding fried foods for several months, should they taste a piece of fried chicken or a French fried potato, it doesn't taste nearly as good as they remember. In fact, the greasy taste and feel can actually turn off their appetite. This has been my experience—even as I write about the taste of fried potatoes or chicken, my stomach begins to feel just a little queasy! On the other hand, a good cheddar cheese, Asiago, or Gruyère has always retained its attraction, and I must be careful to cut exactly what I intend to eat—that is, one standard serving—and put the rest away before I begin. Just as in my own case, I think that for many successful people there will still be certain foods that retain their "turn on," and in our plentiful eating environment, some restraint is likely to remain necessary forever. I hope to show you that this restraint does not mean deprivation—it just means making healthful choices and learning how to include some of those foods that turn you on, as a good cheese does for me, in quantities that won't endanger your success.

A large percentage of successful weight losers find that the kind of life they lead as thinner people is so rewarding that it makes maintaining their lower weight easier than it was to lose weight in the first place, but it takes time to reach that stage, and there are many barriers to cross. As you set out to do this, perhaps my own experiences as a former fat man can be of value.

HOW I LOST 75 POUNDS IN 1963

When I look back at my own many attempts at weight loss before I finally found the way to lose 75 pounds in 1963, I can point to several things that sabotaged my efforts.

Right at the top of the list was my inability to find an approach to losing weight that I could live with until I reached my goal. I was impatient. I wanted, just as you might, to lose a great deal of weight in a hurry—like all 75 extra pounds in one fell swoop. At times I went to extremes, from no plan at all, except to "eat less," to stuffing capsules with gelatin and swallowing them with one or two glasses of water in place of a meal.

Nothing I tried lasted more than a few days. Whatever I did—before I found my personal solution—something would occur that propelled me off whatever diet I was on at the time. I would begin to overeat in response to stress or feelings of frustration and anger. Or I might find myself in some social situation, at a friend's home for dinner or at a restaurant, and simply choose not to restrain myself when delicious high-fat foods, beautifully presented, were placed, unasked, on the table before me. Since I love to cook, I could be my own worst enemy. At that period of my life, I liked porterhouse steaks, along with a large baked potato smothered not with one but with several pats of butter, and 3 or 4 ounces of sour cream. Every so often I would make a chuck roast (that's about the fattiest cut of meat you can get for a roast) or a cheesecake made with the full-fat variety of cream cheese, heavy cream, and eggs! Up until 1963, the year I finally got serious, it never occurred to me that I ought to stop tempting myself with my own cooking, and that it might be to my advantage to rid my pantry and refrigerator of the high-fat foods that were, repeatedly, my undoing.

But something happened in 1963 that showed me just how dangerous my overweight condition really was, and intensified my motivation to do something about it. It took a critical, triggering event.

I knew I was terribly out of shape. I weighed 230 pounds, which is about 70 pounds more than was best for me. I had high blood pressure. It was so high that I had to lie down on a couch for an hour in order to bring it down to 140/90 so that an examining physician would OK me for an insurance policy to cover the new house I had just purchased on moving to Nashville. I had absolutely no endurance for even the slightest physical activity. I used to postpone my trips across the street, from my office to the library, because I would get out of breath just climbing the single flight of stairs from the street to the library entrance.

Then, one hot summer day, at the age of thirty-five, while attempting to play a game of Ping-Pong, something I hadn't done in almost twenty years, I had a heart attack. Fortunately, it was a minor coronary, but as my doctor, Ed Tarpley, showed me my cardiogram, he said something for which I will be forever grateful because it changed my life. The look on his face and the sound of his voice are as clear today as they were over thirty-five years ago: "Dick," he said, using my nickname, you've got to lose that weight. I don't care what kind of a diet you use, but you *have got to get active*. That's the only way you will keep the weight off and possibly prevent another occurrence." Dr. Tarpley was way ahead of his time because he put his finger on the key to weight maintenance long before anyone in the obesity field had researched and proven the point.

In the days that followed I thought long and hard about what I was going to do. I had two children, eight and ten years old, and I certainly did not want to chance another heart attack if I could avoid it. The thought of dying and leaving my wife alone with sole responsibility for the kids was terrifying to me. This was the kind of motivation that started me on my way to losing 75 pounds, which was, in fact, a few pounds more than I felt was best suited for me once I had done it. So, except for a period in which I was injured and temporarily regained some weight when I cut back on physical activity, I have been content to stay just 70 pounds lighter for the past thirty-five years. I will tell you more about how I have been able to change my food preferences and make physical activity a part of my daily life, as well as show you what other successful people are doing, as we go along putting the T-Factor 2000 Diet to work.

Now, what about you?

What is motivating you? The great majority of people who have been successful in losing weight and keeping it off report that it took rather extreme circumstances to motivate them to do what it takes to achieve permanent weight management. Among the successful losers in the National Weight Control Registry (now numbering over 3000), fully 77 percent were motivated by a triggering event that threatened either their health, as in my case, or their emotional well-being, such as a divorce.

I hope that this kind of a trigger is not operating in your situation. If it isn't, however, you may find that just wanting to look better may not prove motivation enough to sustain the kind of real work it's going to take. So consider what there is to be gained in your life by losing weight even if the triggering circumstance is not an immediate threat to your life or well-being.

If you are more than just a few pounds overweight, you *will* undoubtedly like the way you look after losing weight. I can vouch for the satisfaction that follows when one can fit into clothing a few sizes smaller. But there are some real physical and emotional benefits, too. By losing weight you lessen whatever your present risk is for heart disease, high blood pressure, diabetes, arthritis, and several kinds of cancer. Even if you suffer from none of these things now and bear little familial predisposition for any of them, the emotional benefits can be great. With the loss of just a few pounds, you will experience an increase in energy as it becomes easier to move a lighter body around. One of the best ways to see this improvement is to climb one or more flights of stairs daily. (In fact, as you will see in Chapter 9, the extra carbohydrate burning required by adding a few flights of stairs to your daily routine will help make sure you are burning the best mix of carbohydrate and fat to facilitate weight loss and make weight maintenance easier.) Sustain your motivation by keeping the benefits of losing weight at the forefront of your consciousness. Every time you follow through with a behavior or positive thought that can bring you closer to your weight-loss goal, enter it in your "won" column.

WHAT WILL IT TAKE TO SURMOUNT YOUR PERSONAL BARRIERS?

Making a change in the way you eat and replacing inactive times in your day with physically active pursuits is going to have an impact on just about everything and everybody in your life. You probably are well aware of this if you have tried to make some changes in the past. Let's talk first about changing your food choices and make some plans in advance to head off the obstacles that might arise.

To begin with, whether you live alone or in a family setting, changing your eating habits will be much easier if you change the eating environment in your home. As Dr. James Hill* expressed it, successful people create a "mini-environment" in their homes where only foods they feel they can safely handle are allowed to enter. So take a look around in your own kitchen, refrigerator, freezer, and pantry. What do you see? Are there a lot of high-fat foods, energy-dense imitation foods, a large supply of processed and convenience foods, and a nice variety of sugar or fat-laden snack foods that are easy to grab and easier to consume? Ask yourself whether some of these foods have been tempting you to overeat. I'll show you how

*Dr. Hill is professor of pediatrics and medicine at the University of Colorado Health Sciences Center and one of the principal investigators on the National Weight Control Registry research project.

I overcame my own tendency to overeat on certain high-fat foods later in this chapter. I now can keep them in the house and not overeat. But I can assure you that *it is much easier and much more effective to limit the availability of the foods that are keeping you fat than to hold your hands behind your back or mentally glue your mouth shut every time you lay eyes on them!*

But don't leave a void. Replace the foods that tend to be your undoing with a more wholesome, varied, and lean selection that you can turn to whenever you're hungry. This will require a certain amount of planning, and, at first, it may take more time. Don't try to play it by ear. Before you start the T-Factor 2000 Diet, take a look at the lists of foods that pose no threat to weight management and at the menus and recipes in the next chapters. Plan which recipes you will use, make up a shopping list to fit either the menus you find in the next chapter or the menus you create for yourself using T-Factor guidelines.

Virtually everyone with whom you come in contact can be affected by changes in your diet because so many things in our lives are associated with food. This will be especially true of the people you live with. If everyone in your family is not on board, you may find it tough sledding! At the second meeting of one of our weight groups, one woman told us that when she announced her intention to "improve the family diet" her twelve-year-old son complained, "You mean I have to go on a diet because you're trying to lose weight?"

If you are responsible for all or most of the food preparation in your family, you will find it very hard, if not impossible, to prepare different foods for yourself and the other members of the family. And, if they demand high-fat foods, and you agree, thinking you can *always* restrain yourself, it's likely to be your first step on the road to failure. Before you start a weight-loss diet, you must convince everyone that the changes you are about to make will be of benefit to them all. Take time to work together to find foods and ways of preparing them that everyone enjoys and can live with. If your family remains resistant or resentful, don't force the issue. Instead, begin to incorporate subtle modifications into familiar recipes by using leaner meats, lower-fat ingredients, and lower-fat preparation methods. Try some of the new vegetable or grain side dishes, soups, and meatless entrées once or twice each week. If there are children in the family, do everything you can to involve them in the selection and preparation of food. Jamie will have more to say about this in Chapter 10, on weight management for children.

I think it is unfortunate that women are not as likely to obtain the cooperation of the male members of the family in weight-management efforts as the male members are from the women when they decide to go on a diet. Just as in my own case, most of the time, when men decide to lose weight, the wives select and prepare foods that will tend not to undermine their efforts. When men fail, it's usually due to their own willingness to deviate from their announced intentions. This sends a signal to everyone else that they are not serious and results in more temptations.

Women, on the other hand, find that their husbands can be resentful when their food preferences are not being satisfied. Sometimes their dissatisfaction is conveyed rather subtly. New dishes are greeted with a notable lack of enthusiasm, or such faint praise you know they never want to see them again. Feelings are hurt, to say the least. The men (and the children) often insist on having high-fat snacks and desserts around in spite of agreeing to experiment with main meals. And sometimes it will be the husband who gives the "just this once, it won't hurt" invitation to share a high-fat treat. If the woman doesn't, it's taken as a personal rejection, and not simply a desire to avoid something she doesn't want to eat!

If you are a woman and these are the kinds of things that happen to you, it's a good idea to talk them over before you start on the T-Factor 2000 Diet. If you can't get your husband to read this book before you begin so that he will understand its rationale and what you are trying to do, try to explain it to him verbally.

Jamie told me how a woman in her class in weight management finally made an impression on her husband and got his complete cooperation. This woman does all the cooking in her home, and her husband had been resisting any change in the way food was being prepared for the family. In addition to being overweight, she suffered from high blood pressure and had not been able to make any progress dealing with either problem while cooking in the southern style that the family had been accustomed to. She finally asked her husband, "Do you want high-fat southern food, or a thin wife?" He chose the thin—and healthier—wife. By cutting the fat in cooking, she lost 15 pounds over the next several weeks and had a dramatic reduction in her blood pressure.

Even if the changes you wish to make require absolutely no

change on the part of other people, they are likely to note what you are doing and comment on it. Often, persons whose health might benefit if they, too, lost some weight undermine others' efforts. Most of the time it is not done consciously or with a mean intent, but sometimes it is. Your family, colleagues, or friends may be jealous or fearful of how the changes you are making might affect them or reflect on them. One woman in a weight-management group that I was leading reported finding a candy bar—her favorite—on her desk every morning when she came to work. Another severely over-weight person in her office was putting it there. It started to appear each day only after the other woman found out she had joined a weight-management program! A gentle request to stop didn't work. Our participant needed to take firm action to put an end to this kind of behavior. On our advice, she waited until the other person ap-peared at her desk later one day, after having deposited her gift in the morning. Then she explained that the candy bar did not fit into her dietary plans and she threw it into the garbage so that the other person could see her doing it. That was the last candy bar to be placed on her desk.

In another instance, a participant reported that, where she worked, it was customary for one of the office personnel to bring a dozen doughnuts to serve at the morning coffee break. Only one of the several women working in the office was at or near desirable weight, but our participant was not able to prevail on the others to forgo the doughnuts even though it would have been to almost everyone else's benefit. We suggested to our participant that she take her break in another area of the building, which she did halfheart-edly for a short time. We suggested she bring her own snacks for coffee break, which she also did halfheartedly for a short time. The pressure to be part of the group turned out to be too great, and, ul-timately, so did the attractiveness of the doughnuts. Her inability to deal with this situation was reflected in other such situations in-volving high-fat foods and she did not do well in the program.

Another woman solved a similar problem at her coffee break by keeping an insulated take-out container at her office, and bringing a banana to work. The banana went well with coffee, and was, for her, almost as satisfying as the pastries that were part of the daily fare at her office coffee breaks. She ate her banana, and took her coffee mug with her on a walk around the building or in the park-ing lot. Although coffee and a banana were not as satisfying in the actual eating as coffee and a Danish, coffee and a banana plus a fifteen-minute walk around the area resulted in a much more satis-fying post–coffee break. In the hour that followed, she realized how much better she felt, physically and emotionally, compared with the feeling she used to have following coffee and a Danish. In fact, she said it made her feel better about herself the entire day, which is why she kept on doing it.

Learn to ask for the kind of support you need. Don't expect oth-ers to read your mind. If your spouse's "Should you be eating that?" drives you to want to eat more, kindly reinforce his interest, but sug-gest that an encouraging word or compliment does more for your motivation. Your spouse may truly, but mistakenly, believe that a watchdog stance helps and would welcome other ways he can sup-port you.

So, think about the kinds of social pressures that have, in the past, worked against your intentions, and see if you can't develop a plan of action to deal with them before you begin to make any changes in your eating behavior. Here is how I discovered a plan to deal with the social pressures I faced when eating out.

During the period back in 1963 when I was losing weight, we so-cialized frequently, including dinners at friends' homes and at our fa-vorite restaurants. I always tried to make it clear when necessary that I was serious about losing weight, but many times I faced the "just this once won't hurt" invitation. It was on the spur of the moment that I invented the "4-S Diet," which proved from that time forth to be a perfect protection against such invitations. We were out with friends at a restaurant when one of them asked why I was limiting myself to a shrimp cocktail, salad, and a London broil, together with passing on the alcoholic beverages. I put a few "S"s together and said, "I'm on this new diet—it's the 4-S Diet. He asked what that was, to which I replied, "Unlimited indulgence in shrimp, steak, salad, and sex." It got a few laughs, but I noticed that no one pressured me to deviate from my plans for the rest of the night. So, I kept on referring to my 4-S Diet on future occasions whenever I needed its help to stick with my resolution, and it never failed me.

You, too, may need to have some response ready for social situ-ations in which, for whatever reason, someone may do something to undermine your plans. Here are a few useful strategies.

Some people find that just saying, "No, thank you," when food is offered, with a smile to the person's face, and *then looking quickly away* and resuming whatever activity or conversation was in progress, works just fine. This is most effective when performed in a nonchalant, offhanded way, as though the food has no interest for you. If you linger, looking longingly at proffered food, your body language sends a different message than your words.

Be careful about saying, "No, I'm on a diet." This can put the other person in an awkward position—they can't very well agree with you and say, "Oh, yes, you do need to go on a diet!" The natural response is usually, "Oh, you look just fine," or "Just this once won't hurt." So, stay clear about your intentions, but watch your wording and body language.

Some people let friends and colleagues know that they have a health reason for changing their eating habits. This may prove awkward if you don't want to disclose the reason or keep on discussing it. But once everyone understands, they may all participate in maintaining a protective environment when you are eating together.

Many successful people tell a little white lie and just say "Oh . . . no thanks. It looks really good, but I've just eaten," when offered a snack, even when they haven't just eaten. Some successful people learn to take small portions, and to *always leave something on their plates* when serving themselves appetizers at cocktail parties or after being served and finishing their first portions during dinner parties. Leaving something on your plate discourages your hosts from asking if you want more, or attempting to serve you more as they walk around the room or table, offering seconds. But do remember: when you give yourself permission to deviate from your plan for any reason at all, other people may come to the conclusion that you are not serious. This may only encourage them to continue to encourage you, in perhaps the festive spirit of the occasion, to keep on deviating!

Watch out for alcohol!

Alcohol prevents the burning of fat. It's burned in place of fat. So, since it replaces fat in your fuel mixture, you must count alcohol just as though you had eaten the same number of calories in fat in your diet! (It may displace about 7 grams of fat in your fuel mixture per 1½ ounces of whiskey or 4 ounces of wine.) Alcohol also interferes with decision making. You are much more likely to overeat after a drink or two. If you can handle a glass of wine with dinner (perhaps two if you are a man), count it as fat, and make sure it doesn't otherwise interfere with your weight-management plans. If it does, you better pass it up. I know from experience that it does for me, so that's why I passed it up when I was losing weight.

Here I must warn you of a fact that contradicts some of the advice you might get from many well-meaning weight-management leaders. You have probably been told that occasional lapses from a low-fat weight-management diet are not particularly dangerous. In fact, before the research appeared that showed how detrimental to your overall efforts they could be, I used to suggest that people just strive for a "B" grade in their weight-management diets. You don't have to be perfect. I believed, like many others, that eating appropriately 80 or 85 percent of the time was all that was necessary to insure weight-management success. Many health experts still seem to feel that after taking in more calories than you need at one meal, natural physiological processes are set in motion that lead at least to some compensatory reduction in energy intake at later meals. As I showed in the last chapter, this is not necessarily true, especially for fat calories. But, at the same time, trying to be too perfect on a diet might prove stressful and only increase the risk of failure for many people.

I'll tell you how successful people deal with their occasional high-fat lapse after explaining another consequence that appears to be especially detrimental for individuals predisposed to obesity. After a weight loss, your adipose tissue lipoprotein lipase (AT-LPL) begins to work overtime. This is the enzyme that facilitates getting the fat circulating in your blood into your fat cells. A surplus of fat in a single meal goes directly to the fat cells, which seem to be especially hungry after they have lost a part of their fat stores. If an increase in dietary fat continues, as it might for a few days should you be, for example, on vacation, naturally thin folks, not being predisposed to obesity and not having been on a diet, begin to respond quickly by increasing the amount of fat burned in their fuel mixture. Their bodies begin to burn it off and prevent the accumulation of more body fat. This quick increase in fat burning is likely to be lacking in persons predisposed to obesity. In persons predisposed to obesity, the body takes longer to adjust its fuel mix to an increase in fat intake. So, an increase in their fat intake results in an increase in total fat mass. *The threat to individuals predisposed to obesity from increasing fat in the diet appears to increase following weight loss, when AT-LPL becomes even more active than normal!*

What you need to learn from this, and from the studies that I described in the previous chapter, is that indulgence in a high-fat meal requires *conscious* compensation if you don't want to allow excess dietary fat *from even a single eating episode* to take up permanent residence in your fat depots. Successful weight management requires *intentionally* cutting back on fat in subsequent meals, and possibly spending a few minutes more in physical activity for good measure. You must have a compensation strategy in place before these high-fat occasions take you by surprise. As you will see in Chapter 11, where successful people describe what they are doing to remain successful, some of them take action after a single lapse, while others give themselves a certain leeway in terms of how much weight they allow themselves to gain. I give myself a two-pound limit. But whatever strategy you decide to use, it must be part of your plan to make sure you don't suffer a setback while losing weight and it must be part of your strategy for maintaining your weight following weight loss.

TWO T-FACTOR APPROACHES TO SUCCESSFUL WEIGHT LOSS

In view of the research I've just described, you may be asking the question, "How perfect do I have to be to succeed in the weight-management game?" It depends on your definition, or application, of the word "perfection." I prefer to think of it in terms of a tennis match or a football game rather than as a test of marksmanship. In target shooting, perfection requires a bull's-eye with each shot. In a tennis game or football game, the winner usually prevails in spite of many errors. The important thing is to have a game plan such as I have been talking about in this chapter, and to work hard at its execution. Of course, in weight management your opponent is not another person or team but the whole set of circumstances, genetic and environmental, that fight to keep you fat. With two T-Factor 2000 approaches to weight loss, I think I can give you a game plan that will suit your situation to a "T."

The T-Factor 2000 Diet

From day one in the basic plan you begin to make the changes in your diet that lead simultaneously to weight loss *and* weight maintenance. That is, we do from day one what successful people do. We cut the fat. In the research that laid the groundwork for the original T-Factor Diet over ten years ago the participants cut their fat to about 19 or 20 percent of calories during the period in which they were losing weight. On follow-up one year later, they were maintaining at 24 percent of calories in fat. This percent of calories in fat is exactly what has been reported by successful people who have submitted data to the National Weight Control Registry.

The easiest way to be sure you are following a low-fat diet is to count fat grams, not calories or percent of calories in fat for each food or meal, which are more complex operations and difficult to do. We will show you how to count fat grams in the way that easily meets the targeted percent of calories in fat in the next chapter, where we also supply you with an assortment of menus and point you to recipes that meet the criterion.

On the T-Factor 2000 Diet you can consume all you want of *un-refined* carbohydrates—that is, any and all fruits, vegetables, and whole grains (including minimally processed grains such as you find in 100 percent whole-wheat bread and cereals). You need never be hungry and you need never feel deprived. *You can include some of your favorite high-fat foods, as long as you don't exceed the fat gram limits.* While you cannot eat unlimited quantities of energy-dense imitation fat-free desserts, cookies, snacks, etc., because of their potential for lowering your fat-consumption threshold, we will show you how they can be included with minimal threat to your weight-management efforts.

In Chapter 5 I will also show you how weight loss and mainte-nance proceed when you follow this basic plan. I used it myself after regaining some weight following my injury and reduction in physi-cal activity several years ago.

The T-Factor 2000 Rotation Plan

The T-Factor 2000 Rotation Plan is an updated version of the very effective quick-weight-loss diet that I devised for myself when it became apparent after my heart attack that I had to find a way to lose 70 to 75 pounds in 1963. If you have a great deal of weight to lose, as I did, losing weight slowly is likely to be quite unappealing. With the Rotation Plan, you decide either 1) how long you wish to follow the menus we will lay out for you or 2) how much weight you would like to lose while following them. All of the menus meet the same low-fat goals of the basic T-Factor 2000 Diet, so even though you are losing weight more quickly, you will be following the principles of the T-Factor Diet, which insure maintenance. And, of course, we will show you how to make substitutions for our menu suggestions in order to meet your taste preferences.

You can follow the plan for one, two, or three weeks. It's up to you. In three weeks, which was normally the time I used it myself on each rotation, you can expect to lose up to 10 or even 15 pounds, depending on your initial starting weight. If you are 70 pounds overweight, you may even lose close to 20 pounds, as I did on my first rotation. If you are only 10 or 20 pounds overweight, you may lose about 2 or 3 pounds a week.

Instead of a time-limited period for following the diet, you can set a reasonable, reachable weight goal. If you choose a weight goal, I suggest 5 percent of your initial body weight—for example, 10 pounds for a person who weighs 200 pounds. This amount of weight loss is usually reachable in a reasonable period of time, and it's an excellent goal to aim for, because losing just 5 percent of your body weight has significant health benefits.

When you reach your time or weight-loss goal, you stop using the quick-weight-loss version and rotate over to the basic T-Factor 2000 Diet. You expand your choices, eat more, but still make absolutely sure you do not regain any weight. You rotate back to the quick-weight-loss version if you wish to lose more weight. I did not keep track of how many times I used my rotation approach in 1963 and the early part of 1964 to lose those 75 pounds (my interest in helping other people manage their weight did not surface until we started the Vanderbilt Weight Management Program in 1976). I believe it took me five or six rotations, usually three weeks at a time. An important factor in my long-term success with the rotation plan was that I was able to discover and "practice" what it took to maintain my losses between rotations. The plan turned out to be a very easy way to lose weight, I had a great deal of fun doing it, and I felt proud of myself with each 10- or 15-pound loss on the way to my ultimate goal.

I suggest you read about both the basic T-Factor 2000 Diet and the T-Factor 2000 Rotation Plan in the next few chapters before you decide which way suits you best. Study the menus and look over the recipes. Since I feel so strongly that it is important to cut back on the amount of red meat in your diet if you have been consuming meat on a daily basis, you will find that our menus and recipes emphasize the inclusion of plant foods, and more poultry and fish. However, we do include instructions for how to prepare low-fat cuts of beef and pork, and you will find options for including meat or vegetable dishes at various meals on our menus. Ever since its original publication in 1989, we have had many requests to develop a vegetarian version of the T-Factor Diet. We are happy to be able to provide such a version in Chapter 7.

NOW STOP HERE
AND DO THE FOLLOWING TWO EXERCISES
BEFORE YOU BEGIN THE T-FACTOR 2000 DIET

The following two exercises can guarantee your success on the T-Factor 2000 Diet. They are designed to give you complete, conscious control over your eating behavior. Their impact has never failed to surprise—in fact, astonish—*everyone* who has faithfully followed my instructions for how to perform them.

It's important to do them both *before* you begin the T-Factor 2000 Diet.

Exercise I: Knowledge Is Power

The goal of this exercise is to give you insight into, and command over, your eating behavior. As I pointed out earlier, overweight people tend to underestimate the number of calories and amount of fat that they consume by 30 to 55 percent. Although you do not have to count calories or fat grams in this exercise, it will show you whether you are truly aware of how much you eat. In fact, if you were in my presence I'd give you ten to one odds that you don't know, and that this exercise will prove it. It will reveal how food can short-circuit that part of the brain where better judgment resides, and, so to speak, lead you around by your nose and salivary glands. We are going to turn that situation around. This exercise is the first step toward putting better judgment in command of your appetite.

For just one day, I want you to write down, *in advance of each and every eating episode,* what you intend to eat at that time.

You must weigh and/or measure every single item *before* it is eaten.

This is a tedious thing to do. I know because I have done it myself. But the payoff is huge.

If you persevere for just one day, by the time evening rolls around I think you will know why I insist that you do it, and why I am so confident that the insight and control it will give you can make a powerful contribution to your success.

When should you do it? I suggest that you do this exercise when you have the opportunity to choose or prepare food yourself or can examine labels before eating, which means it is best done on a day that you are not eating out and have the time to weigh and measure everything.

What materials do you need? In order to do this correctly, you can use either a plain sheet of paper for the day or a 3 × 5–inch spiral notebook that opens from the side and which you can keep in your pocket. I prefer the little notebook because it can be used to keep other records, such as your daily weight if you decide to keep a weight record as you go along, and any eating records that you decide to keep.

You will need measuring implements, including a food scale, a measuring cup, and spoons. I use a Cuisinart Precision Portion Scale, but any accurate food scale will do.

Watch your reactions to this exercise as you do it. If you are tempted not to complete it, ask yourself why. It's important that you understand whether you have been hiding something from yourself or whether you really already know what this exercise can tell you. If you already know, fine. Skip it. But here's a fact: people who say they have trouble losing weight invariably *do* lose weight when they enter a metabolic ward in a hospital and are fed the number of calories they claim won't lead to weight loss!

Step-by-step directions.

At every eating episode during the day:

1) decide in advance what you are going to eat;
2) weigh or measure each item;
3) open your little notebook so that you can write on both left- and right-hand pages, and write down on the page to the left what you are about to eat, including the weight and any other appropriate measurement;
4) go ahead and eat.
5) After you have finished eating, think for a few moments about what you might have eaten had you not weighed, measured, and written everything down in advance.
6) If you would have eaten differently, record what you would have eaten on the page to the right.
7) If you did eat something other than what you originally intended, record what you ate on the right and indicate whether it was a case of food "taking over" and subverting your better judgment

or whether you made what you consider to be a nutritionally equivalent substitution.

Do not worry about keeping track of calories, fat grams, or anything else for now. We are concerned only with measured quantities of food. And, for the purposes of this exercise, it is unimportant whether you are trying to make any kind of modification in your eating habits at this time, or whether you decide to eat in the way you have been eating before you tried the exercise. *However, before you begin, it's important to decide which it will be*—a day of "normal" eating, or one in which you are trying to restrain yourself and lose weight. Note your choice at the top of the page on the left. Whatever you decide, you will gain an important insight into your relationship with food.

Let me give you an example, using breakfast, of the kind of measurement we need and of how this exercise should be done.

Suppose you decide you intend to have fruit juice, cereal, milk, and coffee with half-and-half. Write down the amounts exactly. For example:

6 ounces of orange juice
¾ cup cereal
½ cup of 1% milk
1 cup of coffee
1 teaspoon of half-and-half

If you don't have a 6-ounce glass for the juice, it must be measured. Measure the amount of cereal and milk, etc.

When you think for a moment about what you might have eaten had you not measured and written it down, write down what you think you would have eaten on the page to the right. Of course, if you did vary from your original intention, be sure to record what you ate with a note on why.

Be prepared for lunch, between-meal snacks, dinner, and after-dinner snacks to be a bit more complicated than breakfast. Be patient and take your time because the insight you will obtain, and the control over your eating that you will experience, will be worth every moment of the effort you put into it.

Evening snacks are often a source of excess consumption, especially if you eat while watching TV or during any other evening activity. An accurate record of your nighttime eating intentions and behavior can prove to be the most valuable part of your record.

What normally happens when overweight people do this exercise?

The most significant thing that I hear from overweight people who have never done an exercise of this kind before is that there is a substantial difference between what they consciously decide to eat *in advance of eating* and what they would have eaten if they had not written it down. They tell me that the impact is much different from keeping the more common type of eating record where they try to recall, sometime late in the day, what and how much they have eaten since getting up in the morning. This is true whether or not they are attempting to lose weight. Most of the time, people who do this exercise eat quite differently just because they are consciously trying to direct their behavior and are observing themselves. You will sense whether this is happening as you do the exercise, and it is an important insight.

Whether you have eaten differently in a way that has an effect on your weight may be immediately apparent if you habitually weigh yourself each day. But I think you may have discovered two important things about your eating behavior as a result of weighing and measuring food and recording intentions and consumption. You may not have been aware of the size of the portions of food you generally consume, and you may not have had an accurate idea of the total quantity of food you normally eat on a given day.

You might want to use the Fat Gram Counter in Appendix D to calculate your fat grams and total calories when you finish the day. Do it three ways: Compare the totals for your intentions, what you actually ate, and what you imagined you might have eaten if you had not performed this exercise.

By the end of the day, most people who do this exercise feel a clear change in the way they approach eating. They are slowing down and considering whether what they are about to eat is consistent with their goal for the day—that is, "normal" eating or restraint to lose weight. People who sometimes feel driven, a little out of control, or even frenzied in their eating behavior note that they feel calmer when they start to eat as a result of taking time to consider what they want to eat and writing down their intentions. By the second eating episode in the day, many people already sense a difference in their mental attitude toward food. By the end of the day, the entire process of intending and selecting as they approach time to eat begins to become second nature. Of course, this is what I intend. The goal is to achieve the kind of conscious control over your eating behavior that you can go through mentally, whenever you choose to, without having to write your intentions down, and still carry out your intentions successfully.

Just one day of this exercise will change the way you approach food. You will feel a greater degree of control over your appetite, and one day may be enough for you to pursue this exercise. If you don't feel that the change in your attitude and behavior toward food is significant in just one day, I strongly advise you to do the exercise for one or two more days. With three days of practice, you will have discovered a whole new possibility in your relationship with food!

Suppose you were unable to carry out your eating intentions? Occasionally, food "gets the better of them" the first time people try this exercise, especially if someone in their eating environment distracts them from the task, or they are hungry and come face to face with a particularly enticing food. *But this can be informative.* If it happens to you, you know the kind of situations that can interfere with your intentions. Repeat the exercise another day and use some of the suggestions I am making throughout this book to change those situations or your behavior in response to them.

Exercise II: Taking Control

This exercise is one that was particularly helpful to me in changing my own eating behavior, and it may be just as helpful to you.

When I was overweight there were certain foods that seemed to possess an overwhelming power to control my appetite. While I might overeat on any occasion when one of my favorite high-fat foods was available, there was one high-fat food that I included frequently in my diet and which inflamed my appetite and produced some compulsive eating behavior—peanut butter!

My approach to peanut butter was what my son, who once observed me in action, called that of a "food consumption engineer." I would sit down at the table with a quart of milk, a box of crackers, a jar of peanut butter and a jar of jelly, and start to eat. When my better judgment told me it was time to stop, I would proceed to try to make everything come out even. That is, I had to finish my glass of milk, have eaten all the crackers I had put on my plate, and have eaten peanut butter in a way that made it come out level and smoothed over in the jar. (I didn't have any requirement for the jar of jelly!) If I still had milk left when the peanut butter was leveled,

I'd have to have another cracker and a bit more peanut butter and jelly. But then when the milk was finished, the peanut butter invariably would not be in the desired state. So, I'd pour another quarter-glass of milk. Then I might find that I had put one too many crackers on my plate. And so on it would go. Quite often, I would end up eating half the jar of peanut butter before I had everything evened out to my satisfaction. That's a half-pound of peanut butter and 112 grams of fat! According to the label on the jar of my favorite brand of peanut butter, Smucker's, that's 1050 calories in fat alone, and 1400 total calories. (Peanut butter contains 25 percent of its total calories in carbohydrate and protein and it contains a high percentage of monounsaturated fats—it's really a great food to include in your diet once you learn how to live with it in healthful quantities!)

After losing weight in 1963 I insisted that peanut butter stay out of the house, and it did for twenty years! Then, one day, several years after I became director of the Vanderbilt Weight Management Program and had become experienced with helping people use behavior-change strategies to change their eating habits, I decided to put one of these strategies into action myself.

I had been telling participants in the program that if they repeatedly found that they could not resist consuming more than they thought best of certain high-fat foods, they should keep them out of their eating environment. This is what I had done with peanut butter and it had worked very well. After all, you can only eat something if you have access to it! Constructing a healthful eating environment is still one of the most important steps you can take to assure that you and your family eat a nutritious diet.

But to allow peanut butter to have such control over my eating behavior?

I told myself that was ridiculous.

What I did broke the spell that peanut butter had over me in about ten minutes.

As I had planned when I bought a jar of Smucker's, I took it to the dining room table together with a slice of bread. Smucker's is the kind of "natural" peanut butter that contains only peanuts and salt and is not homogenized. It requires several minutes of mixing and stirring to blend in the oil on the top of the jar with the solid block of ground peanuts below. Even while mixing, I recall that I felt my confidence growing.

When the mixing task was completed, I challenged myself to see how thinly I could spread the peanut butter on the bread and still taste it. I put a film of peanut butter so thin on a corner of the bread that I could almost see through it, and took a bite. The result was a surprise greater than I had anticipated. I could taste it! Even this small amount. In fact, the flavor seemed to jump out at me. I had not eaten peanut butter in twenty years, so maybe my taste buds had become more sensitive. Twenty years earlier, if I had made a peanut butter and jelly sandwich, I would have layered the peanut butter almost as thick as the bread itself.

I spread another little dab on the bread, and slowly took another bite. I chewed more slowly than usual, and paid close attention to my taste sensations. I could not believe that I could taste peanut butter spread so thinly!

I finished the one piece of bread and peanut butter, and felt no desire to have another or to make a peanut butter and jelly sandwich. After that little exercise, my relationship with peanut butter changed. My taste for it changed so much that it no longer remains very high on my list of food preferences. I did make myself some peanut butter and jelly sandwiches during the following weeks. But, in contrast with the speed that peanut butter used to disappear from our house in the past, this time it was around for several months.

After that little experiment, we have continued to keep peanut butter in the house. But these days, it's kind of a fallback food. If there are no good leftovers for lunch, I may make a peanut butter and jelly sandwich. A one-pound jar continues to last several months. In fact, the jar I looked at a few moments ago to make sure that my fat-gram and calorie counts were accurate has already sat for several weeks, harmlessly, right in front of my nose on the top shelf on the door of our refrigerator! It's not even half-gone, even though both Enid and I have made peanut butter sandwiches, or spread it on sliced apples (which, by the way, is a good combination) whenever we felt like it.

This exercise had a large-scale effect. I began to see how little mayonnaise I could use on sandwiches and in salads and still fully enjoy the flavor. I did the same with the olive oil I use in cooking and baking. But for health reasons, because of the saturated fat, I have never done the same with butter and have eliminated it almost entirely from my diet.

I strongly advise you to use this exercise with one of the foods that has in the past tempted you to overeat. It is most easily and successfully done with a spreadable fat like peanut butter, butter or margarine, cream cheese, or mayonnaise. Your success with any one of these is likely to carry over to all high-fat spreads.

Your new-found feeling of self-control may also prove to be helpful when you are dealing with high-fat or energy-dense baked goods, snacks, and confections, but these may require a slightly different kind of practice. If any food in these categories has been more than an infrequent problem, I suggest you do a similar exercise, but with some slight modification because these foods are different from spreads and eaten in a different way.

With desserts, cookies, pastries, snacks, and candy, it is best to serve yourself exactly the amount you intend to eat. The serving should never be larger than the portion size indicated on the package, or what is a standard serving size—for example, one-eighth of a commercial pie. Then, put the package the food came in away so that it is not in clear sight, go to another room, and make sure that you are in a calm frame of mind.

The reason I say that the exercise must be done in a calm frame of mind is that many people who overeat on the foods we are talking about become highly aroused at their sight and smell. They feel driven to eat quickly until every single morsel has disappeared from sight. Only then can they relax. So, take a few minutes to let whatever heightened impulse to eat that you experience quiet down. Then begin to eat slowly and savor every bite.

You may find that this exercise is even more effective if you do it with another person. The social context adds to its potency, and a public display tends to increase commitment. It can be done with someone who has joined you with a desire to accomplish what you are trying to accomplish or who just wishes to be of help to you.

With these exercises under your belt, you will be well prepared to make a complete success of the T-Factor 2000 Diet.

So, don't just read about them—do them!

The Road to Permanent Weight Management: Putting the T-Factor 2000 Diet to Work

The T-Factor 2000 Diet is an easy diet to follow. It's based on certain guidelines for the amount of fat in your diet and the kind of foods that can be *freely* included. These guidelines can insure success in your quest for permanent weight management. *Permanent* is the key word. While any diet that results in a reduction in calories below your energy needs leads to weight loss, it's what happens after the diet that's the critical issue.

I think that one of the reasons so many people fail in maintaining the weight they have lost on various low-calorie diets is that the diet they use to lose weight has no relationship to what they will have to do to keep it off after they have lost it! This is particularly true of the high-protein diets that have cycled in and out of popularity for the last hundred years and which have recently become popular again. These diets lead to a quick weight loss (which is almost entirely water, as I have explained previously), and you can't continue to eat the way they require for losing weight for the rest of your life. In fact, if you did, you might encounter some serious liver and kidney problems.

The T-Factor 2000 Diet is a way to lose weight that is absolutely harmonious with the way you have to keep it off. The principles are one and the same. The only thing you must consider is the amount of fat in your diet.

Let's review the core principles.

1) Control over the amount of fat in your diet is central.

2) As long as you stick with unrefined carbohydrates you are free to eat as much as you want. Fruits, vegetables, and whole grains hold no danger to *permanent* weight management because they are capable of generating physiological signals that are strong enough to "turn off" your appetite before you outeat your energy needs.

3) This brings us to the refined, imitation, fat-free carbohydrates in the dessert, cookie, snack food, pastry, and confection category—foods that are engineered to simulate the taste and texture of fat. Just like the original fat-containing foods that these are designed to replace, they can stimulate your appetite to the point where you outeat your energy needs, and the carbohydrate they contain can depress your fat-consumption threshold (that is, they prevent your body from burning fat in its fuel mixture).

What this means is that because carbohydrate has priority over fat in your fuel mixture, if you take in a large load of carbohydrate your body switches to carbohydrate burning and cuts back on the fat it burns in its fuel mix. Keep in mind my illustration comparing an unrefined carbohydrate food and a refined fat-free carbohydrate: one 5-ounce apple contains 80 calories, while 5 ounces of a fat-free dessert or pastry such as an apple streusel can squeeze in over 300 calories. Apples hold no danger to weight management, but a piece of fat-free apple streusel of the same weight is a potential catastrophe! By the time turn-off signals to your appetite arrive from a fat-free apple streusel or any other fat-free dessert or pastry, you are quite likely to have consumed three or four times the calories that you would have had you eaten a fresh apple or any other fresh fruit. The excess of carbohydrate calories in the streusel is quite likely to divert to storage 100 or more calories of fat that you might have consumed in other foods during the day. If you had stuck with the apple you would have been home free.

The degree to which this suppression of fat burning by excess carbohydrate in the diet will either result in the expansion of the fat depots in a person who is gaining weight or prevent weight loss will vary from person to person. Recent research suggests that this kind of suppression of fat burning occurs more frequently in persons with a genetic predisposition to gain weight easily.

Does this mean you can never eat a fat-free cookie or any other fat-free food in the dessert, pastry, etc., categories without endangering your weight-management efforts?

Not at all. But you should not kid yourself. These foods are so energy-dense that they cannot fit into the "all you can eat" category.

In the guidelines below I am going to give you a simple formula to use when you include these in your diet. The formula will protect you.

While I prefer never to include these fat-free foods in my own diet, Jamie does on occasion. For Jamie, as a working mother of a three-year-old, they are convenient when she is unable to bake something herself. Jamie knows how to satisfy her appetite with appropriate-size portions. I don't include these imitation fat-free foods simply because I don't like them! I prefer fresh fruit for a sweet, or the low-fat desserts you will find among the recipes in Chapter 8. Besides tasting a great deal better, the ingredients in these recipes are far more nutritious than the refined flours, artificial ingredients, and large amount of sugar used in commercial products. (For an example, take a look at the recipe for Berry Crisp, which can be used with a wide variety of fruit.)

What about *reduced-fat* versions of dessert foods, cookies, etc.?

I have noticed that many of the companies that quickly jumped on the fat-free food bandwagon during the past decade have switched their marketing emphasis away from fat-free to reduced-fat versions. This seems to be the case especially in the case of desserts, cookies, and pastry. I think that there are two reasons for this. They taste better with a few grams of fat among the ingredients and, at the same time, benefit from the psychological impact of the reduced-fat label. People tend to exercise less restraint with reduced-fat foods, just as with fat-free foods. While I don't know of any research that proves this, I suspect that people who eat commercial reduced-fat baked goods may often consume larger portions or more servings of these foods, and possibly even more fat, than if they had eaten a single serving of the full-fat versions. Participants in the Vanderbilt Weight Management Program often tell us this, and, as you will see in Chapter 11, most permanently successful weight losers have come to the same conclusion.

Below, I'll give you some simple formulas for the consumption of fat-free and reduced-fat foods in the baked goods and candy categories if you wish to continue to include them in your diet.

What about dairy products?

You do not have to be as concerned with reduced- or low-fat versions of dairy products as you do with the baked goods and snacks.

The fat that is removed from these products is not replaced with sugar or other carbohydrates, so the food is not as packed with calories as it was initially. As you go from rich whole milk (4% fat), which contains about 160 calories per cup, down to 2%, 1%, and skim (almost completely free of fat), the calorie content is reduced to about 120, 100, and 80, respectively. We strongly encourage you to include reduced-fat and fat-free dairy products in your diet if you are not lactose intolerant, since they are among your best sources of calcium.

THE "MAGIC" NUMBERS*

Because of the great inaccuracy of self-reports, it is difficult to say with certainty how much fat the average person in the United States is consuming. *The percent of fat in the food supply has gone up from 42 to 43 in the last decade.*[†] Even with the fat that is trimmed or otherwise wasted, however, it is certain that the average person is consuming closer to 40 percent of calories in fat than the 34 percent reported in the most recent National Health and Nutrition Examination Survey.

Our own studies and a number of others' have shown that the average American woman is eating close to 100 grams of fat each day. Overweight women who are high fat eaters may be averaging 150 grams a day. With 9 calories per gram of fat, these figures add up to about 900 and 1350 calories in fat each day. Men average about 20 grams more than women.

---

*I continue to use the word "magic" in quotation marks, as I did in the original *T-Factor*, so as not to be misunderstood. There is no magical cure for obesity. Permanent changes in diet and almost always in physical activity are necessary to achieve a permanent change in weight. The quotation marks are meant to communicate an "as if by magic" quality, because controlling fat intake is so much easier than calorie counting. Research studies show that people who follow a low-fat diet tend to be more successful in weight maintenance than those who try to restrict intake by counting calories.

†This includes foods prepared for pets as well as for humans, but pet foods are generally lower in fat than the average daily diet of a person in the United States. For example, Milkbone Biscuits are only 18% fat. Pets are almost always thinner when fed animal chow than when fed foods consumed by humans. In fact, there is a strong correlation between obesity in owners and their pets—obese owners tend to have obese pets. I think you can guess why. It's not because their pets overeat on animal chow.

This is simply too much fat! It's too much for weight management, and it's way too much if you have any interest in reducing your risk for both heart disease and cancer.

The T-Factor formula for weight loss is:

20 to 40 grams of fat per day for women
30 to 60 grams of fat per day for men

Men can eat more fat than women and still lose weight because they have higher energy needs. The range is large to allow for flexibility. At the upper limit of 40 grams of fat a day, most women will be cutting fat by half, and will lose weight, although not as quickly as they would at the lower limit.

Only fat grams are limited.

When you have reached your quota of fat grams for the day, you may substitute natural, unrefined, no-fat foods for foods with fat at any time until your appetite is satisfied. I'll give more details on how to implement this formula as we go along.

It's not wise to go below the ranges that I suggest for fat consumption, because fat supplies some essential nutrients that cannot be obtained from other foods, and a minimal amount is necessary for the transport of fat-soluble vitamins. Besides, fat makes food taste good! If you don't get enough fat, you are likely to feel deprived. The latitude in the guidelines allows you to construct a fully enjoyable diet.

With respect to protein, the T-Factor 2000 Diet recommends levels and kinds of protein foods that are common in this country, although I hope you will follow my recommendation to switch a portion of your animal protein intake to vegetable sources. If you follow my menu suggestions (or devise your own according to T-Factor guidelines), protein intake will be adequate. This leaves you free to compensate for the reduction of fat in your diet with whatever increase in *unrefined* carbohydrate foods satisfies your appetite.

Because of the greater weight and volume of unrefined carbohydrate foods compared with fatty foods, which helps to give them their greater ability to turn off your appetite before you have overeaten, virtually everyone experiences an automatic cutback in calories. This automatic reduction in calories takes place without conscious effort, and it serves to foster a speedier loss of weight.

Since you don't have to cut fat to unreasonable levels, food still tastes good. You obtain yet another big plus because your diet will improve immensely in its nutritional value. Calorie for calorie, unrefined carbohydrate foods (fruits, vegetables, and whole grains) have far more vitamins and minerals than fatty foods. In addition, plant foods are the only sources of thousands of other valuable phytochemicals that help reduce your risk of cancer and heart disease. The T-Factor 2000 Diet, with its emphasis on plant foods, does more than just assure you of weight loss and maintenance. It builds your body's defenses to lower your risk of both heart disease and cancer—the two leading causes of death in the United States.

GUIDELINES FOR THE INCLUSION OF FAT-FREE AND REDUCED-FAT, ENERGY-DENSE FOODS

Because of the likelihood that energy-dense fat-free and reduced-fat foods in the dessert, pastry, snack food, and confection categories can lead to overconsumption of carbohydrate and result in a suppression of fat burning, *a portion of their caloric content should be counted as fat in the diet.* But science has yet to determine exactly the degree of suppression that the average person who is predisposed to obesity might experience. I have, however, devised a good rule of thumb, based on the metabolic processes that are involved. The rule will give you a ballpark figure and protect you from both a physiological and psychological perspective if you use it.

First, here is how to apply it to fat-free foods.

When you look at the label on a fat-free food of the kind to which I refer, **count a fat gram for every 10 calories over 50 per serving!**

I arrived at this figure in the following way:

The majority of fruits, vegetables, and grain foods have a caloric content that runs between 20 and 80 calories. You can check this out for yourself in the Fat Gram Counter in Appendix D. The average will run around 50 calories if you eat a wide variety. All of these foods are low in energy density because of their high fiber content and, in the case of fruits and vegetables, their high water content. A serving of these unrefined carbohydrates results in a feeling of fullness, which is an important appetite turn-off signal. When only 50 calories of an imitation fat-free but energy-dense carbohydrate has been consumed, this turn-off signal is likely to be lacking. These energy-dense foods are acting on your appetite and, to a large extent, on your ability to burn the fat in your diet, **just as if they were high-fat foods!**

The way to combat this, from both a psychological and physiological standpoint, is to **treat them like high-fat foods.**

For every 10 calories above the 50 that you might have taken in if you had chosen an unrefined carbohydrate instead of an energy-dense refined carbohydrate—for example, a piece of fruit instead of a fat-free cookie—**add a fat gram to your daily total.**

In practice, this means adding about 2 to 3 grams of fat to your daily record whenever you choose to eat a serving of fat-free cookies, cake, etc., that contains between 70 and 80 calories. This caloric content is typical of these foods (and it's also the reason the serving size is so small—it's the processor's strategy for making you think the food is low in calories even though people rarely eat such a small serving). By adding fat back into your calculations, the metabolic impact with respect to your weight is accounted for in part, and you will be more likely to treat these foods with the same mental attitude with which you approach foods that contain fat.

Of course, I think you are wasting fat grams and calories when you include these junk foods in place of natural, unrefined, nutrient-rich fruits and vegetables. You are also maintaining your preference for the taste and texture of high-fat foods, rather than changing those tastes in a way that would further your enjoyment and protect your health with more natural, unrefined foods.

Now, how should you apply the rule to reduced-fat foods?

The best way to handle reduced-fat foods in the categories I'm concerned with is: **put the fat back into your count!** The reason for this is that the reduction in fat—for example, 33 percent less fat—is usually almost completely compensated for by an increase in sugar or other carbohydrate calories. Thus if a reduced-fat food says it contains 4 grams of fat and that this is a 33 percent reduction from the original recipe, the original recipe contained 6 grams of fat, and you need to put 2 grams back into your count! (If the product says that it contains only 50 percent of the original fat, then just double the remaining fat-gram count.)

If you follow the rule, you will slightly overestimate the impact on fat burning and the possible storage of other fat from your diet should you be overeating on reduced-fat foods, but it will serve an important psychological purpose in helping you restrain yourself when you decide to include them in your diet.

These guidelines do not apply to dairy products, as I have already indicated, or to meat products, mayonnaise, or margarine. The reduction in fat in these products is not compensated for by an increase in sugar or other carbohydrates. For example, when turkey franks state that they contain 33 percent less fat, it also means 33 percent fewer calories from fat in the product *that have not to an appreciable extent been replaced by other calories.* The same holds true for the most part with reduced-fat or fat-free mayonnaise and salad dressings, or reduced-fat margarine. Fat grams can be counted as they are listed on the label.

FIRST STEPS FIRST

I think you will find it easier to succeed if you take these steps before you begin:

1) Study the fat-substitution guide in Table 4-1. This list contains our latest suggestions for making low-fat substitutions for high-fat foods that are in your present diet. It will also give you an overall feeling for foods that fall in the low-fat category. Keep in mind, however, my warnings about fat-free and reduced-fat baked goods, etc.

2) Study my suggestions for reducing the amount of fat in food preparation and menu design. I will give you some "standard" menus for breakfast, lunch, and dinner below, as well as detailed menus for twenty-one days of the T-Factor 2000 Diet and twenty-one days of the T-Factor Rotation Plan in Chapter 6. I encourage you to look at all the recipes in Chapter 8, and I want especially to encourage you to try every one of the plant food–based recipes in the Meatless Main Course/Vegetarian Entrées, Pasta, and Vegetable and Grain Side Dishes sections. If you are accustomed to including a meat dish daily, you will do yourself a healthy favor if you begin to include at least one meatless day. Study the menus in the vegetarian version of the T-Factor 2000 Diet in Chapter 7 for some meatless day menu suggestions.

3) Until you have a good idea of how to construct a diet that falls in the 20- to 40-gram fat limit for women or the 30- to 60-gram limit for men, you must count fat grams every day. People who continue to record their fat grams until they reach their goal tend to be far more successful than those who don't. But after you have assured yourself of success and have established the full selection of foods

that fit your personal, day-to-day low-fat diet, you may find it no longer necessary to keep counting anything. I don't. Nevertheless, remember that about one-third of the people in the National Weight Control Registry who have been successful in maintaining a significant weight loss for an average of five years *continue to count fat grams.*

CUTTING BACK ON FATS

The T-Factor 2000 Diet gives you the option of including foods from all the foods groups as long as you stay within the guidelines of 20 to 40 grams of fat a day (30 to 60 if you are a man). You can use your preferred oil. However, for other health reasons in addition to losing weight, I would suggest that you eliminate most of the butter and margarine from your diet. The saturated fat in butter and *trans*-fatty acids* in margarine have an adverse effect on blood cholesterol and put you at greater risk of heart disease and certain cancers. I also suggest that you switch from polyunsaturated oils (for example, safflower, sunflower, corn, soybean oils) to monounsaturated oils (olive, canola, peanut). Monounsaturated oils tend to lower bad cholesterol (low-density lipoprotein cholesterol, or LDL) without lowering the good cholesterol (high-density lipoprotein cholesterol, or HDL), and are therefore helpful in lowering your risk of heart disease. In addition, there is less risk of promoting the growth of certain cancers with the use of monounsaturated fats than with polyunsaturated fats.

On the right-hand side of Table 4-1 you will find a list of high-fat foods that are often found in the diets of overly fat persons. On the left-hand side are some good low-fat substitutions. Take a careful look at the right-hand side of the table and see if you can identify those high-fat foods that might contribute to your own weight problem. You may find several that apply to you. For men, it tends most often to be meat, meat products, and the methods of their preparation. For women it is often foods in the dessert, confection, or snack categories. Just following the "use . . . instead of" suggestions alone can cut the fat in your diet by half!

---

*Trans-fatty acids are created when hydrogen atoms are attached in an unnatural way to the fatty acids in polyunsaturated fats in oils like corn and soybean during hydrogenation, in order to harden them for margarine and use in baked goods.

Table 4-1.
Substitutions to Trim Fat and Calories

Use	*Instead of*
Nonfat or 1% milk	Whole or 2% milk
Evaporated skim milk (canned)	Cream, whipping cream, coffee creamers
Reduced-fat sweetened con-densed milk	Sweetened condensed whole milk
Nonfat dry milk	Whole or 2% milk, coffee whiteners, or creamers
Plain nonfat yogurt	Sour cream, mayonnaise, whole-milk yogurt
Nonfat yogurt "cheese" (made by draining liquid from yo-gurt) or blenderized 1–2% cottage cheese	Sour cream, cream cheese
Fat-free or Neufchâtel cream cheese	Regular cream cheese
Nonfat or light sour cream al-ternative	Sour cream
Reduced-fat, light, or fat-free cheeses	Regular cheeses
Fat-free or 1–2% cottage cheese	4% fat cottage cheese
Nonfat or light ricotta	Whole-milk ricotta
Part-skim cheeses in moderate quantities (farmers, sapsago, mozzarella, and others with ≤ 4 grams fat per ounce)	Regular whole-milk cheeses
Extra-sharp cheeses in smaller quantities	Regular, milder cheeses
Reduced-calorie or fat-free mayonnaise	Regular mayonnaise
Mustard, catsup, barbecue sauce as condiment	Mayonnaise
Reduced-fat dips or salsa	Sour cream or mayonnaise-based dips
Reduced-calorie margarine	Margarine, butter
⅓ to ½ less fat and/or oil in recipes	Amount original recipe calls for

Use	Instead of
Applesauce, mashed bananas, fruit purée, or juice	Part of fat called for in muffins or baked goods
Prune or other fruit "butter" (purée)	Part of fat called for in cookies or other baked goods
Nonstick cooking spray	Oil, shortening, butter, other fats
No- or low-fat salad dressings	Regular salad dressings
2 egg whites or ¼ cup egg substitute	Whole egg
Cocoa powder (3 tablespoons + 1 tablespoon water or low-fat milk)	Chocolate in recipes (= 1 ounce)
Sherbet, low-fat frozen yogurt, ice milk, light ice cream	Ice cream
Popsicles, fruit bars, reduced-calorie	Regular ice cream
Angel cake, light cake mixes	Higher-fat cakes
Lower-fat cookies	Higher-fat or chocolate cookies
Puddings made with nonfat or 1% milk	Puddings made with whole or 2% milk
Graham cracker or crumb crust (1½ cups crumbs, 2 tablespoons honey, 1 tablespoon oil)	Pastry crust
Bagels, English muffins, raisin bread	Croissants, biscuits, pastries, doughnuts
Reduced-fat muffins or pastries	Regular muffins or pastries
Pretzels, unbuttered popcorn, fat-free or baked chips, rice cakes	Regular chips, nuts,* buttered popcorn
Low-fat crackers with < 3 grams fat per ounce	High-fat crackers, chips
Toasted Grapenuts cereal	Nuts* as dessert topping
No added fat to packaged rice, pasta, or hot cereals	Added fat in directions
Chopped water chestnuts	Nuts* in vegetable dishes
Broth-based soups	Cream or cheese-based soups
Reduced-fat cream soups	Regular cream soups
Low-fat sauces and marinades	Cheese or cream sauce, high-fat gravies

Use	*Instead of*
Meatless spaghetti sauces	Spaghetti sauce with meat
Legumes, beans, peas, tofu	Meat
Water- or juice-packed fruits	Sweetened or syrup-packed fruits
Fresh or dried fruit	Sweet snacks or desserts
Vegetables seasoned with herbs, spices, bouillon, low-fat sauces, or small amounts of olive oil	Vegetables seasoned with margarine/butter, or meat fat, in cheese or cream sauce; fried vegetables
Frozen entrées with < 8 grams fat per serving	Higher-fat frozen entrées
Frozen dinners with < 12 grams fat per serving	Higher-fat frozen dinners

*Because nuts and seeds are so high in fat, individuals who are losing weight need to exercise caution in their use. Nuts are, however, an extremely valuable addition to the diet because they are an excellent source of monounsaturated fatty acids. Monounsaturated fats, such as are found also in olive, canola, and peanut oils, have proven helpful in reducing cholesterol and the risk of heart disease. In addition, as the source of new life for the parent plants, they are loaded with antioxidants that protect them from deterioration and keep them capable of germination for hundreds of years. These antioxidants appear to protect against cancer in human beings. A serving of nuts (generally two tablespoons or about half an ounce) will contain from 7 to 10 grams of fat. As long as you stick within T-Factor 2000 guidelines for total fat consumption, nuts are an excellent substitute for meat in the diet, and there is no reason not to include nuts in your diet as a garnish in vegetable dishes and as an occasional snack. Your diet will increase its nutritional value if you replace the saturated fats found in animal products with monounsaturated fats.

Table 4-2 lists grains, fruits, and vegetables that contain no more than a trace of fat—that is, they contain less than five-tenths of a gram in the case of the fruits and vegetables and less than 1 gram in the grains. There is generally a small amount of fat in a whole-grain food, and it resides in the germ or husk. Even dry cereal products made without added fat but which contain whole grains usually contain about half a gram of fat per serving, but anything half a gram or over must be rounded up to 1 gram on the label. Watch out for certain cereals, however, which contain considerable added fat in spite of their healthy-sounding names. Granola, for example, may contain 5 or more grams of fat for only a ⅓-cup serving. Other high-fiber cereals, such as raisin bran, may contain just 1 gram of fat and two to three times the fiber in a serving size that is three times as large as a granola! If you like to include cereal in your diet, read the labels to find the best values, health-wise and money-wise.

Table 4-2.
Fruit, Vegetables, and Grain Foods
Having Little or No Fat*
(you do not need to control your consumption of these foods)

Fruit

(fresh)

Apple	Honeydew melon	Persimmon
Banana	(and other melons)	Pineapple
Blackberries	Kiwi	Plum
Blueberries	Mango	Raspberries
Canteloupe	Orange	Strawberries
Cherries	Papaya	Tangerine
Grapefruit	Peach	Watermelon
Grapes	Pear	

(dried)

Apples	Mango	Pineapple
Apricots	Papaya	Prunes
Dates	Peach	Raisins
Figs	Pear	

Vegetables

Asparagus	Dandelion greens	Rhubarb
Bean sprouts	Eggplant	Rutabaga
Beets	Endive	Spinach
Beet greens	Escarole	String beans
Broccoli	Green pepper	Summer squash
Brussels sprouts	Kale	Tomatoes
Cabbage	Lettuce	Turnips
Carrots	Mushrooms	Turnip greens
Cauliflower	Mustard greens	Watercress
Celery	Okra	Wax beans
Chard	Onions	Winter squash
Chicory	Parsley	Zucchini
Collards	Pumpkin	
Cucumbers	Radishes	

Grains, Legumes, and Other Starchy Foods

Breads

Bagel	Hard dinner rolls	Tortilla
Bread (per slice)	Melba toast	Zwieback
English muffin	Pita bread	

Breakfast Cereals

Except for granola-style cereals, most cold and hot breakfast
cereals contain no fat to 1 gram of fat per serving.
Check the labels of your favorite brands.

Crackers

Animal crackers	Oyster crackers	Saltines
Bread sticks	Pretzels	Venus (brand)
Graham crackers	Rice cakes	crackers

Grains and Grain Foods

Corn	Noodles	Spaghetti
Macaroni	Rice	Wheat (bulgur, etc.)

Legumes and Other Starchy Foods

Kidney beans	Peas, chick	Red beans
Lentils	Peas, green	White beans
Lima beans	Pinto beans	Yams
Navy beans	Potatoes, sweet	
Peas, blackeye	Potatoes, white	

*Fruits and vegetables that contain only trace amounts (less than 0.5 gram) of fat
per serving. The grain and other starchy foods usually have less than 1 gram of fat
per serving. Be sure to check the labels on all commercially prepared foods for
added fat.

ADDITIONAL HINTS FOR CUTTING FATS

Here are some additional hints for cutting fats. In part, these explain
and amplify some of the suggestions in Table 4-1. I expand on them
because they constitute the dietary modifications most often reported by people who have maintained significant weight losses. I

can vouch for them personally because I follow all of them. They work!

1. If you are eating more beef, lamb, or pork than you are fowl or fish, you should at least reverse that ratio. Many successful weight losers have drastically cut their consumption of red meat or eliminated it altogether. If you prefer to include beef, lamb, or pork in your diet, use the leanest cuts and trim all fat. The Fat Counter in Appendix D lists the fat content of various cuts of meat. We have included recipes (Chapter 8) that can make lean meats taste just as satisfying as the fattier cuts.

2. *Don't eat fried foods. Period.* This is another rule adopted almost universally by permanently successful weight losers. Frying can turn a wonderfully healthy food into a junk food! For example, a potato contains no fat. But turn even a small potato into just one cup of French fries and you end up with about 24 grams of fat. That's about 200 calories of fat that could come out of your fat cells instead of going in! It's even worse when you fry chicken or fish with a crumb or batter crust. So, when it comes to these foods, bake, broil, steam, poach, or occasionally stew or grill in place of frying.

3. Cultivate your taste for meatless dishes. We have made a great effort to show you how to do this with the many recipes we include in the Meatless Main Courses/Vegetarian Entrées, Pasta, and Vegetable and Grain Side Dishes sections of Chapter 8.

4. Switch from whole milk to either low-fat or skim milk. Use low-fat cottage cheese and yogurt, and part-skim cheeses whenever possible. Successful people almost universally change to low-fat dairy products. As for processed lowered-fat cheese foods, if you like them use them, but watch out for any tendency to increase the amount you use. I prefer the best-tasting hard cheeses—for example, cheddar, Parmesan, Romano, Asiago, Gruyère—over less satisfying, reduced-fat varieties; of course, use the former moderately.

5. Substitute fruit or unbuttered popcorn for most of your desserts and sweets. For most people, dried fruits and fresh fruits send powerful physiological signals that tend to turn off appetite before energy balance has been exceeded. If you prefer popcorn made with oil, as I do, 2 tablespoons of oil used to pop enough corn to fill a 12-cup popper will add less than 2 grams of fat to each cup of popcorn.

6. Do not use gravies and sauces made with more than minimal

amounts of fat or oil. See the recipes in the Sauces section of Chapter 8 for some low-fat suggestions.

7. Experiment to see how little fat or oil you can use in your own recipes and still end up with the taste and texture that satisfy you.

But what about diet spreads and commercial calorie-reduced salad dressings? Whether you use these or not is a matter of personal choice. I don't use these products myself. I prefer to use less of the full-bodied, full-flavored product when a fat is called for in any recipe. However, Jamie prefers to use them, as do a majority of the participants in the groups at the Vanderbilt Weight Management Program. Therefore, we include many recipes that do use calorie-reduced products that received excellent ratings from our tasters. As for mayonnaise and salad dressings, many people are able to find a commercial reduced-fat variety that they like, with no more than three grams of fat and just 35 calories or less per tablespoon. I have recently discovered Nayonnaise, a nicely flavored low-fat soy product that is almost as satisfying to me as my favorite Hellmann's Mayonnaise (also known as Best Brands). You will find some excellent low-fat recipes for dressings in the Salads and Salad Dressings section of Chapter 8.

HOW TO DEVELOP YOUR DAILY MENU PLAN

Most people alternate among several standard breakfasts and lunches. If you eat your main meal at night, I think it's a good idea to include no more than half the fat you plan to eat in a given day in these first two meals of the day, combined. Remember, however, that most health experts recommend against eating a large meal before going to sleep. It can interfere with sleep and it may be dangerous for people with cardiovascular disease. The size and fat levels of the dinners in our menus are well within good health limits.

Basic Breakfasts

A satisfying breakfast need not be loaded with fat, and I think you should feel free to eat any kind and combination of foods for breakfast that appeal to you. I very often just eat something left over from the night before. For example, this morning when I looked in the refrigerator I found a container containing about 2 cups of broccoli that had been steamed for dinner last night. It took 2 minutes to heat in the microwave. I sprinkled 2 tablespoons of Parmesan cheese over it (just 3 grams of fat) together with a little garlic powder and had a satisfying breakfast. Yesterday it was a bowl of leftover vegetable soup.

For more traditional breakfast fare, take a look at the many different breakfasts we suggest in the twenty-one days of T-Factor 2000 menus. Most people find just one or two basic breakfasts that they eat on weekdays, saving more elaborate meals for the weekends. Try the ones we suggest on our menus, but feel free to choose those you like best and rotate them. If you prefer a cold cereal, you can greatly increase its nutritional value by adding fruit and soy nuts, and if your preference is one of the cereals that's relatively low in fiber, try mixing it with a high-fiber variety. You will find some great bread and muffin recipes in the Breads and Muffins section of Chapter 8. Any of these will serve to make a satisfying breakfast food, but watch out for commercial muffins. Some national brands contain 10 grams of fat per muffin, while local bakeries may produce "quarter-pounders" that have 25 grams of fat. If a muffin feels heavy and sticky to the touch, it contains plenty of fat! Normally we recommend you drink coffee or tea without cream, but if you like half-and-half (as I do) it contains 0.5 gram of fat per teaspoon. Be sure to count it in your fat gram total.

Basic Lunches

Lunches pose a bit of a problem if you have to eat out every day and cannot carry your own. While I frequently order salads when I eat out, or soup and salad or a sandwich, I prefer to make my own lunches. The tuna, chicken, or shellfish salads in restaurants will often contain between 12 and 24 grams of fat unless they have been specifically designed as low-fat recipes. If you pour additional dressing on the lettuce and other vegetables that accompany these salads, it's 9 to 10 grams of fat per tablespoon of the regular varieties.

Hearty soups—I mean with potatoes, lentils, rice, and plenty of vegetables—are great for lunches. You will find ten delicious soup recipes in the Soups section of Chapter 8. Remember, when you have soup at a meal you tend to take in fewer calories, so give soup a place in the creation of your own menus.

Here are some generic fat-gram figures to help you plan your own luncheon combinations. Once again, be sure to check the labels of commercial products.

1. Tuna fish, packed in water, contains only 1 gram of fat per 3-ounce serving (packed in oil it contains about 20 grams).

2. Low-fat varieties of cottage cheese contain from 2 to 3 grams of fat per half-cup.

3. Soups, bouillon-based with added vegetables and potatoes, are practically fat-free.

4. Vegetable or vegetable beef and chicken soups will contain about 3 grams of fat per cup (the popular cream of broccoli and cheddar/potato soups served in restaurants and on salad bars may contain up to 25 grams of fat).

5. Sardines, oil all drained off, will contain about 6 grams of fat per half-tin (about 2 ounces).

6. Fruits and vegetables that are virtually fat-free (see the lists in Table 4-2), can be added to any luncheon menu in unlimited quantities.

7. Bread for sandwiches contains about 1 gram of fat per slice.

8. Mayonnaise, regular varieties, contain 4 grams per *teaspoon*.

9. Use catsup and mustard for flavoring.

10. Use lemon juice and vinaigrette dressings, or my own low-fat salad dressings (Chapter 8).

11. My sandwich spreads (Chapter 8) contain little or no fat.

12. White meat of chicken or turkey contains about 1 gram of fat per ounce.

13. Sliced beef, extra lean, contains about 2.5 grams per ounce; regular cut, about 6 grams per ounce.

14. Baked beans, vegetarian style, are a good substitute for meat dishes and contain less than 1 gram of fat per half-cup serving.

15. Venus (brand) wafers have 2 grams of fat per 1-ounce serving, while saltines contain 1.5 grams per serving of 5 crackers.

Check out the various luncheon suggestions in the twenty-one different daily menus later in this chapter. They will introduce you to many new recipes (found in Chapter 8). I hope you will find several that you would like to include among your own selections on a regular basis. Substitute the recipes you like best for any that don't appeal to you any day of the week. If you must eat out most days of the week, choose a restaurant that offers items that approximate the ones we suggest in our menus. As you will see when I describe my own experience eating out while using my original rotation plan in 1963 (Chapter 6), you may have to find a restaurant that you can depend on to offer at least a few of the foods on a regular basis that meet your needs. This may mean that you have to repeat the same limited selection of lunches on those days, which in turn means that you should seek greater variety in your other meals and snacks.

Basic Dinners

It is easy to design a low-fat dinner if you include a standard serving of a lean meat, poultry, or fish. Just add all the vegetables you like, plus a starch (potatoes, rice, other grains, or pasta), plus fruit or unbuttered popcorn for dessert. This is an approach most in line with the typical American diet. Just remember that butter and margarine contain about 12 grams of fat per tablespoon, so, when preparing vegetables, allow 1 tablespoon of added fat per recipe for four servings—that's just 3 grams of fat per serving if none sticks to the pot. However, many vegetables can be seasoned satisfactorily without added fat through the judicious use of herbs and spices. When I began to lose weight, I discovered that a baked potato tasted just fine with salt and pepper. Later on a participant in one of our weight-management groups suggested salsa. Neither of us has returned to the use of butter and sour cream.

Once again, I want to encourage you to limit your consumption of red meat, and make a serious effort to include more meatless dishes in your diet. You will greatly reduce the fat content of your diet, as well as increase the nutritional value when you increase the variety and amounts of plant foods. You will see a strong emphasis on meatless main courses in our menus. Give them a try, but if the success of your weight-loss efforts depends on it, feel free to construct your own version of dinner in the more traditional American style. Even under these conditions, I strongly encourage you to emphasize poultry and fish rather than red meat.

HOW TO USE THE T-FACTOR 2000 MENUS

The T-Factor 2000 Diet menus below are meant to introduce you to the wide variety of foods and styles of food preparation that will make your diet interesting and satisfying. You can, as I have said, substitute freely once you have found the particular meals and recipes you like best. If one of my suggestions doesn't appeal to you, just substitute a similar food prepared in the manner I suggest among my other recipes in Chapter 8. You may also substitute a basic menu of a serving of lean meat, poultry, or fish, plus vegetable, starch, and fruit, whenever circumstances make such a meal more convenient than the meal I have suggested.

Choosing a wide variety of foods helps assure sound nutrition. Our main concern is with fat. Just hold to the range of fat grams, 20 to 40 for women and 30 to 60 for men, and you have complete freedom in your choice of *unrefined* low-energy-dense carbohydrates—that is, all fruits, vegetables, and grains.

Add fat-free unrefined carbohydrates at main meals or for snacks until your appetite is satisfied. Don't go hungry!

Use the fat gram counter in Appendix D when you make substitutions or create your own menus.

Keep track of fat grams each day in the manner I suggest in Appendix D.

If you are both overweight and suffer from noninsulin-dependent diabetes mellitus (NIDDM), please see the note on dietary recommendations in Appendix C, show it to your physician, and tailor the following menus to suit your individual requirements.

DAILY T-FACTOR 2000 MENUS

Many of these daily menus come out at the low end of the spectrum of 20 to 40 grams of fat for women. This was done to leave room for some low-fat snacks, or desserts, including nuts, that do contain some fat. Men may increase the portion sizes of the foods that contain fat up to half to meet their goal of 30 to 60 grams of fat per day. *Do not go below 20 grams of fat per day if you are a woman, 30 if you are a man.* Symptoms of a deficiency in fat intake include chapped lips, dry skin, and brittle hair. A serving of nuts will prevent a deficiency of fat in your diet and many nutritionists are suggesting that people include a serving of nuts as a more healthful substitute for meat in the diet. The nutritional analyses listed at the end of each day use the first item listed if alternatives are offered (for example, if the alternatives non-fat or 1% milk are offered, non-fat milk will be used in the analysis). You can safely use the higher-fat alternative, or use more fat in the preparation of any of the foods for that day, on days when the fat count is at the lower end of the range. For example, on Day 1 below, using all the alternatives would still leave you well below 40 grams of fat for the day, but weight loss would not proceed quite as quickly.

Average weekly weight loss among participants who are 40 to 50 pounds overweight in the Vanderbilt Weight Management Program is 1 pound, with heavier participants losing an average of as much as 1½ pounds a week. Of course, if you are under medical care, you should not make any changes in your diet without consulting your physician.

Day 1

Breakfast
1 toasted whole-grain bagel or English muffin; 2 tablespoons fat-free or light cream cheese; jelly or jam; 1 cup nonfat or 1% milk; 1 cup blueberries or other seasonal fruit; coffee or tea

Lunch
2 ounces lean ham; 1 ounce low-fat Swiss or other cheese with 2 pineapple slices on ½ whole-grain pita bread; alfalfa sprouts; mustard or reduced-calorie mayonnaise; 1 ounce pretzels or fat-free chips; no-cal beverage

Dinner
1 serving Chicken Picante*; ½ cup brown or wild rice; ½ cup black beans or canned refried beans; 1 cup steamed broccoli; 1 piece Corn Bread* (or 2 corn tortillas); 1 cup cantaloupe; no-cal beverage

Total for Day 1:   1490 calories, 24 grams of fat (18%), 9 grams saturated fat, 130 mg. cholesterol, 3770 mg. sodium, 33 grams fiber

Day 2

Breakfast
1 ounce ready-to-eat cereal; banana, sliced; 1 cup nonfat or 1% milk; 1 slice whole-grain toast; 1 teaspoon light margarine; jelly or jam if desired; coffee or tea

---

*Recipes for items with asterisks (used at first mention only) can be found in Chapter 8. Serving sizes are as given in recipe.

Lunch

Spinach salad: 2 cups fresh spinach, sliced fresh mushrooms, ½ hard-boiled egg, 1 ounce no- or reduced-fat cheese, chopped red onion, 3 tablespoons reduced-fat salad dressing; Apricot Muffin* or other low-fat muffin; orange; no-cal beverage

Dinner

3–4 ounces Baked Flank Steak*, 1 serving Potatoes Au Gratin*, 1 serving Asparagus with Mustard Sauce*; tossed vegetable salad; 2 tablespoons reduced-fat salad dressing; whole-grain roll; 1 serving Gingerbread*; no-cal beverage

Total for Day 2: 1450 calories, 31 grams of fat (19%), 6 grams saturated fat, 226 mg. cholesterol, 3420 mg. sodium, 25 grams fiber

Day 3

Breakfast

Refrigerator Bran Muffin*; 1 cup nonfat yogurt (plain or 100-calorie variety); grapefruit; coffee or tea

Lunch

Fast-food restaurant broiled chicken sandwich (hold the mayo!) with lettuce, tomato, and mustard or barbecue sauce; 1 ounce fat-free chips or pretzels; small side salad; fat-free salad dressing; no-cal beverage

Dinner

1 serving Eggplant Parmesan*; 1 cup pasta of choice; 1 slice garlic toast (Italian or other bread broiled with 1 teaspoon light margarine and garlic powder); tossed vegetable salad; 2 tablespoons reduced-fat salad dressing; 2 pineapple slices; no-cal beverage

Total for Day 3: 1400 calories, 20 grams fat (14%), 10 grams saturated fat, 162 mg. cholesterol, 3310 mg. sodium, 22 grams fiber

Day 4

Breakfast

1 ounce ready-to-eat cereal; ½ cup sliced peaches or other seasonal fruit; 1 cup nonfat or 1% milk; 1 slice whole-grain toast; 1 teaspoon light margarine; jelly or jam if desired; coffee or tea

Lunch

Medium baked potato stuffed with ½ cup non- or low-fat cottage cheese, chopped green onions, chopped tomatoes, and salsa; apple; no-cal beverage

Dinner

1 serving Tuna Teriyaki*; ½ cup brown or wild rice; 1 cup green beans; ½ cup cherry tomato halves; 1 slice French or Italian bread; 1 citrus fruit cup, ½ cup orange sherbet; no-cal beverage

Total for Day 4:   1520 calories, 24 grams fat (14%), 7 grams saturated fat, 97 mg. cholesterol, 1900 mg. sodium, 27 grams fiber

Day 5

Breakfast

1 slice Spiced Banana Bread*; 2 teaspoons apple butter; 1 poached or boiled egg; 1 cup melon or other seasonal fruit; 1 cup nonfat yogurt (plain or 100-calorie variety); coffee or tea

Lunch

1 cup Minestrone* or broth-based soup; cheese toast: 1 ounce low-fat cheese on 1 slice whole-grain bread; assorted raw vegetables; 2 plums; no-cal beverage

Dinner

1 serving Shepherd's Pie*; 1 Light Wheat Biscuit*; ½ cup applesauce; 2 reduced-fat cookies; no-cal beverage

Total for Day 5:   1280 calories, 33 grams fat (27%), 7 grams saturated fat, 226 mg. cholesterol, 2650 mg. sodium, 19 grams fiber

Day 6

Breakfast

1 ounce ready-to-eat cereal; 2 tablespoons raisins; 1 cup nonfat or 1% milk; 1 slice whole-grain toast; 1 teaspoon light margarine; jelly or jam if desired; coffee or tea

Lunch

Tomato stuffed with ½ cup tuna salad (made with water-packed tuna, fat-free mayo, pickles, chopped onion); 1 ounce breadsticks or low-fat crackers; 1 cup grapes; no-cal beverage

Dinner

1 serving Broccoli Pesto* with pasta; whole-grain roll; tossed vegetable salad; 2 tablespoons reduced-fat salad dressing; ½ cup low-fat frozen yogurt with 1 cup sliced strawberries; no-cal beverage

Total for Day 6:   1370 calories, 25 grams fat (16%), 4 grams saturated fat, 35 mg. cholesterol, 2550 mg. sodium, 20 grams fiber

Day 7

Breakfast

1 serving Bran Cakes*; ¼ cup Fruit Topping* or 3 tablespoons light syrup; 1 ounce reduced-fat sausage (≤ 3 grams fat) or 1 ounce Canadian bacon; ½ cup orange juice or fresh orange; 1 cup nonfat or 1% milk; coffee or tea

Lunch

2 ounces sliced turkey or chicken on 6-inch whole-grain sub roll; lettuce, tomato, and mustard or fat-free mayo; 1 ounce fat-free chips or pretzels; banana; no-cal beverage

Dinner

1 serving Cream of Portabella Soup*; ½ whole-grain bagel or pita pocket, 2 tablespoons hummus, tossed vegetable salad; 2 tablespoons reduced-fat salad dressing; 1 serving Berry Crisp* with 2 tablespoons light whipped topping (or angel cake with sliced peaches); no-cal beverage

Total for Day 7:   1590 calories, 24 grams fat (15%), 7 grams saturated fat, 70 mg. cholesterol, 3790 mg. sodium, 29 grams fiber

Average for Week 1/Days 1–7:   1440 calories, 26 grams fat (18%), 7 grams saturated fat, 135 mg. cholesterol, 3060 mg. sodium, 25 grams fiber

Day 8

Breakfast

1 ounce ready-to-eat cereal; 1 cup raspberries; 1 cup nonfat or 1% milk; 1 slice whole-grain toast; 1 teaspoon light margarine; jelly or jam if desired; coffee or tea

Lunch

½ cup canned refried beans (spice them up as desired!); 1 ounce shredded low-fat cheddar cheese, 2 medium soft flour tortillas; shredded lettuce; chopped tomatoes; chopped onion; salsa; orange; no-cal beverage

Dinner

1 serving Baked Chicken with Tarragon and Fennel*; ½ cup brown or wild rice; 1 serving Parmesan-Dill Brussels Sprouts*; whole-grain roll; tossed vegetable salad; 2 tablespoons fat-free salad dressing; seasonal fruit of choice; no-cal beverage

Total for Day 8: 1350 calories, 22 grams fat (15%), 5 grams saturated fat, 105 mg. cholesterol, 2525 mg. sodium, 38 grams fiber

Day 9

Breakfast

1 bagel or English muffin; 1 tablespoon peanut butter, 2 teaspoons jelly or jam; 1 cup nonfat yogurt (plain or 100-calorie variety); 1 cup V8 or tomato juice; coffee or tea

Lunch

2 ounces turkey on 2 slices whole-grain bread with ¼ cup cranberry sauce and alfalfa sprouts; 1 ounce pretzels or fat-free chips; 1 cup grapes; no-cal beverage

Dinner

1 serving Meatless Meatloaf*; 1 serving Potatoes and Spinach*; 1 serving Cauliflower Sauté* (or 1 cup steamed cauliflower); whole-grain roll; tossed vegetable salad; 2 tablespoons reduced-fat salad dressing; seasonal fruit of choice; coffee or tea

Total for Day 9: 1545 calories, 26 grams fat (14%), 5 grams saturated fat, 31 mg. cholesterol, 4540 mg. sodium, 36 grams fiber

Day 10

Breakfast

1 serving Fruity Breakfast Barley*; 1 cup nonfat or 1% milk; 1 sliced whole-grain toast; 1 teaspoon light margarine; jelly or jam if desired; tangerine; coffee or tea

Lunch

1 serving leftover Meatless Meatloaf on whole-grain sandwich roll; lettuce; tomato slices; 1 ounce fat-free or baked tortilla chips; pear or peach; no-cal beverage

Dinner

1 serving Salmon Loaf*; 1 serving Couscous, Chickpeas, and Vegetables*; 1 slice Oatmeal Molasses Bread*; tossed vegetable salad; 2 tablespoons fat-free salad dressing; banana; ½ cup pudding prepared with nonfat or 1% milk; no-cal beverage

Total for Day 10:   1400 calories, 20 grams fat (14%), 5 grams saturated fat, 30 mg. cholesterol, 2850 mg. sodium, 31 grams fiber

Day 11

Breakfast

1 slice Carrot Pineapple Bread*; 1 teaspoon light margarine, 1 cup nonfat yogurt (plain or 100-calorie variety); ½ cup orange or other juice; coffee or tea

Lunch

1 2-ounce vegetarian/"garden" burger; 1 ounce low-fat cheese; 1 whole-grain hamburger bun; lettuce, tomato slice; mustard or reduced-fat mayonnaise; 1 cup tomato soup; 1 ounce low-fat crackers; no-cal beverage

Dinner

1 serving Sassy Salsa Beans* or other beans of choice; ½ cup brown or wild rice; 1 serving Mixed Greens with Oranges and Olives*; whole-grain roll, tossed vegetable salad; 2 tablespoons reduced-fat salad dressing; 2 kiwi fruit; no-cal beverage

Total for Day 11:   1470 calories, 21 grams fat (13%), 3 grams saturated fat, 40 mg. cholesterol, 3420 mg. sodium, 39 grams fiber

Day 12

Breakfast

1 ounce ready-to-eat cereal; sliced banana; 1 cup nonfat or 1% milk; 1 slice whole-grain toast; 1 teaspoon light margarine; jelly or jam if desired; coffee or tea

Lunch

1 cup nonfat yogurt (plain or 100-calorie variety) or ¾ cup 2% cottage cheese; 1 slice Carrot Pineapple Bread; 2 tablespoons no- or low-fat cream cheese, ½ cup grapes; no-cal beverage

Dinner

3 ounces grilled flank or round steak (Steak Marinade*); 1 medium baked potato; 1 cup green beans, 1 slice French or Italian bread; tossed vegetable salad; 2 tablespoons reduced-fat salad dressing; ½ cup citrus fruit cup; 2 gingersnap cookies; no-cal beverage

Total for Day 12:   1520 calories, 20 grams fat (13%), 7 grams saturated fat, 104 mg. cholesterol, 1890 mg. sodium, 24 grams fiber

Day 13

Breakfast

1 egg (boiled, poached, or scrambled without added fat), 1 slice whole-grain toast, 1 teaspoon light margarine; jelly or jam if desired, 1 cup nonfat or 1% milk; grapefruit; coffee or tea

Lunch

Chef salad: assorted raw vegetables, 2 ounces lean ham or turkey breast, ½ ounce shredded reduced-fat cheese, ¼ cup croutons; 3 tablespoons reduced-fat salad dressing; ½ ounce low-fat crackers; apple; no-cal beverage

Dinner

1 serving Spinach Lasagna*; 1 serving Glazed Orange-Spice Carrots*; 1 whole-grain roll; 1 piece Pumpkin Cheesecake* (or plain variation); 1 cup sliced strawberries; no-cal beverage

Total for Day 13:   1390 calories, 31 grams fat (20%), 11 grams saturated fat, 340 mg. cholesterol, 3120 mg. sodium, 24 grams fiber

Day 14

Breakfast

1 serving Whole-Wheat Pancakes*; ¼ cup Fruit Topping* or 3 tablespoons light syrup; 1 cup sliced peaches or other fruit; 1 ounce Canadian bacon or lean ham; 1 cup skim or 1% milk; coffee or tea

Lunch

1 serving Fresh Vegetable Soup* or other broth-based soup; 1 bagel; 1 serving Salmon-Herb Spread*; 1 cup melon or seasonal fruit; no-cal beverage

Dinner

1 serving Fragrant Pork Roast*; 1 serving Lemon Broccoli Risotto*; 1 medium baked sweet potato; 1 whole-grain roll; tossed vegetable salad; 2 tablespoons reduced-fat salad dressing; orange; no-cal beverage

Total for Day 14:   1455 calories, 22 grams fat (16%), 7 grams saturated fat, 160 mg. cholesterol, 3690 mg. sodium, 29 grams fiber

Average for Week 2/Days 7–14:   1450 calories, 23 grams fat (15%), 6 grams saturated fat, 115 mg. cholesterol, 3150 mg. sodium, 32 grams fiber

Average for both weeks, Days 1–14:   1445 calories, 25 grams fat (17%), 7 grams saturated fat, 125 mg. cholesterol, 3100 mg. sodium, 28 grams fiber

Day 15

Breakfast

1 ounce ready-to-eat cereal; sliced banana; 1 cup nonfat or 1% milk; 1 slice whole-grain toast; 1 teaspoon light margarine; jelly or jam if desired; coffee or tea

Lunch

Herbed Pinto Bean Spread*; toasted bagel; tomato slices; ½ cup baby carrots; peach or other seasonal fruit; no-cal beverage

Dinner

1 serving Savory Turkey Loaf*; 1 serving Macaroni and Cheese*; 1 cup French style green beans; whole-grain roll; ½ cup applesauce; no-cal beverage

Total for Day 15:   1425 calories, 28 grams fat (17%), 7 grams saturated fat, 101 mg. cholesterol, 2765 mg. sodium, 38 grams fiber

Day 16

Breakfast

1 serving Mixed Grain Cereal*; 1 cup V8 or tomato juice; 1 cup non-fat or 1% milk; 1 slice whole-grain toast; 1 teaspoon light margarine; jelly or jam if desired; coffee or tea

Lunch

3 ounces leftover Savory Turkey Loaf; whole-grain bun; lettuce; tomato slices; onion slices; mustard; 1 ounce pretzels or fat-free chips; 1 cup grapes; no-cal beverage

Dinner

1 serving Spaghetti Sauce with Tempeh and Broccoli*; 1 slice Italian bread; tossed vegetable salad; 2 tablespoons reduced-fat salad dressing; nectarine; no-cal beverage

Total for Day 16:   1390 calories, 21 grams fat (13%), 4 grams saturated fat, 35 mg. cholesterol, 3770 mg. sodium, 24 grams fiber

Day 17

Breakfast

1 ounce ready-to-eat cereal; 1 cup sliced strawberries; 1 cup nonfat or 1% milk; ½ whole-grain bagel or English muffin; 1 teaspoon light margarine; jelly or jam if desired; coffee or tea

Lunch

1 serving Tuna with Chickpeas* salad; whole-grain pita pocket; alfalfa sprouts; apple; no-cal beverage

Dinner

1 serving Barbecue Chicken*; ½ cup brown or wild rice; 1 serving Roasted Mushrooms, Peppers, and Onions*; tossed vegetable salad; 2 tablespoons reduced-fat salad dressing; ½ cup pineapple; ½ cup low-fat frozen yogurt or ice milk; no-cal beverage

Total for Day 17:   1510 calories, 29 grams fat (17%), 5 grams saturated fat, 120 mg. cholesterol, 2970 mg. sodium, 34 grams fiber

Day 18

Breakfast
1 slice Date-Bran Bread*; 2 teaspoons honey; 1 cup nonfat yogurt;
½ cup orange juice or fresh orange; coffee or tea

Lunch
1 serving Fresh Pea Soup*; 1 piece Corn Bread; 1 cup cherry tomatoes; pear; no-cal beverage

Dinner
1 serving Orange Roughy with Spinach*; 1 serving Baked Beets and
Potatoes*; 1 whole-grain roll; tossed vegetable salad; 2 tablespoons
reduced-calorie salad dressing; 1 serving Cocoa Zucchini Cake*; ¼
cup light whipped topping; no-cal beverage

Total for Day 18: 1430 calories, 27 grams fat (21%), 7 grams saturated fat, 66 mg. cholesterol, 3120 mg. sodium, 27 grams fiber

Day 19

Breakfast
1 ounce ready-to-eat cereal; 1 cup sliced peaches; 1 cup nonfat or
1% milk; 1 slice whole-grain toast, 1 teaspoon light margarine; jelly
or jam if desired; coffee or tea

Lunch
1 serving Sweet 'n' Savory Chicken Salad*; 1 ounce low-fat crackers
or breadsticks; celery sticks; 2 Dikkie's Chocolate Chip Meringue
Cookies*; no-cal beverage

Dinner
1 serving Hearty Vegetarian Chili*; 1 slice Quick Mustard-Rye Bread*;
tossed vegetable salad; 2 tablespoons reduced-fat salad dressing; 1
cup melon or other seasonal fruit; 1 cup nonfat yogurt; no-cal beverage

Total for Day 19: 1370 calories, 20 grams fat (15%), 5 grams saturated fat, 51 mg. cholesterol, 2525 mg. sodium, 32 grams fiber

Day 20

Breakfast

1 serving French Toast*; ¼ cup Fruit Topping or 3 tablespoons light syrup; ½ cup apple or other juice; 1 cup nonfat or 1% milk; coffee or tea

Lunch

1 serving leftover Hearty Vegetarian Chili; 1 slice Quick Mustard-Rye Bread; 1 cup baby carrots; 2 kiwi fruit; no-cal beverage

Dinner

1 serving Pot Roast* with vegetables; tossed vegetable salad; 3 tablespoons reduced-fat salad dressing; 1 citrus fruit cup; no-cal beverage

Total for Day 20:   1535 calories, 22 grams fat (17%), 6 grams saturated fat, 85 mg. cholesterol, 2700 mg. sodium, 43 grams fiber

Day 21

Breakfast

1 ounce ready-to-eat cereal; ½ cup blueberries; 1 cup nonfat or 1% milk; 1 slice whole-grain toast; 1 teaspoon light margarine; jelly or jam if desired; coffee or tea

Lunch

Toasted pita pocket: ½ cup Veggie Sandwich Spread*; 6-inch whole-wheat pita pocket; tomato slices; alfalfa sprouts or shredded lettuce; raw vegetables of choice; orange; no-cal beverage

Dinner

1 serving Royal Indian Salmon*; 1 serving Mashed Carrots and Parsnips*; 1 serving Tri-Color Pepper Sauté*; 1 slice French or Italian bread; 1 serving Elegant Pears*; no-cal beverage

Total for Day 21:   1505 calories, 31 grams fat (18%), 8 grams saturated fat, 99 mg. cholesterol, 2195 mg. sodium, 32 grams fiber

Average for Week 3:   1460 calories, 26 grams fat (17%), 6 grams saturated fat, 80 mg. cholesterol, 2860 mg. sodium, 33 grams fiber

Average for Weeks 1–3:   1450 calories, 25 grams fat (17%), 6 grams saturated fat, 110 mg. cholesterol, 3020 mg. sodium, 30 grams fiber

Other nutrient averages for Weeks 1–3:   70 grams protein, 210 grams carbohydrate, 1880 RE vitamin A (235% RDA), 253 mg. vitamin C (422% RDA), 485 mcg. folic acid (269% RDA), 900 mg. calcium (90% RDA), 17 mg. iron (113%), 11 mg. zinc (95%)

CHAPTER 5

What to Expect When You Use the T-Factor 2000 Diet

When we designed the original T-Factor Diet in 1987 and 1988, our research groups averaged a loss of approximately 1 pound a week, just as I did when I tried the diet myself along with the very first group. Even though I was right smack in the middle of the desirable weight range at the time (5' 10½" tall, and 160 pounds), I was not going to recommend an approach that I didn't think would be effective. I lost 7 pounds in 7 weeks, just like the average of the group.

But even more important than short-term effectiveness was the interest of everyone on the research staff in whether the T-Factor Diet offered an easy-to-use and permanent solution to the weight-management problem. Just counting fat grams with no restriction on the consumption of carbohydrates led to an average percent fat intake of 19 percent of calories,* and comments like "I can't believe I'm eating like this and losing weight!"

Of course, at that time, imitation highly processed, energy-dense, fat-free desserts, snacks, pastries, and candies were not easily available. Foods of this kind were not included in their diets by research

---

*Participants in the original T-Factor study, almost 90 percent of whom were women, consumed an average of 30 grams of fat and 1427 calories a day. This amounts to 19 percent of calories from fat during the period in which they were actively losing weight. In follow-up one year later on maintenance, fat grams averaged 24 percent of calories, as in the National Weight Control Registry.

participants. Eating *unrefined* carbohydrates, our participants made comments that included:

"It's great being able to eat at any time—all you want—so long as you watch the fat. It's wonderful for munchers like me."

"The flexibility is a strong point. No rigid rules about substitutions and I'm learning the fat content of foods."

"I was surprised to see how many good things there are that do not contain fat."

"It's a lifestyle I can live with for the rest of my life. I never need to feel hungry or deprived. It's a logical, rational, good-health program."

All of the participants agreed that counting fat grams was easier than counting calories or attempting to monitor the percentage of fat in their diets on a meal-by-meal or day-by-day basis.

Our good results were aided by a significant increase in the physical activity of the group members. The women in the group averaged 60 pounds overweight. When they came into the group, in the preliminary fitness assessment, few of them were able to walk a mile at the moderate pace of three miles per hour (twenty minutes per mile). By the end of twelve weeks the women were averaging three miles of walking a day, at paces alternating between three and four miles per hour, six days a week.

Now, some ten years later, research on over 3000 successful people in the National Weight Control Registry confirms the effectiveness of the principles that remain the foundation of the T-Factor 2000 Diet. The average fat intake among the registrants who now average a weight loss of 67 pounds for a period of five years is 24 percent of total calories. This is exactly the percentage of total calories from fat that we found on follow-up among the original T-Factor research subjects. Although over half the participants in the registry lost weight in commercial or medically directed programs, almost one-third of them report that counting fat grams is among their ongoing strategies for maintaining their weight loss.

The energy expenditure in physical activity among successful people is, however, even higher than what we suggested as a goal in our original research. Just a word about that here, since I will go more into how successful people manage their weight and the *key* role that physical activity plays in maintenance in Chapter 9.

Our participants engaged almost exclusively in moderate to brisk walking as their exercise and averaged an energy expenditure of approximately 2000 calories per week. Participants in the National Weight Control Registry are averaging 2800 calories per week in physical activity (about 3500 for men, and 2600 for women). But, in large part, this heightened energy expenditure is due to many of them participating in medium- and high-intensity exercise, such as stationary and road cycling, running and jogging, weight lifting (especially the men), and stair stepping. About half of the successful women in the Registry are exceeding the 2000 calories per week expenditure that our subjects attained, and half are below that level. Sixty-two percent of the men in the registry, however, exceed that level, mainly as a result of high-intensity activity.

LATEST RESULTS FROM THE VANDERBILT WEIGHT MANAGEMENT PROGRAM

The Vanderbilt Weight Management Program was closed to the public and offered only to staff and faculty of the university on an occasional basis after I retired from the university in 1991. Jamie has been directing the staff program since that time, offering weight-management groups about twice a year. Results from the latest complete program, finished in the spring of 1998 and consisting only of women participants, demonstrate exactly what women can expect when they follow T-Factor 2000 guidelines—that is, 20 to 40 grams of fat a day for women, with no restrictions on the consumption of fruits, vegetables, and whole grains. The average weight loss among the women was approximately 1 pound per week. Since speed of loss is highly correlated with initial starting weight, heavier participants lost more than lighter ones. By the end of the sixteen-week program, the average weight loss was 7 percent of initial body weight. This is a couple of percentage points above the 5 percent goal that many experts suggest as a reasonable goal in a weight-loss effort. If you would like to lose more than 5 percent of your body weight, you might find it easier to set an initial goal of just 5 percent and, once you reach that goal, set a new one. From a health standpoint, a weight loss of just 5 percent of your body weight can lead to a significant reduction in the risk factors for heart disease, including a reduction in serum cholesterol and blood pressure, an increase in insulin sensitivity, and better control over blood sugar.

HOW WEIGHT LOSS PROCEEDS ON
THE T-FACTOR 2000 DIET

If you stick within T-Factor 2000 guidelines, weight loss should proceed at a steady pace, week by week, with only slight up-and-down variability due to fluctuations in your water balance. Notice I said, "steady pace, *week by week,*" because daily variations of one or two pounds, up and down, around the downward trend are to be expected.

How often should you weigh yourself?

I wish I could say to everyone who wants to lose weight permanently, "Throw away your scale. Let your body adjust to your biologically ideal weight by eating a healthful low-fat diet and increasing your activity level so you can burn all the fat you would like to eat in physical activity rather than through an expansion of fat mass." While this advice can work for some people, it doesn't work for most. I, for one, find that daily weighing keeps me on track. When I didn't do it, it led to problems, as I'll show you in a moment. Weighing every day alerts me to upward deviations that need immediate compensation in order to prevent a more serious weight gain.

Let me give you an illustration of why I have returned to weighing every day.

One evening last week I went with friends to Caesar's, one of my favorite Italian restaurants. I know I can get low-fat dishes there, although, as in many restaurants, you sometimes have to ask for a particular dish to be prepared with less fat than is customary. This night I chose "Pasta a la Puttanesca." This pasta is served with a thick tomato sauce containing canned artichokes (quartered), sliced green and black olives, onions, and bell peppers. Caesar himself works the kitchen and sees to it that portions are generous—just as he would like himself! So, the oversize dinner plate arrived with generous double-size portions of pasta and sauce—I estimate 2 cups of pasta and more than a full cup of sauce to which the vegetables had been added. In the spirit of the occasion, I sprinkled an ample 2 tablespoons of Parmesan cheese over my feast. In addition, I had two glasses of Chianti, but at Caesar's, a glass of wine is not a 4-ounce serving. It's 6 ounces. Thus, in reality, I had three glasses of wine, not two!

I almost forgot to mention that the meal began with a house salad, served with blue-cheese dressing on the side (I just dip the tines of my fork in the dressing before spearing the vegetables so that I use about a teaspoon of dressing, total). Oh, yes—and I helped my wife finish her pizza. Just a slice and a half of a small vegetarian pizza blanketed with mozzarella and more green and black olives among the toppings.

I mention these details because portions in the meal I was served, as in most restaurants, were far larger then the "standard serving" for which fat, calories, and other nutrients are measured and reported in nutrient counters. In addition, while I had no trouble remembering that I had helped my wife finish her dinner, I really did almost forget the salad. Circumstances like these keep people from being fully aware of how much they are eating and account, in part, for serious underestimates of food consumption in surveys.

I also go into detail because the next morning I was 2 pounds heavier!

After checking the sodium content of the foods I had eaten, I realized that I had had over 2500 milligrams of sodium in that one meal. That would, of course, lead to considerable water retention. But, in addition, while the meal contained at least 25 grams of fat, the three glasses of wine could contribute to a suppression of about 21 grams of fat that my body might otherwise have burned from the rest of the day's food consumption. *Remember: Alcohol must be counted as fat in the diet because it prevents your body from burning fat in your fuel mixture (about 7 grams of fat per serving)!*

While a bathroom scale can show you the impact of a meal like this on your total body weight, there's no way one can be exact outside of the laboratory about the actual impact of a wonderful feast like this on body fat stores. It's clear, however, that between total calories, the amount of actual fat in the meal, and the wine's impact on fat burning, within that 2-pound weight gain, about 20 to 25 grams of fat were in danger of being permanently deposited in my fat cells.

This is the kind of eating and overnight weight gain that requires a compensatory reaction. Should this happen to you and your scale show a 2-pound weight gain, there might be half-an-ounce or an ounce of fat that ends up permanently in your fat cells. That's how occasional meals of this kind, just once or twice a week, without compensation, can result in a weight gain of several pounds a year.

So I do suggest weighing every day. While you can compensate anytime after a meal that leads to the kind of gain I'm talking about, the sooner the better, or the damage may be compounded by another "occasional" festive meal. I took immediate compensatory action after this meal, with less fat and more fruit and water in my diet the next two days. That's how long it took for the balance beam on my scale to return to where it had balanced the morning of my Italian dinner.

How should you gauge your true progress?

Your true progress is indicated by the trend that your weight is following, week by week. I suggest you choose one day of the week, and compare the weight on that day each week to judge how well you are doing. Many people use Mondays because it gives them an idea of what they might need to do during that week to compensate for a festive weekend.

I had occasion to gauge my own progress losing weight on the T-Factor Diet after an injury to my shoulder in the fall of 1993. I tore my rotator cuff, which made it impossible to serve or hit overheads in a game of tennis. It had been my custom to play singles tennis for one and a half hours daily, plus several hours of doubles during the week, ever since I lost 70 pounds in 1963. I also typically jogged an additional two to three miles with my dogs each evening.

Rather than have the shoulder operated on, I decided I would just add a few miles to my jogging routine, since I found jogging just as satisfying as tennis. Cutting back on the time spent in physical activity would allow me to spend more time in my many other interests.

I was not accustomed to weighing myself at that time, since I had never experienced a noticeable weight gain. It had been years since I had gotten on a scale, but then, during those years, there had been no significant change in my life or level of physical activity. But, little by little, I noticed my pants getting a bit tighter. Finally, one day (three years later) I had to take a really deep breath and pull in my stomach to get my pants buttoned. I turned and took a good look at myself in the mirror, and indeed my stomach was protruding a bit over the belt buckle. Obviously, my new routine of jogging five miles a day did not equal the energy expenditure of tennis combined with two or three miles of jogging, to which I had been accustomed for many years. In fact, when I took the time to calculate the difference, it was probably about 300 calories less each day. I was not compensating by a suitable reduction in energy intake.

I got on the scale, and the results of what I saw and what the sight motivated me to do are illustrated in the graph in Figure 5-1.

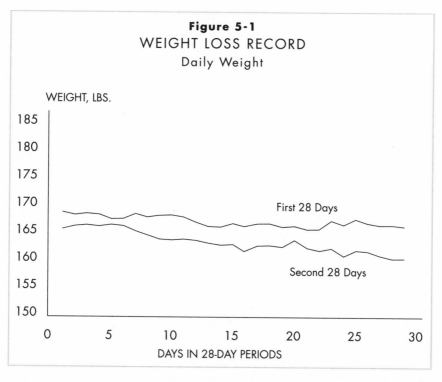

Figure 5-1
WEIGHT LOSS RECORD
Daily Weight

I lose 7.5 pounds in eight weeks on the T-Factor 2000 Diet after gaining weight due to an injury.

The first thing I did was to take make sure I was aware of what I was eating. I followed the advice I would give to others: I wrote down in advance what I intended to eat at each meal of the day and for snacks for just one day. I didn't get any big surprises, but I did find out, had I not been writing down my intentions and thinking of what I might have done otherwise, that I very likely would have had doubles at dinner and served myself somewhat larger than standard portions.

As I went along with the weight-loss effort, I also noted that while Enid and I rarely watch television, when we did, we made a big batch of popcorn to keep us company. We were, of course, doing just what many people do when they watch TV: **EATING!**

I was a little disappointed with my early results. I wanted to see a nice substantial weight loss to reward me for my efforts, which were to stay below 60 grams of fat a day. However, my experience was similar to what people who have the last 5 to 15 pounds to lose experience. It's slow, and you just have to stick with it! The more you weigh, the more you lose on any diet during the initial stages. And for most people who would like to lose weight, the motivation for the final 5 to 15 pounds is not as great as when you are faced with 50 or more pounds. The initial loss on any diet for a person 15 pounds or less overweight is not as likely to be as great or as satisfying as the initial loss for a person 50 or more pounds overweight, even though the effort is equal.

Like everyone else who elects to follow a gradual weight-loss program that's designed to result in an average loss of a pound or so a week, I experienced many day-to-day ups and downs. You can see the peaks in the graph. I can't explain all of them, but I can for what happened in the last week of the first twenty-eight days, and the first week of the second twenty-eight days. I was walking with two of the dogs that are part of our family, a German shepherd and an Akita. Together they weigh over 200 pounds. I walk them on a pair leash that has two branches at the dog's end. On this occasion, another dog in the neighborhood, which was allowed to roam freely, charged into our midst. While nothing serious happened to the dogs, by the time the little tussle was terminated I had twisted my back. The pain kept me from doing anything more than standing around in my own yard watching the dogs amuse each other for several days, and it was several more days before I got back up to full steam in our walks. But I did get within a half-pound of my goal at the end of eight weeks.

Women who are in the 40- to 50-pound overweight range can expect to lose an average of about a pound a week on the T-Factor 2000 Diet, just as I did. Heavier persons will average a little more. While women only 5 to 15 pounds overweight may lose more slowly, we do not have results for such persons because they do not participate in the weight-management program.

Expect to see some ups and downs when you look at your progress on a day-to-day basis. These will occur on any long-term weight-management program that includes the wide array of foods you are accustomed to eat and will continue to eat when you reach your goal. Along the way, or when you reach your goal, a single meal like my Italian feast can result in a temporary weight gain of two pounds. A couple of them during a week can put you both up a couple of pounds and on a higher plateau for a week or two. Only on very-low calorie diets (under 800 or 900 calories a day) is there likely to be a steady loss, and even on these diets there is a dramatic decline in the rate of loss and some days without any loss, as time goes on.

When you do have a day of eating that leads to a weight gain, don't wait—deal with it quickly. Compensate, and get right back on track. Now at my desired weight, I use a two-pound guideline. When I see the beam on my scale balance at 162, I take corrective action because I don't intend to let my weight get out of hand as it did a few years ago. If you are still trying to lose weight and hit a plateau for two weeks, go back to keeping an accurate record once again if you have stopped doing it. Repeat Exercise I from Chapter 3 to make sure you know that what you are eating is really in line with T-Factor guidelines.

When you reach your goal you will be free to add more fat to your diet. In follow-up, our research subjects added about 5 percent more fat to their diets, and ended up with around 24 percent of total calories in fat. This matches the average intake among successful people in the National Weight Control Registry.

Whenever you decide to stop losing weight, be sure to stick with T-Factor 2000 principles for maintenance. By emphasizing low-fat foods, a wide variety of fruits, vegetables, and grains, with minimal animal products, and replacing saturated fats with monounsaturated fats, you will be following a diet that is more than just a weight-management diet. It's a diet that can cut your risk of both heart disease and cancer in half. Besides being thinner, when you stick with it, you will be twice as likely to enjoy a healthier, happier, and longer life. Think about the long-term benefits, as well as the short-term outcome, and let these thoughts help sustain your motivation. And be sure to try a variety of plant-based recipes in Chapter 8, especially those that introduce new foods for you. You will see that a healthful weight-management diet can taste good, too.

BUT—

If you ever become discouraged with the speed of loss on the slow-but-steady route to permanent weight management that I have described in these last two chapters, there is an effective alternative. It's one that you might want to use if you have 50 or 75 pounds to lose, as I did in 1963, and if, right from the start, a diet that yields a pound-a-week loss doesn't suit your temperament. You can jump-start the process and achieve a quick, initial 10- to 15-pound weight loss with a rotation on the T-Factor 2000 Rotation Plan, which I describe in the next chapter.

CHAPTER 6

The T-Factor 2000 Rotation Plan

The T-Factor 2000 Rotation Plan is an updated version of the quick-weight-loss Rotation Diet that created a national sensation in 1986, when upwards of fifteen million people rotated, three weeks at a time, and untold millions of pounds were lost. Unfortunately, advances in the fields of biochemistry and physiology that the T-Factor 2000 Diet anticipated had not yet been made. So, I was not able to formulate the guidelines that are now proven to be essential for weight maintenance—namely, a low-fat diet and the need, on average, for about 80 minutes a day of some kind of physical activity. The new T-Factor Rotation Plan is a more nutritious adaptation based on the T-Factor principles that I have explained in the previous chapters of this book. If I can show you how to incorporate these principles into your lifestyle, I can assure you that you will not regain any of the weight that you lose on each rotation.

The T-Factor 2000 Rotation Plan will lead to a weight loss of up to 10 or 15 pounds in a three-week period for most overweight people. I designed it as my personal weight-loss plan in 1963 and made several rotations on the plan to go from 230 pounds to 155 pounds.* On the first of the several occasions that I used it I lost al-

*Over the next several years I found that I felt and looked best at 160 pounds, and that is the weight I have maintained, except for occasions when I have experimented with different diets or suffered a physical injury. At one point in a research project I went down to 148 pounds, but at that weight I looked and felt terrible. On two occasions I gained several pounds during periods when I had to reduce my level of physical activity as a result of injuries.

most 20 pounds, as I did on one other occasion when I stayed on it for four weeks instead of three out of just plain enthusiasm!

But, **do not even think of using the T-Factor Rotation Plan unless you have studied the previous chapters and are prepared to maintain your losses by following the dietary guidelines I've laid out in *The T-Factor 2000 Diet.*** It's a must. Why go through the struggle to lose a great deal of weight, only to experience the anguish of putting it all back on again? And, if you are a sedentary person and physically capable, a *serious* increase in physical activity may be *the key* to keeping it off. I insist on this because the diet will likely do you no permanent good unless you make T-Factor principles a part of your life. Our own follow-up studies on the Rotation Diet, the T-Factor Diet, and research conducted by the National Weight Control Registry prove the point: No matter what diet people use to lose weight, the way successful people keep it off is to follow a low-fat, high complex carbohydrate diet (about 24 to 25 percent of total calories in fat) and make a significant increase in their level of physical activity. My goal in *The T-Factor 2000 Diet* is to show you exactly how to do that and how to *sustain* whatever changes you need to make in your life in order to stick with it.

HOW MY ORIGINAL ROTATATION DIET WAS BORN

In the week that followed my heart attack in 1963 I spent a great deal of time thinking about how to get my excess weight off. I had tried many diets in my lifetime. I tried grapefruit diets and egg diets. I tried fasting and even devised my own version of a powdered, high-protein diet. I would stuff ten gigantic capsules with a package of plain gelatin and swallow them all with two glasses of water for breakfast. Then I would swallow another package of capsules for lunch, with yet another two glasses of water. (You can imagine what I did for the rest of the day.) I could lose weight as fast as anyone. And put it back on just as fast. I really didn't know how to design a healthful diet for weight loss in those days, and I wasn't at all certain that I would be able to keep it off if I did succeed in losing as much weight as I needed to lose.*

---

*At the time of my heart attack and subsequent diet I was researching the effects of anxiety on learning. It was not until 1975 that I became interested in the problem of obesity, and the Vanderbilt Weight Management Program did not come into existence until 1976.

But I did know that *something had to change!* I knew that I could not eat fatty foods or a lot of sweets and lose weight easily. And while I knew nothing about how alcohol interfered with fat metabolism, I knew that my resolve might dissolve after a couple of drinks and my weight-loss efforts could go down the drain.

So, I cut all of these things out of my diet. I told myself that I could be perfect for three weeks, and I was. Then I would stop dieting and return for a certain period of time to a less restrained eating pattern, which included more food, some higher-fat foods, and occasional alcoholic beverages. Whenever the time seemed right and I felt motivated, I would go on my diet again. Without realizing it at the time, I was consciously plotting a strategy for losing a lot of weight that became the Rotation Diet some twenty-two years later, after we had proven its effectiveness as a weight-loss strategy in the Vanderbilt Weight Management Program.

What exactly did I do and what did I learn as I went along?

The diet was simple. I cut out all desserts other than fresh or dried fruit. Except for a smidgen of butter added to make cooked greens more palatable, a teaspoon of half-and half in my coffee, and perhaps a teaspoon of salad dressing, I cut out all added fat. I did not consume any alcoholic beverages.

I alternated between several menus for breakfast.

1. 2 slices of dry toast (whole grain, rye, or pumpernickel), sometimes with jelly, sometimes without, coffee with half-and-half, and a piece of fruit or a glass of fruit juice at breakfast or later in the morning;
2. Cold cereal, with fruit and milk (at that time we were already using low-fat milk);
3. A slice of toast with one or two hard-boiled eggs, coffee with half-and-half, and juice with the meal or later in the morning.

The reason I usually drank the juice later in the morning was that my stomach did not react well to citrus juices first thing. And if I were to modify these original breakfasts, it would be to not include any eggs for breakfast more than a couple of times a week. I still like half-and-half with my coffee!

For lunch I had to find a place that would make exactly what I wanted every day because it was more convenient to eat out than to prepare something to take with me to the office. The Campus Grill right next to the psychology building had just what I wanted. For five days during the week, I ate one of two different lunches.

1. My most frequent lunch was the dieter's special that was popular in those days: ground beefsteak (it was really just a large, lean hamburger patty, no more than about 4 or 5 ounces, cooked weight), a scoop of cottage cheese (full fat, I'm sure), and usually sliced tomato and lettuce, but sometimes a small dinner salad, coleslaw (the creamy version, but I don't recall it being overly fatty), or canned fruit. The meal came with a small roll on the side, which I ate plain—I stopped using butter altogether during this period except for the tiny bit I would put on cooked vegetables.

2. For variety once or twice a week I would have "soup of the day" (chicken noodle, vegetable or vegetable beef, tomato, etc.— these were all canned, individual servings heated to order) and a house salad. It came with two small packages of saltines. Sometimes I skipped the soup and had a large salad. At first I used the whole small package of dressing that came with it but then I learned to just dip the tines of a fork in my salad dressing. I like the full-fat versions of salad dressings, especially blue cheese. It amazed me how little it took to make salad greens taste good. You can eat a large salad this way, end up using less than a teaspoon of dressing, and still enjoy it.

If I were to design two basic lunches for a diet of this kind today, I would keep my soup and salad lunch pretty much like it was in 1963, only I would stick with plant-based soups, since I don't eat red meat anymore. And in my dieter's special, I would substitute broiled or poached fish, a broiled skinless breast of chicken, or a bowl of vegetarian chili.

Dinner at home almost always followed the same formula: a standard serving of either meat (for example, a London broil or well-trimmed cut of steak), poultry or fish, a cooked vegetable, rice or potatoes, and sometimes a salad. This is when I discovered I could eat baked potatoes with just salt and pepper. Sometimes I would substitute a slice or two of a whole-grain bread for the cooked starch. Dessert was either fresh or dried fruit, or, on occasion, one of my favorites: two fig bars.

These basic dinner suggestions are as good today as they were in 1963 for someone who wishes to stick close to the typical American diet. If you do, my original menu for dinner can be used as a substitute for any dinner in the menus for the twenty-one-day Rotation Plan in this chapter. Today, since I don't eat red meat, I would be limiting myself to fish or poultry along with plant-food side dishes. Of course, the reason we have devised the kind of menus that we have for the twenty-one-day Rotation Plan is to introduce you to a much wider assortment of plant-based foods and recipes, and to encourage you to cut back on your consumption of animal foods. We think that is best for long-term maintenance and for your health in general.

THE "SAFE FRUIT"—AN ORIGINAL IDEA TO KEEP ME FROM EVER BECOMING SO HUNGRY THAT I COULD BLOW MY DIET

When I designed my personal rotation plan back in 1963, I also decided that I needed something to fall back on as a snack. I knew that I might get hungry at times I couldn't predict in advance, so I wanted something I could always turn to if I felt hungry, whether as part of a meal or not. I chose grapefruit, perhaps because of its reputation as a diet food. I called it my "safe fruit" and I really did eat only grapefruit as a snack each time I went on one of my three-week rotations. I would sit, peel it, and eat it in sections. It's amazing how full you can get with just one whole grapefruit when you include the roughage. In fact, when many people decide to use grapefruit as their "safe fruit" they find it's so filling they can eat only half of one at a sitting; save the other half for later in the day.

Although I didn't count anything—calories or fat grams—in my original Rotation Plan, it is obvious that I made a great reduction in both fat and calories compared with my usual diet. I had eliminated bacon, sausage, scrambled eggs in butter, cheese omelets, chuck roasts, apple pie with cheddar cheese or ice cream, ice cream sundaes, cheesecake, the thick blanket of butter and sour cream on my potatoes, peanut butter, alcohol, etc. Since I wasn't keeping track of anything, I have no idea of how many calories I consumed on average each day, but it was at least a couple of thousand less than I had been used to eating.

While I no longer eat red meat and rarely poultry, I still believe that an approach that severely limits the variety of foods one uses in a short-term weight reduction effort is a viable one. As you will see in Chapter 11, many successful people have used this strategy. If you wish to design your own personal version of my original Rotation Diet, then, in place of red meat and two servings of any animal product on a daily basis, I would recommend that you substitute some of the easy-to-prepare bean, soy, and pasta recipes in Chapter 8.

Later in this chapter you will find three weeks' of menus and recipes to be followed in the T-Factor 2000 Rotation Plan. These will introduce you to the many different foods and styles of cooking that we think should become a permanent part of your diet. They are not likely to pose a threat to weight management. In addition, our suggestions embody the latest nutritional recommendations for a diet that can help protect you against heart disease, cancer, and diabetes. However, it is important for your success that you end up with a plan that suits your personal tastes. So, in the introduction to these menus I will give you some guidelines to make sure that when you construct your own personal Rotation Plan it will be compatible with T-Factor principles.

How did I keep my weight off between rotations?

Here we get to discuss the most important factor involved in whether the Rotation Plan will help you succeed in achieving permanent weight management.

Back in 1963 when I used the Rotation Plan, I did not go hog-wild over food, but neither did I deny myself in between rotations. I rarely ever added butter and sour cream to my baked potatoes, but I must admit I still could go overboard when I did! However, I never resumed buttering my bread. And I continued my light breakfasts six days of the week, reserving the omelets and bacon or sausage for Sunday, and not always then.

I knew from past experience, however, that I was not capable of restricting myself to the kind of low-calorie diet that, by itself, without physical activity, could prevent me from regaining weight. So, just as Dr. Tarpley had ordered, I searched for some physical activity that might help me keep the weight off and prevent another, possibly more serious, heart attack.

The real key to my weight maintenance proved to be tennis!

It was through my new-found enthusiasm for the game of tennis that I discovered just how physical activity can be a sure guarantee of weight maintenance after a significant loss of weight.

I had, since childhood, always wanted to learn to play tennis. My uncle, Jules Daniels, was the top player in upper New York State when I was a child. Since he ran his own little jewelry store for a living, he was never free to prepare for and enter Forest Hills and play for the national championship. But he was tops. He was good enough to play competitively with Don Budge in practice sessions, and I watched him lose a close match to Vinnie Richards (Don Budge was United States Champion and Richards was ranked right behind him in the 1930s). Jules was the best in central New York State and he was perennial City Champion in Utica, New York, where I grew up. He was my childhood idol!

But the most he would do was to show me how to hold a tennis racket. He would never get on the court with me. I was such a fat kid, 50 pounds overweight by the time I was twelve years old, that I think he felt there wasn't an athletic bone in my body.

But with the consent of my physician, I decided after my heart attack that I would take up the game of tennis. The first thing I did was to test myself to see how easily I could learn to hit a ball. I remember the first time I went on the court after the heart attack. The wife of one of my colleagues had two tennis rackets. I told her what I wanted to do. Together, both in street clothes, we went onto the tennis courts behind Vanderbilt University's Wesley Hall (the old psychology building). Within minutes I found I could hit the ball. I never knew where it would land that day, but I could hit it!

I decided, then and there, that I would become a tennis player.

I took it seriously. Tennis became as essential a part of my weight-management plan as my diet. I started taking lessons. I played singles for an hour and a half every day and added several hours of doubles on the weekends. And, much to my satisfaction, I discovered that with only minimal restraint, with that level of physical activity, I never regained any weight in between rotations on my 4-S Diet (which as you may recall, is what I called it at that time). Each time I rotated on the diet, I would lose between 10 and 15 pounds, and once I stayed on it for four weeks and lost almost 20 pounds again.

MAKE SURE YOU DO NOT REGAIN WEIGHT AFTER EACH ROTATION

There is one thing you must understand whenever you lose weight on a quick-loss plan. *A large part of the initial loss is water!* While you do start losing fat weight immediately, it's only after excess water is flushed from your system that fat becomes the major part of the loss you see on your scale. Indeed, in the first week of the diet, if you have been retaining water, you can see a weight loss of as much as 7 to 10 pounds, but only a couple of pounds are fat! If you see a two-pound loss in week three after a big water loss in week one, it's much more likely to be almost entirely fat. So it's important that you make sure you don't start retaining more water than your system needs as you begin to increase your food intake after you finish a rotation. For morale's sake, this may be as important as making sure you don't start out-eating your energy needs and begin to regain some of the fat you have lost.

When you finish a rotation on the plan, add food gradually over several days and make sure you do not exceed the T-Factor fat gram range (20 to 40 for women, 30 to 60 for men). While you might find yourself retaining a small amount of water the first day or two, by adhering to T-Factor fat gram guidelines, *you will not begin to refill your fat cells.* Staying active will also help prevent you from retaining too much water. Just in case you are not aware of this, the more water you drink (and the more fruits and vegetables that you eat that have a high water content), the less likely you are to suffer from excessive water retention. It's also a good idea to limit your sodium intake.

MENUS FOR THE T-FACTOR 2000 ROTATION PLAN

Below are three weeks of menus for the T-Factor 2000 Rotation Plan. You do not have to follow the plan for the full three weeks. Some people prefer to use it one week at a time, others for two weeks instead of three. Some people prefer to set a weight goal, such as 5 percent of their body weight. This is an excellent goal from a health standpoint. If you are 20 or 30 percent above your desired weight, as I was, just rotate on the plan for a 5 percent weight loss several times. Many people find that rotating either by time or by a percent weight loss is much more satisfying from a psychological standpoint than attempting to lose 50 or 75 pounds in one long, slow grind. A reasonable time limit or an attainable weight-loss goal will prevent your becoming frustrated should you set an impossibly large weight-loss goal and then hit a plateau. Practice in maintaining small losses for a planned period of time as you progress toward a larger goal will help assure future maintenance at a much lower weight.

The menus below follow T-Factor guidelines for fat consumption and introduce you to styles of food preparation and menu planning that can become part of your permanent eating plan after each rotation and when you reach your weight-loss goal. Each day's menus tend to average between 1000 and 1100 calories. Consider this your "core diet." By this I mean that there is room to add a "safe fruit" as a snack at any time so that you never feel hungry. The core diet has been designed to bring you as close as possible to the Recommended Daily Allowances of major vitamins and minerals at a minimal fat intake. This leaves room for adding, either in the preparation of foods or in snacks, between 1 teaspoon and 1 tablespoon of fat or a serving of nuts each day to meet the lower limit of the recommended fat-gram count. Remember that a serving of nuts is a recommended substitute for meat in your diet.

Once again, the daily guidelines for fat consumption are 20 to 40 grams for women, and 30 to 60 grams for men.

Feel free to substitute similar recipes so that you end up eating the foods you like. If necessary for matters of convenience, remember the menus that I used back in 1963. While I don't consider the choices I made at that time to be as nutritious as the ones we have designed today for the Rotation Plan, a fallback dinner that includes the following:

1) a standard serving of meat, poultry or fish,
2) a cooked vegetable,
3) with or without a salad,
4) a starchy plant food, and
5) fruit for dessert,

is a good one to have in your repertoire if you include animal products in your diet. If you do not include animal products, look to legumes and grains and the recipes in Chapter 8.

While each of the menus includes a snack, I think you would do well to choose a fruit to be your "safe fruit" or a vegetable to be your "safe vegetable" from Table 4-2 in Chapter 4. As you may recall, mine was grapefruit, and I chose only grapefruit on each rotation. I'm sure if I chose a different fruit or vegetable every day, I would have ended up eating more because variety stimulates appetite. Successful people often tell me that they really do choose carrot and celery sticks! Even if you choose a variety of fruits and vegetables, and eat more than you would if you limited yourself to one selection, the difference won't amount to much—maybe 50 to 100 calories each day. I think the improvement in the nutritional value of your diet would be worth it, and you would be laying the groundwork for safe snacking when it's time for maintenance. Make the choice that suits you.

Day 1

Breakfast
½ banana; 1 ounce ready-to-eat cereal; 1 cup nonfat or 1% milk; coffee or tea

Lunch
2 ounces turkey or chicken breast; mustard or fat-free mayonnaise; 1 small whole-grain bagel; alfalfa sprouts and assorted raw vegetables; apple; no-cal beverage

Dinner
1 serving Orange Roughy with Spinach*; ½ cup couscous; 2 cups tossed vegetable salad; 2 tablespoons fat-free salad dressing; no-cal beverage

Snack
1 cup strawberries; 1 cup plain, nonfat yogurt

Total for Day 1: 1105 calories, 12 grams fat (10%), 2 grams saturated fat, 81 mg. cholesterol, 2880 mg. sodium, 23 grams fiber

Day 2

Breakfast
½ grapefruit; 1 whole-grain English muffin; 1 teaspoon light margarine; 1 cup nonfat or 1% milk; coffee or tea

Lunch
2 ounces water-packed tuna, ½ whole-wheat 6-inch pita; 2 teaspoons fat-free mayonnaise; sliced tomato; lettuce; assorted raw vegetables of choice; small pear; no-cal beverage

---

*These recipes appear in the recipe section that follows (but are marked at first mention only). Serving sizes are as noted in recipe.

Dinner
1 serving Zucchini Nut Skillet*; 1 cup steamed carrots; 2 cups tossed vegetable salad; 2 tablespoons fat-free salad dressing; ½ cup grapes; no-cal beverage

Snack
4 cups air-popped or microwave "light" popcorn

Total for Day 2:   1055 calories, 17 grams fat (14%), 3 grams saturated fat, 25mg. cholesterol, 2040 mg. sodium, 28 grams fiber

Day 3

Breakfast
½ cup blueberries or other seasonal fruit; 1 ounce ready-to-eat cereal; 1 cup nonfat or 1% milk; coffee or tea

Lunch
Cheese toast (1 ounce reduced-fat cheese, 1 slice whole-grain bread); 1 serving Chilled Celery Soup* or 1 cup broth-based soup; assorted raw vegetables; no-cal beverage

Dinner
3½ ounces skinless baked chicken; ½ cup boiled potatoes; 1 teaspoon light margarine; 1 cup asparagus; 2 cups tossed vegetable salad; 2 tablespoons fat-free salad dressing; ½ citrus fruit cup; no-cal beverage

Snack
½ cup 1–2% cottage cheese; 2 pineapple slices

Total for Day 3:   970 calories, 16 grams fat (15%), 5 grams saturated fat, 100 mg. cholesterol, 2325 mg. sodium, 18 grams fiber

Day 4

Breakfast
½ cup hot cereal of choice; 2 tablespoons raisins; 1 cup nonfat or 1% milk; coffee or tea

Lunch
2 ounces leftover chicken for sandwich; 1 whole-grain sandwich roll or 2 slices bread; tomato slices; lettuce; 2 teaspoons fat-free mayonnaise; 1 kiwi fruit; no-cal beverage

Dinner

1 serving Pork Tenderloin with Orange Marmalade*; 1 serving Cauliflower Sauté* or steamed cauliflower; ½ cup applesauce; 2 cups tossed vegetable salad; 2 tablespoons fat-free salad dressing; no-cal beverage

Snack

1 ounce baked or fat-free tortilla chips; 2–3 tablespoons salsa

Total for Day 4: 990 calories, 18 grams fat (16%), 5 grams saturated fat, 130 mg. cholesterol, 1600 mg. sodium, 17 grams fiber

Day 5

Breakfast

1 cup honeydew melon or other seasonal fruit; 1 poached or boiled egg; 1 slice whole-grain toast; 1 cup nonfat or 1% milk; coffee or tea

Lunch

1 serving Fresh Vegetable Soup* or other broth-based soup; chef salad: 2–3 cups tossed vegetable salad, 1 ounce turkey or lean ham, 1 ounce reduced-fat cheese, ¼ cup croutons, 2 tablespoons fat-free salad dressing; no-cal beverage

Dinner

1 serving Chicken and Vegetables Alfredo*; 1 slice Italian bread; 2 cups tossed vegetable salad; 2 tablespoons fat-free salad dressing; no-cal beverage

Snack

orange; 2 small gingersnaps

Total for Day 5: 1055 calories, 19 grams fat (22%), 6 grams saturated fat, 275 mg. cholesterol, 3370 mg. sodium, 12 grams fiber

Day 6

Breakfast

½ cup peaches; 1 ounce ready-to-eat cereal; 1 cup nonfat or 1% milk; coffee or tea

Lunch

1 serving Salmon Herb Spread* or 2 ounces canned salmon; 5 low-fat crackers; assorted raw vegetables; apple; no-cal beverage

Dinner

1 serving White Chili*; 1 whole-wheat roll; 1 cup baby carrots (raw or steamed); 2 cups tossed vegetable salad; 2 tablespoons fat-free salad dressing; no-cal beverage

Snack

6 ounces V8 or tomato juice; rice cake

Total for Day 6:   1105 calories, 15 grams fat (16%), 4 grams saturated fat, 81 mg. cholesterol, 2080 mg. sodium, 28 grams fiber

Day 7

Breakfast

½ grapefruit; 1 small bagel or whole-wheat English muffin; 1 teaspoon light margarine; 1 cup nonfat or 1% milk; coffee or tea

Lunch

½ cup 1–2% cottage cheese; ½ cup assorted fresh fruit; Zucchini Muffin*; raw vegetables of choice; no-cal beverage

Dinner

3½ ounces flank or lean round steak (Steak Marinade*); 1 medium baked potato; 1 cup French style green beans; 2 cups tossed vegetable salad; 2 tablespoons fat-free salad dressing; no-cal beverage

Snack

4 cups air-popped or microwave light popcorn

Total for Day 7:   1165 calories, 19 grams fat (16%), 7 grams saturated fat, 78 mg. cholesterol, 1870 mg. sodium, 22 grams fiber

Average for Week 1 (Days 1–7):   1060 calories, 17 grams fat (16%), 5 grams saturated fat, 110 mg. cholesterol, 2310 mg. sodium, 21 grams fiber

Day 8

Breakfast

1 small whole-grain bagel; ½ cup sliced seasonal fruit; 1 cup nonfat yogurt; coffee or tea

Lunch

2 ounces sliced turkey; 2 slices whole-grain bread; tomato slices; lettuce; mustard or fat-free mayonnaise; small pear; no-cal beverage

Dinner

1 serving pasta (1 cup) with Red Clam Sauce*; 1 cup steamed broccoli; 2 cups tossed vegetable salad; 2 tablespoons fat-free salad dressing; no-cal beverage

Snack

orange; 2 vanilla wafers

Total for Day 8:   1075 calories, 16 grams fat (12%), 2 grams saturated fat, 48 mg. cholesterol, 2295 mg. sodium, 26 grams fiber

Day 9

Breakfast

½ cup sliced seasonal fruit; 1 ounce ready-to-eat cereal; 1 cup nonfat or 1% milk; coffee or tea

Lunch

English pizza: 1 split English muffin, ¼ cup meatless spaghetti/ pizza sauce (or leftover Red Clam Sauce), 2 ounces reduced-fat mozzarella cheese (bake or broil until cheese is bubbly); ½ cup grapes; no-cal beverage

Dinner

1 serving Polenta with Spaghetti Squash*; 1 cup turnip greens or other greens; 2 cups tossed vegetable salad; 2 tablespoons fat-free salad dressing; no-cal beverage

Snack

¼ cup dried apricots; 2 gingersnaps

Total for Day 9:   980 calories, 21 grams fat (18%), 8 grams saturated fat, 37 mg. cholesterol, 3435 mg. sodium, 21 grams fiber

Day 10

Breakfast

½ cup hot cereal of choice; 2 tablespoons raisins; 1 cup nonfat or 1% milk; coffee or tea

Lunch

1 cup Fresh Pea Soup* or split pea soup; 1 cup baby carrots; 1 slice Quick Mustard Rye Bread*; 1 cup melon; no-cal beverage

Dinner

1 serving Oven-Stewed Chicken and Vegetables*; 2 cups tossed vegetable salad; 2 tablespoons fat-free salad dressing; no-cal beverage

Snack

4 cups air-popped or microwave light popcorn

Total for Day 10:   1065 calories, 13 grams fat (10%), 3 grams saturated fat, 90 mg. cholesterol, 2530 mg. sodium, 26 grams fiber

Day 11

Breakfast

2 slices raisin toast; 2 teaspoons peanut butter; ½ banana; 1 cup nonfat or 1% milk; coffee or tea

Lunch

Spinach salad: 2 cups fresh spinach, ½ boiled egg, 1 ounce reduced-fat shredded cheese, red onion slices, fresh mushroom slices, ¼ cup croutons; 2–3 tablespoons fat-free salad dressing; 1 tangerine; no-cal beverage

Dinner

1 serving Dikkie's Roasted Salmon with Herbs and Pepper*; ½ cup couscous; 1 cup steamed cabbage; 2 cups tossed vegetable salad; 2 tablespoons fat-free salad dressing; no-cal beverage

Snack

½ cup 1–2% cottage cheese; 2 pineapple slices

Total for Day 11:   1155 calories, 31 grams fat (24%), 7 grams saturated fat, 227 mg. cholesterol, 2360 mg. sodium, 13 grams fiber

Day 12

Breakfast

½ cup raspberries; 1 ounce ready-to-eat cereal; 1 cup nonfat or 1% milk; coffee or tea

Lunch

1 serving Minestrone Soup* or other broth-based soup; ½ whole-grain pita pocket; 2 tablespoons hummus; alfalfa sprouts; tomato slices; 1 kiwi fruit; no-cal beverage

Dinner

1 serving Basic Better Beans*; ½ cup brown rice; 1 serving Spinach Casserole*; 2 cups tossed vegetable salad; 2 tablespoons fat-free salad dressing; no-cal beverage

Snack

1 cup nonfat yogurt

Total for Day 12: 1125 calories, 16 grams fat (12%), 3 grams saturated fat, 12 mg. cholesterol, 3105 mg. sodium, 34 grams fiber

Day 13

Breakfast

1 serving French Toast*; ¼ cup Fruit Topping*; 1 ounce Canadian bacon or lean ham; ½ cup orange juice; coffee or tea

Lunch

1 small baked potato; ½ cup 1–2% cottage cheese; chopped green onions; 2 tablespoons salsa; apple; no-cal beverage

Dinner

1 serving Baked Flank Steak*; 1 serving Mashed Carrots and Parsnips, 1 serving Parmesan-Dill Brussels Sprouts*; no-cal beverage

Snack (or dessert)

½ cup frozen yogurt; ½ cup berries

Total for Day 13: 1105 calories, 20 grams fat (16%), 7 grams saturated fat, 89 mg. cholesterol, 1800 mg. sodium, 23 grams fiber

Day 14

Breakfast

½ cup sliced fruit; 1 ounce ready-to-eat cereal; 1 cup nonfat or 1% milk; coffee or tea

Lunch

Stuffed tomato: 1 whole tomato, 2 ounces water-packed tuna, 2 teaspoons fat-free mayonnaise, assorted chopped vegetables; 1 ounce low-fat crackers or breadsticks; no-cal beverage

Dinner

1 serving Spinach Lasagna*; 1 slice Italian bread; 2 cups tossed vegetable salad; 2 tablespoons fat-free salad dressing; ½ cup grapes; no-cal beverage

Snack

4 cups air-popped or microwave light popcorn

Total for Day 14: 1010 calories, 11 grams fat (10%), 3 grams saturated fat, 36 mg. cholesterol, 2335 mg. sodium, 19 grams fiber

Average for Week 2 (Days 8–14): 1075 calories, 18 grams fat (15%), 5 grams saturated fat, 75 mg. cholesterol, 2550 mg. sodium, 23 grams fiber

Day 15

Breakfast

½ cup blueberries; 1 whole-grain English muffin or small bagel; 1 teaspoon light margarine; 1 cup nonfat or 1% milk; coffee or tea

Lunch

1 serving leftover Spinach Lasagna; 1 cup baby carrots; peach; no-cal beverage

Dinner

1 serving Savory Turkey Loaf*; 1 serving Potatoes Au Gratin*; 1 serving Braised Cabbage and Leeks*; 2 cups tossed vegetable salad; 2 tablespoons fat-free salad dressing; no-cal beverage

Snack

nectarine

Total for Day 15: 1129 calories, 24 grams fat (21%), 6 grams saturated fat, 103 mg. cholesterol, 2990 mg. sodium, 23 grams fiber

Day 16

Breakfast

½ cup hot cereal of choice; 2 tablespoons raisins or other dried fruit; 1 cup nonfat or 1% milk; coffee or tea

Lunch

4 ounces leftover Savory Turkey Loaf; 2 slices whole-grain "light" bread; tomato slices; lettuce; mustard or barbecue sauce; orange; no-cal beverage

Dinner

1 serving Asparagus-Nut Stir Fry*; 1 small baked sweet potato; 2 cups tossed vegetable salad; 2 tablespoons fat-free salad dressing; no-cal beverage

Snack

1 cup strawberries; 1 cup nonfat yogurt

Total for Day 16: 970 calories, 23 grams fat (20%), 4 grams saturated fat, 48 mg. cholesterol, 1975 mg. sodium, 20 grams fiber

Day 17

Breakfast

½ banana; 1 ounce ready-to-eat cereal; 1 cup nonfat or 1% milk; coffee or tea

Lunch

Toasted pita pocket: 1 ounce reduced-fat cheese, ½ 6-inch whole-grain pita; tomato slices; chopped lettuce; assorted raw vegetables; 1 cup melon; no-cal beverage

Dinner

1 serving Dijon Swordfish*; 1 serving Roasted Mushrooms, Peppers, and Onions*; ½ cup brown or wild rice; 2 cups tossed vegetable salad; 2 tablespoons fat-free salad dressing; no-cal beverage

Snack

1 ounce fat-free tortilla chips; 2–3 tablespoons salsa

Total for Day 17: 1060 calories, 20 grams fat (16%), 5 grams saturated fat, 81 mg. cholesterol, 1890 mg. sodium, 17 grams fiber

Day 18

Breakfast

½ cup orange juice; 1 cup nonfat yogurt; 1 Refrigerator Bran Muffin*; coffee or tea

Lunch

1 cup tomato soup; ½ cup cottage cheese or reduced-fat cheese; 1 ounce low-fat crackers; assorted raw vegetables; no-cal beverage

Dinner

1 2-ounce vegetarian burger; 1 whole-grain sandwich roll; tomato slices; lettuce; mustard and catsup; 1 serving Oven-Fried Potato Sticks*, 2 cups tossed vegetable salad; 2 tablespoons fat-free salad dressing; no-cal beverage

Snack

½ cup grapes

Total for Day 18:   1145 calories, 13 grams fat (11%), 6 grams saturated fat, 21 mg. cholesterol, 2455 mg. sodium, 21 grams fiber

Day 19

Breakfast

½ cup sliced peaches; 1 ounce ready-to-eat cereal; 1 cup nonfat or 1% milk; coffee or tea

Lunch

1 serving Creamy Crab Spread* on ½ 6-inch whole-wheat pita; tomato slices; lettuce or alfalfa sprouts; mustard or fat-free mayonnaise; tangerine; no-cal beverage

Dinner

1 serving Oven-Fried Chicken*; ½ cup corn; ½ cup sugar snap peas; 2 cups tossed vegetable salad; 2 tablespoons fat-free salad dressing; no-cal beverage

Snack

½ banana; ½ cup pudding made with nonfat or 1% milk

Total for Day 19:   960 calories, 13 grams fat (14%), 3 grams saturated fat, 101 mg. cholesterol, 2010 mg. sodium, 19 grams fiber

Day 20

Breakfast

½ grapefruit; 1 slice Carrot Pineapple Bread*; 1 cup nonfat yogurt; coffee or tea

Lunch

1 small baked potato; ½ cup 1–2% cottage cheese; chopped green onions; 2–3 tablespoons salsa; apple; no-cal beverage

Dinner

1 serving Once-A-Week Pasta*; 1 slice Italian bread; 2 cups tossed vegetable salad; 2 tablespoons fat-free salad dressing

Snack

4 cups air-popped or microwave light popcorn

Total for Day 20:   1080 calories, 14 grams fat (13%), 3 grams saturated fat, 46 mg. cholesterol, 1530 mg. sodium, 18 grams fiber

Day 21

Breakfast

2 tablespoons raisins; 1 cup ready-to-eat cereal; 1 cup nonfat or 1% milk; coffee or tea

Lunch

1 serving Curried Squash/Cauliflower Soup*; 1 whole-grain roll; assorted raw vegetables; orange; no-cal beverage

Dinner

1 serving Baked Fish Fillets*; 1 serving Bessie's Lima Bean Casserole*; 1 serving Glazed Orange-Spice Carrots; 2 cups tossed vegetable salad; 2 tablespoons fat-free salad dressing; no-cal beverage

Snack

1 cup berries of choice; 1 cup nonfat yogurt

Total for Day 21:   1110 calories, 20 grams fat (18%), 4 grams saturated fat, 120 mg. cholesterol, 2400 mg. sodium, 27 grams fiber

Average for Week 3 (Days 15–21):   1065 calories, 18 grams fat (16%), 4 grams saturated fat, 75 mg. cholesterol, 2180 mg. sodium, 21 grams fiber

Average for Weeks 1–3 (21 days):   1070 calories, 18 grams fat (16%), 5 grams saturated fat, 87 mg. cholesterol, 2350 mg. sodium, 22 grams fiber

Other nutrient averages for Weeks 1–3:   63 grams protein, 158 grams carbohydrate, 1975 RE vitamin A (247%), 215 mg. vitamin C (360%), 420 mcg. folic acid (233%), 840 mg. calcium (84%), 14 mg. iron (96%), 10 mg. zinc (82%)

Note: It is difficult to achieve all recommended intakes of vitamins and minerals within calorie levels below 2000 without careful planning and attention to variety and balance. A multivitamin-mineral supplement (100% RDA) can help but should not be viewed as a replacement for choosing nutrient-rich foods.

CHAPTER 7

The Vegetarian T-Factor Diet

More and more people are cutting back on their consumption of animal foods and placing plant foods at the core of their diets. There are a number of reasons for this change in eating preferences. While consumption of red meat has been linked to heart disease and certain cancers, people who have been successful in losing a significant amount of weight and keeping it off also mention a reduction in their consumption of red meat right at the top of their list of dietary changes. This is understandable, since for large numbers of people, especially men, red meat is a major source of fat in the diet.

Many people become part-time vegetarians as they begin to sample different plant foods and different styles of preparation. I place myself in this class because, while I eliminated red meat from my diet several years ago, I still include fish quite frequently and poultry on certain occasions—for example, when I have been invited out to dinner. Jamie still chooses to include lean red meat, poultry, or fish several times per week, although most of her meals center around grains or vegetables.

Even though it's true that vegetarians as a group weigh less than meat eaters, they are as likely to share the same genetic factors that predispose them to obesity as the rest of the population. When vegetarians combine a predisposition to obesity with a diet which, although vegetarian, is still just as high in fat and energy-dense foods as the typical American diet, they can end up just as obese as persons who include meat in their diets. I suspect it's for this reason that I have received many requests for a vegetarian version of the original T-Factor Diet.

You will find below a week's worth of T-Factor 2000 vegetarian menus, with reference to a number of my favorite recipes. These are in the lacto-ovo vegetarian eating style (see the box below for a comparison of the three vegetarian eating styles). Even if you are not a vegetarian and have no desire at this time to become even a part-time vegetarian, I still want to encourage you to try one or more of these menus and begin to increase your intake of plant foods. Start by having at least one meatless day each week. Both your health and efforts to manage your weight will benefit.

VEGETARIAN EATING STYLES:

- **Lacto-ovo vegetarians** avoid meat, poultry, and fish but include dairy products ("lacto") and eggs ("ovo") among their food choices. Lacto-ovo vegetarians comprise the largest percentage of vegetarians in the United States and Canada.
- **Lacto-vegetarians** also avoid meat, poultry, and fish as well as eggs or any foods containing eggs or derivatives of eggs (like egg whites or egg albumin). Lacto-vegetarians may eat dairy products like milk, cheese, and yogurt.
- **Vegans** avoid all animal products or foods with ingredients derived from animals.

Of course, you can design your own vegetarian menus. See Table 7-1 for a daily food guide for vegetarians. If you already include many vegetarian dishes in your diet, feel free to substitute your favorite recipes for those we suggest whenever you like. But be sure to stick with recipes that use similar food groups so that you assure yourself of meeting daily nutritional requirements and stay within the fat-gram limits we advise. And remember the guidelines for daily fat consumption: 20 to 40 grams of fat for women and 30 to 60 grams of fat for men.

Table 7-1.

A General Daily Food Guide for Vegetarians

Food Group	Suggested Daily Servings	Serving Sizes
Breads, cereals, and other grain foods	6 or more	1 slice of bread ½ roll, bagel, or English muffin ½ cup of cooked cereal, rice, or pasta 1 ounce of dry cereal
Vegetables	4 or more*	½ cup cooked or 1 cup raw
Fruits	3 or more	1 piece of fresh fruit ¾ cup of fruit juice ½ cup of canned or cooked fruit
Legumes and other meat alternatives	2 to 3	½ cup of cooked beans 4 ounces of tofu (soybean curd, rich in protein and often fortified with calcium) or tempeh (a fermented soybean food that's rich in protein and fiber) 8 ounces of soy milk 2 tablespoons of nuts or seeds† 1 egg or 2 egg whites
Milk and milk products	2 to 3‡	1 cup of nonfat or low-fat milk 1 cup of nonfat or low-fat yogurt 1½ ounces of low-fat cheese

*Include 1 cup of dark green vegetables each day to help meet iron requirements.
†Nuts and seeds are generally high in fat, and you should pay attention to the serving size. Two tablespoons of most small nuts or seeds weigh about ½ ounce, while serving sizes for larger nuts like macadamias and Brazil nuts go by numbers of pieces. In general, a serving of most nuts and seeds will contain between 7 and 10 grams of fat.
‡Vegetarians who do not use milk or milk products should use soy milk fortified with calcium, vitamin D, and vitamin B_{12}.

Here are some additional tips for plant-based eating.

▪ Eat a wide variety of plant foods to provide all essential nutrients, including sufficient protein. If you are eating a good mix of vegetables, grains, and legumes each day and meeting your caloric needs, there is no need to "complement" proteins at each meal. The complementary protein theory, which is no longer considered to be accurate, contended that for vegetarians to get sufficient usable protein they had to be careful to combine certain foods like beans and rice or nut butters with bread.

▪ Getting started:
  • Whatever your ultimate goal may be in increasing your plant-food intake, most people find that it is easiest and most enjoyable to eliminate animal products gradually as they experiment with new vegetarian products and recipes.
  • Pick up a vegetarian cookbook or pick up a copy of a vegetarian magazine to see if something strikes your fancy. Among our favorite cookbooks are *The Occasional Vegetarian* by Karen Lee (Warner Books), *The TVP Cookbook* by Dorothy Bates (The Book Publishing Company), and *Tofu Quick and Easy* by Louise Hagler (The Book Publishing Company). Another excellent vegetable cookbook that uses some animal products as garnish in certain recipes is *Greene on Greens* by Bert Greene (Workman Publishing).
  • Look through the specialty food sections of your favorite supermarket for new plant-based products and browse through a natural food store and experiment with a few of the products that seem interesting to you.
  • Substitute meat alternatives for meats in your favorite recipes like spaghetti sauces, chili, or soups. Alternatives readily available in most supermarkets are TVP (textured soybean protein, used in soy burgers and other vegetarian products), tofu, and tempeh.
  • Try different brands of vegetarian burgers, breakfast links, and hot dogs. Sometimes these foods are designed to mimic the taste of the original animal products. Others simply go for a flavor and texture that suits the plant ingredients without any attempt to make them taste like the animal food they're named after. I find that the latter are usually the best. Some of these foods will be found in the freezer section of the store, others in the specialty areas.

- Choose restaurants that offer a variety of pasta dishes, salads, and grain or vegetable-based dishes. I have found that just about all better restaurants offer at least one vegetarian dish, and most offer enough vegetables to make a satisfying vegetarian platter even if it isn't on the menu.
- Prepare enough of your favorite vegetarian dishes at evening meals so that leftovers can be used at breakfast or taken to work for lunches.

■ Think ethnic! Virtually every international cuisine includes vegetarian dishes. For example, Italian tomato-based sauces on pastas, vegetable and cheese pizzas, cheese cannelloni, vegetable lasagnas, and eggplant Parmesan; Mexican bean burrito and cheese enchiladas; Asian vegetable stir-fries and vegetable moo shu; Indian vegetable curries; Greek spinach pie, or spanakopita; and Middle Eastern falafel and hummus.

Here are some special health-oriented tips based on the nutritional needs of all vegetarians.

■ Include plant foods that are good sources of iron on a regular basis: dark green leafy vegetables, dried beans, dried fruits, prune juice, pumpkin seeds, sesame seeds, blackstrap molasses, and iron-fortified cereals.

■ Choose foods rich in vitamin C at meals (citrus fruits, tomatoes, strawberries, cabbage, and broccoli, for example) to help your body absorb the iron contained in the same meal.

■ Meeting zinc needs is a challenge for vegetarians as well as for anyone eating the typical American diet. Plant foods that are good sources of zinc include legumes, nuts, seeds, wheat germ, and fortified cereals.

■ Special considerations for vegans:
- Without dairy foods, vegans should be sure to include calcium-rich foods like green leafy vegetables, broccoli, dried beans, tofu that has been prepared with calcium, calcium-fortified orange juice, and other calcium-fortified plant foods.
- Vegetarians who include milk generally do not have to worry about getting enough vitamin D, as milk has been fortified with the "sunshine" vitamin for many years (except for one or two of the widely available organic brands). Vegans, particularly those living in northern cities and those who do not get regular exposure to the sun, may require a supplement. Check with your physician or registered dietitian.

- Complete avoidance of any animal product warrants supplementation with vitamin B_{12} or regular use of B_{12}-fortified soy milks and vegetarian specialty products. It is important to look for the word *cyanocobalamin,* as this is the reliable and usable form of B_{12}.

T-FACTOR 2000 VEGETARIAN MENUS

These T-Factor 2000 vegetarian menus average about 1450 calories and 28 grams of fat. They are lacto-ovo vegetarian style (that is, they include dairy and egg products but no meat, poultry, or fish). If you get hungry, satisfy your appetite with a snack from the list of foods in Table 4-2.

Day 1

Breakfast
1 grapefruit; 1 serving Fruity Breakfast Barley*; 1 slice whole-grain toast; 1 teaspoon light margarine; 1 cup nonfat or 1% milk; coffee or tea

Lunch
1 serving Cream of Broccoli Soup* or 1 cup other low-fat soup; ½ 6-inch whole-wheat pita; 2 tablespoons hummus; ½ cup raw baby carrots; apple; no-cal beverage

Dinner
1 serving Vegetable Tofu Bake*; 1 whole-wheat roll; 2 cups tossed vegetable salad; 2 tablespoons reduced-fat salad dressing; 1 serving Berry Crisp with ½ cup nonfat frozen yogurt or ice milk (or ¹⁄₁₂ angel food cake with ½ cup fresh berries and frozen yogurt); no-cal beverage

Total for Day 1:   1410 calories, 33 grams fat (22%), 8 grams saturated fat, 22 mg. cholesterol, 2525 mg. sodium, 32 grams fiber

Day 2

Breakfast
1 cup melon of choice; 1 whole-grain bagel or English muffin; 2 tablespoons fat-free or light cream cheese; 1 cup nonfat yogurt; coffee or tea

Lunch

1 serving Easy Bean Burritos* with shredded lettuce, chopped tomatoes, and onions; 1 tablespoon sliced black olives; 2–3 tablespoons salsa; orange; no-cal beverage

Dinner

1 serving Eggplant Parmesan*; 1 cup pasta; 2 cups tossed vegetable salad; 2 tablespoons reduced-fat salad dressing; no-cal beverage

Total for Day 2: 1410 calories, 22 grams fat (15%), 5 grams saturated fat, 29 mg. cholesterol, 3540 mg. sodium, 36 grams fiber

Day 3

Breakfast

1 sliced banana; 1 ounce ready-to-eat cereal; 1 cup nonfat or 1% milk; 1 slice whole-grain toast; 1 teaspoon light margarine; coffee or tea

Lunch

Spinach salad: 2 cups fresh spinach, ¼ cup sliced mushrooms, ½ boiled egg, 1 ounce reduced-fat cheese, chopped red onion; 2 tablespoons reduced-fat salad dressing; Apricot Muffin*; 1 cup grapes; no-cal beverage

Dinner

1 serving Tempeh Barbecue on Mashed Potatoes*; 1 serving Mixed Greens with Oranges and Olives*; 1 cup steamed cabbage or cauliflower; 1 serving Corn Bread; ½ cup nonfat frozen yogurt or ice milk with ½ cup sliced fresh peaches; no-cal beverage

Total for Day 3: 1480 calories, 36 grams fat (25%), 8 grams saturated fat, 135 mg. cholesterol, 2990 mg. sodium, 28 grams fiber

Day 4

Breakfast

1 serving Whole-Wheat Pancakes*; 1 serving Fruit Topping or 3 tablespoons reduced-calorie syrup; 1 ounce low-fat smoked sausage or Canadian bacon; 1 cup nonfat or 1% milk; coffee or tea

Lunch

1 2-ounce vegetarian/garden burger; 1 whole-grain sandwich bun; tomato slices, lettuce leaves, pickle slices, onion slices; 1 ounce low-fat chips or pretzels; 1 pear; no-cal beverage

Dinner

¾ cup beans of choice with 1 cup brown rice ("beans and rice"); 1 serving Parmesan-Dill Brussels Sprouts*; 2 cups tossed vegetable salad; 2 tablespoons reduced-fat salad dressing; 1 serving Cocoa Zucchini Cake* with ¼ cup light whipped topping; no-cal beverage

Total for Day 4: 1570 calories, 25 grams fat (17%), 7 grams saturated fat, 60 mg. cholesterol, 3630 mg. sodium, 38 grams fiber

Day 5

Breakfast

1 cup blueberries; 1 ounce ready-to-eat cereal; 1 cup nonfat or 1% milk; 1 slice whole-grain toast; 1 teaspoon light margarine; coffee or tea

Lunch

Medium baked potato with ½ cup 1–2% cottage cheese, chopped green onions, chopped tomato, 2 tablespoons salsa; 1 cup cantaloupe; no-cal beverage

Dinner

1 serving Asparagus-Nut Stir Fry*; 1 cup macaroni; 1 serving Mashed Carrots and Parsnips*; 2 cups tossed vegetable salad; 2 tablespoons reduced-fat salad dressing; 2 pineapple slices; 2 gingersnaps; no-cal beverage

Total for Day 5: 1420 calories, 26 grams fat (16%), 4 grams saturated fat, 10 mg. cholesterol, 2640 mg. sodium, 28 grams fiber

Day 6

Breakfast

1 cup nonfat yogurt; Refrigerator Bran Muffin*; 1 banana; coffee or tea

Lunch

1 serving Fresh Vegetable Soup*; 1 slice Oatmeal Molasses Bread*; ½ tablespoon peanut butter; assorted raw vegetables; 2 kiwi fruit; no-cal beverage

Dinner

2 slices cheese and vegetable pizza (¼ 14″ pie); 2 cups tossed vegetable salad; 2 tablespoons reduced-fat salad dressing; tangerine; no-cal beverage

Total for Day 6:   1300 calories, 25 grams fat (19%), 10 grams saturated fat, 42 mg. cholesterol, 2840 mg. sodium, 22 grams fiber

Day 7

Breakfast

2 tablespoons raisins or other dried fruit; 1 ounce ready-to-eat cereal; 1 cup nonfat or 1% milk; 1 slice whole-grain toast; 1 teaspoon light margarine; coffee or tea

Lunch

1 serving No-Fry Falafel* with 6-inch whole-wheat pita; alfalfa sprouts; tomato slices; nectarine; no-cal beverage

Dinner

1 serving Super-Easy Angel Hair with Spinach and Feta*; 1 slice Italian bread; 2 cups tossed vegetable salad; 2 tablespoons reduced-fat salad dressing; 1 serving Elegant Pears*; no-cal beverage

Total for Day 7:   1530 calories, 27 grams fat (20%), 11 grams saturated fat, 47 mg. cholesterol, 3300 mg. sodium, 31 grams fiber

Average for Days 1–7:   1450 calories, 28 grams fat (19%), 8 grams saturated fat, 50 mg. cholesterol, 3150 mg. sodium, 31 grams fiber

Other nutrient averages for Days 1–7:   52 grams protein, 214 grams carbohydrate, 1797 RE vitamin A (225%), 230 mg. vitamin C (384%), 505 mcg. folic acid (280%), 905 mg. calcium (90%), 17 mg. iron (110%), 10 mg. zinc (80%)

CHAPTER 8

Recipes

A note about the ingredients you will find in our recipes, and other suggestions:

Where to find unusual ingredients. Certain recipes contain ingredients that may be new to you. They can usually be found in the specialty, gourmet, or ethnic food sections of your favorite supermarket. If you can't find an ingredient, be sure to ask, since different markets shelve foods in different ways. In our experience, all can be found in one local shop or another or at farmers' markets.

Using eggs and egg substitutes. We tend to use egg substitutes in many recipes in place of whole eggs. We use whole eggs, however, when we think the result is so superior that the extra calories, cholesterol, and fat are worth it. A whole egg contains 75 to 80 calories, 5 to 6 grams of fat, and about 200 milligrams (mg.) of cholesterol. One-quarter cup of egg substitute, or 2 egg whites, contains 30 calories, 0 fat, and 0 cholesterol. When you divide up the recipe using a whole egg into its component servings, one egg actually contributes very little extra fat, cholesterol, or calories. Nevertheless, in almost all recipes that originally called for whole eggs, I use Eggbeaters. That's been my brand for many years, but there are now many comparable, less expensive brands.

Nonstick sprays versus oil for greasing. Many recipes call for nonstick sprays, but we do not want to give a mistaken impression that their use contributes no fat, or a great deal less fat than a light greasing with oil. In order to qualify as "no-fat," a spray must contain less than 0.5 gram of fat "per serving." I encourage you to read the label of the nonstick spray you may be using. You will most likely see that what constitutes a serving is the amount accumulated on a surface in a third of a second's worth of spraying. That's the amount that contains just under 0.5 gram of fat. In order to coat a cookie sheet, skillet, or baking pan, you will most likely spray for between one and two seconds. This adds up to almost exactly the same amount of fat you would have contributed had you oiled the pan with a quarter-teaspoon of your favorite vegetable oil (about 3 grams). So feel free (as we do) to oil a pan if you prefer rather than use a nonstick spray.

Which vegetable oil should you use? Many of our recipes reflect a Mediterranean influence. Mediterranean cuisine includes more vegetables and fruits than are found in the typical American diet and, of course, olive oil. We are convinced, as many studies have shown, that these characteristics of the Mediterranean diet, together with a higher level of physical activity and somewhat higher consumption of wine, are responsible for the area's lower incidence of heart disease. For this reason, we have switched almost exclusively to the use of olive oil in our recipes, although if you prefer, canola is equally good.* We use Bertolli Classico brand for all but desserts and baked goods, where Bertolli Extra Light works very well. In your own recipes, where butter might normally be used, try Bertolli Extra Light and add ¼ teaspoon of salt. Our recipes reflect this usage, and we think you will not be able to detect the difference!

Fresh versus dried herbs. Fresh herbs frequently have a much different flavor than dry. I find the fresh to be generally sweeter and fuller flavored (they are more fragrant and seem to stimulate more taste buds) and at the same time less pungent and mellower. But when you have to substitute as a matter of convenience, use 1 teaspoon of the dried for 3 tablespoons of fresh herb, chopped fine.

Fresh versus frozen versus canned vegetables. I can think of very few recipes other than certain sauces in which I prefer frozen or canned vegetables to the fresh. But we are fortunate in having an organic produce distributor who delivers a large box of produce, right from the farmer's truck to our door, once a week. We also have several good supermarkets near our home. If you have a problem keep-

---

*These two oils are predominately monounsaturated, which is the form most associated with a reduced risk of heart disease in many research studies.

ing up with fresh vegetables before they go bad after you purchase them, there is nothing wrong with using frozen or canned. In fact, several studies show that the nutritional value of frozen and canned food is often higher than that of the fresh versions. That's because food to be frozen or canned is generally processed very quickly after harvesting, frequently the same day. Fresh produce may be handled by many people and spend several days in travel and on the store shelf before it is purchased. Water-soluble vitamins tend to dissipate in time when exposed to the air and dissolve in the water that's sprayed on them on produce shelves. For many people, using frozen or canned is simply more convenient. If you do prefer fresh (the flavor and texture are usually superior) but find that much of your purchase tends to go bad before you get to use it, be sure to try my Once-a-Week Pasta recipe. It provides a tasty and healthful way to make sure all your produce is used in a delicious recipe every week.

Reduced-fat and no-fat foods. While I urge you to be cautious in your use of refined fat-free but high-density desserts, pastries, snacks, and candies (if you use them at all), reduced- and no-fat dairy products and certain other foods can play a useful role in your diet. Many people find that fat-free or reduced-fat mayonnaise and other dressings are acceptable. We used reduced-fat mayonnaise in many of our recipes, and the nutritional analysis was performed assuming reduced-fat mayonnaise. If you substitute regular or no-fat, use the fat-gram counter in back of the book to adjust the analysis. We also found at least one brand of sour cream (Daisy's Light) that came close to the flavor and texture of the full-fat versions. It also works well in cooking (where fat-free tends to fail). I use Breakstone's 2% cottage cheese, Prego Part-Skim Ricotta, and Purity Dairies (our local dairy) fat-free (skim) or 1% milk in my own recipes.

Jamie finds that canned reduced-fat cream soups are very convenient to use with vegetables and in rice and noodle-based casseroles. You can improvise a tasty meal quite quickly with frozen vegetables, a reduced-fat cream soup, and rice or pasta.

BEFORE YOU START

Making changes in the way you have been preparing your favorite foods at home and experimenting with new recipes can be an exciting adventure if you approach it correctly. It can also result in a great deal of confusion and inconvenience if you are not properly prepared. So, before you start to experiment with some of these new recipes, I'd like to give you some hints that can make the T-Factor 2000 Diet become a part of your life easily and enjoyably.

I think it's important that you do everything you can to make preparing food just as pleasurable as eating it. I approach cooking in the spirit of an artist working on a fresh canvas. I think of each meal as a new creation, even when I'm preparing dishes I've made many times before. The foods are new, fresh, and colorful, and the urge invariably hits me to vary my seasonings or to add another ingredient that happens to catch my fancy at that moment.

To really enjoy preparing food, you should bear in mind that while certain dishes take more care than others do, recipes are not mathematical formulas. For me, recipes are just convenient guidelines that open the door to my own inventiveness. I hope you will enter into this spirit of cooking yourself, if you haven't already. Some of my favorite dishes are based on complex ethnic recipes that, in their original versions, required lengthy preparation and sometimes ingredients that are not easily available in local markets. My wife, Enid, and I took considerable liberties in shortening the original methods and adapting the recipes to our taste. And, by the way, although coming from many different sources, every one of the recipes included in this book was prepared and tested by Enid and myself or by Jamie. We also introduced them to many of our friends at dinner parties. While you may not like everything we like, you can be certain that no recipe finds its way into this collection that did not pass muster with ourselves and our guests. But think of these recipes as starting points; vary the seasoning to match your taste and be creative about making substitutions if you think one of your favorite ingredients would go better in a recipe than what I have suggested.

Most of our recipes take twenty minutes or less to prepare once you get acquainted with them, but probably a little longer the first time through. Some special dishes may take as much as forty-five minutes, but they are worth every minute of the effort. I suggest you try the more complex recipes on a weekend before scheduling them for a weekday meal. It's a good idea to increase the size of the recipes you like, especially the casseroles, and plan to serve them at two or more meals on succeeding days, or freeze portions for a later time.

While most of the recipes in this chapter were created especially for *The T-Factor 2000 Diet,* based on the fan mail I have received in response to my other books, I have included a number of my all-time favorites. Recipes that have been included in the menu plans have been marked with an asterisk (*).

AN ORGANIZED KITCHEN WILL DOUBLE YOUR PLEASURE

I know from personal experience when both Enid and I were working full time that cooking under pressure can produce a great deal of tension for persons who are away from home most of the day. If you come home close to dinnertime, tired from a day's work, and must start a meal from scratch, it's likely to be impossible to remain calm and enjoy the preparation of a new recipe. This is especially true if you have family members coming into the kitchen every few minutes demanding to know when dinner will be ready. So, here are some hints that might make cooking an easier, more pleasurable task.

First, some basics. You must have the right equipment.

Knives. You need sharp knives that keep their edge and make it possible for you to cut, chop, and mince quickly, with little effort. A minimum set would include (with approximate measurements, since blades may vary a bit among manufacturers):

10-inch slicing knife (a thin blade for slicing turkey, for example)
8- or 10-inch chef's knife (for the chopping jobs, or splitting a winter squash)
6½-inch utility knife (sometimes better on the larger vegetables such as carrots, potatoes, and cabbages than a paring knife or chef's knife)
4-inch paring knife (I like two because they are in constant use)

My favorite knives are Henckels or Wusthof. They hold their edge, fit my hand, and are a pleasure to use.

Keep your knives in a wooden knife block conveniently near the place on your counter or chopping block where you work (but out of the reach of small children) and, by all means, keep them sharp. *More accidents occur with dull knives than with sharp ones because of the difference in effort involved.* And it's no fun to have to fight with your food to prepare it. I like ceramic sharpening sticks or stones for everyday use. Give your knives a few swipes on the stick each time, just before you use them. This is standard procedure for professional chefs. Every so often you should put a new edge on your knives. If you don't know how, and instructions don't come with your stick, ask at your cutlery store for help. Recently I purchased a *Chef's Choice* electric sharpener. I can recommend this brand. But any good electric sharpener can put an edge on a dull knife in a matter of seconds and save you considerable work in comparison with the manual method.

Pots, pans, and casseroles. Big combination dishes, pasta, and casseroles often require large utensils. I suggest, as a minimum:

2- and 3-quart saucepans (with covers)
6-quart covered stockpot (can be used for pasta as well as stew, soup, chili, etc.)
6-, 10- and 12-inch skillets
3½- and 5-quart casseroles (oven and microwave safe)

Also handy are a small assortment of baking dishes and muffin tins, and a roasting pan large enough for chicken and turkey. By all means have a baking dish suitable for lasagna (approximately 8 × 11 × 2 inches for serving six, but, if you like lasagna, it's worth having a special lasagna dish for parties, about 10 × 14 × 4 inches, so that you can serve twelve).

I prefer a skillet to a wok on my electric stovetop for stir-frying, but the product is not quite as crispy and flavorful as you will get with using a wok (my stove's manufacturer warns against using a wok on the electric element). You may be able to find a skillet-wok specially designed for use on an electric stove at your cutlery store, but I haven't tried one.

Miscellaneous. It's a good idea to have an assortment of serving spoons, spatulas (which will not scratch your pots and pans), and other implements handy near the stove. I keep mine upright in a canister, looking like a bouquet, right near the stove. A blender and/or a food processor are indispensable—I think you need both, as well as a big wooden salad bowl (about 4 inches deep and 14 inches across the top for everyday use, larger for company). I prefer wood for my cutting board, but whether you use wood or plastic, be sure to wash it after each use to prevent the growth of harmful bacteria. And finally, you need a pepper mill, and, if not a special spice grinder, at least a mortar and pestle for grinding herbs, spices, and seeds.

Plan your meals ahead of time as much as possible, and be organized in your kitchen and in your cooking technique.

1. Obviously, if you are about to prepare new recipes, you must decide which ones for any given day, and you may have to shop for ingredients—fruits and vegetables are best fresh. You may need a new assortment of herbs and spices. So, a shopping list is called for.

You may have to find a convenient day with a little extra time to cook new recipes since it may take a little longer to put unfamiliar things together. And new recipes usually require some thought about accompanying dishes.

2. It's pleasant to cook in a well-organized kitchen. Just in case you haven't given this much thought, make sure the pots, pans, casseroles, etc., that you are going to use most frequently are in convenient places. You may be pulling out utensils you haven't used much in the past now that you are preparing more combination dishes and casseroles.

3. Keep your preparation space as uncluttered as possible and organize your utensils and your ingrededients before you start to cook. *This ranks right up with the most important advice I can give you for making cooking a pleasant experience.* If you don't already do it for recipes requiring more than a few ingredients and one pot, try this just once: before you begin, lay out (on your uncluttered counter and stovetops) each mixing dish and pot that you will need for the recipe. Then, lay out each ingredient that you will use in the recipe in the order it is called for. If you have been accustomed to playing hide and seek with your ingredients and utensils in the middle of preparation, making an assembly line of this kind is going to make a tremendous difference in your tension level!

Microwave Cooking

Many of our recipes can be converted to microwave cooking. Just check the instruction book that came with your microwave for recipes that are similar to the ones in this book and follow those directions. While microwaves vary somewhat, roasts take around thirteen minutes per pound, chops anywhere from five to twenty minutes, depending on thickness and how many you are microwaving at once, and chicken pieces run about three minutes per piece (four pieces will take about twelve minutes). Muffins tend to take about half the time they would need in a conventional oven, as do fish fillets. Most vegetables sliced will take about eleven minutes per pound, but high-fiber ones, such as broccoli, if you include the stalks, will take more. I usually cut the stalks into small pieces, microwave separately for six minutes, and then add the flowerets for ten or more minutes, depending on quantity. There are special microwave cookers for asparagus that you can find in cookware specialty shops. The asparagus are placed vertically in a covered glass container, with the stalks in water and the tips remaining above in the steam. This avoids having undercooked stalks or overcooked tips with a single cooking time. One of my personal favorites, a medium-size baked potato (about 6 ounces), takes only six minutes.

NUTRITIONAL ANALYSIS

The nutritional content of all recipes was analyzed using the *ESHA* Food Processor Nutrition and Fitness Software computer program, Version 7.1. After each recipe you will find information about calories, cholesterol, dietary fiber, total fat, saturated fat, and sodium content. Cholesterol and sodium values are rounded up or down to the nearest whole milligram, while fat and fiber values were rounded up or down to the nearest gram except in certain cases where the fraction is almost equal to 0.5 gram (for example, 0.47 gram will be rounded up to 0.5).

I normally use my own vegetable stocks saved from their original uses in recipes that call for a stock or bouillon. They are free of added salt. When I use a prepared bouillon, it's Morga Vegetable Broth (a powder that contains 710 milligrams of sodium per teaspoon). You may prefer to use your own favorite brands of low- or no-sodium bouillon if you are controlling your sodium intake. Adjust the sodium content noted for the recipe accordingly.

Meat and fish shrink about 25 percent in cooking. We used cooked weight in our analyses. In combination dishes, total weight of meat or fish, after cooking, is divided by number of servings to arrive at their contribution to the nutritional analysis.

CONCISE GUIDE TO HERBS AND SPICES

I have included this guide to herbs and spices because their judicious use can add a great deal to your cooking and eating pleasure as you reduce the fat and sugar in your recipes. I keep the spices and herbs I use most frequently in a wine-style rack at the rear of my work area. I keep others on revolving shelves in the cabinet above, one shelf for seeds, another for liquids, and a third for infrequently used items. I have compiled the guide from various sources, often from different recipes that looked particularly interesting (although I haven't gotten around to trying all the herbs and spices with the foods they might complement).

I suggest you try each seasoning either one at a time or in simple, limited combinations, to see what you like best. All foods can be seasoned in a variety of ways, each quite distinctive. For example, I have found recipes suggesting that carrots fare well with the addition of all the following: bay leaves, caraway seed, celery seed, chervil, chives, curry powder, dill seed, dill weed, ginger, mace, marjoram, nutmeg, savory, tarragon, and thyme, in addition to pepper and parsley. So, while using pepper and parsley, I might add just one of the others when preparing carrots as a side dish.

Allspice—meats, fish, gravies, relishes, tomato sauce

Anise—fruit

Basil—green beans, onions, peas, potatoes, summer squash, tomatoes, lamb, beef, shellfish, eggs, sauces

Bay Leaves—artichokes, beets, carrots, onions, white potatoes, tomatoes, meats, fish, soups and stews, sauces and gravies

Caraway Seed—asparagus, beets, cabbage, carrots, cauliflower, coleslaw, onions, potatoes, sauerkraut, turnips, beef, pork, noodles, cheese dishes

Cardamom—melon, sweet potatoes

Cayenne Pepper—sauces, curries

Celery Seed—cabbage, carrots, cauliflower, corn, lima beans, potatoes, tomatoes, turnips, salad dressings, beef, fish dishes, sauces, soups, stews, cheese

Chervil—carrots, peas, salads, summer squash, tomatoes, salad dressings, poultry, fish, eggs

Chili Powder—corn, eggplant, onions, beef, pork, chili con carne, stews, shellfish, sauces, egg dishes

Chives—carrots, corn, sauces, salads, soups

Cinnamon—stewed fruits, apple or pineapple dishes, sweet potatoes, winter squash, toast

Cloves—baked beans, sweet potatoes, winter squash, pork and ham roasts

Cumin—cabbage, rice, sauerkraut, chili con carne, ground-beef dishes, cottage or cheddar cheese

Curry Powder—carrots, cauliflower, green beans, onions, tomatoes, pork and lamb, shellfish, fish, poultry, sauces for eggs and meats

Dill Seed—cabbage, carrots, cauliflower, peas, potatoes, spinach, tomato dishes, turnips, salads, lamb, cheese

Dillweed—vegetables, salads, poultry, soups

Ginger—applesauce, melon, baked beans, carrots, onions, sweet potatoes, poultry, summer and winter squash, beef, veal, ham, lamb, teriyaki sauce

Mace—carrots, potatoes, spinach, summer squash, beef, veal, fruits, sauces

Marjoram—asparagus, carrots, eggplant, greens, green beans, lima beans, peas, spinach, summer squash, lamb, pork, poultry, fish, stews, sauces

Mustard—asparagus, broccoli, brussels sprouts, cabbage, cauliflower, green beans, onions, peas, potatoes, summer squash, meats, poultry

Mustard Seed—salads, curries, pickles, ham, corned beef, relishes

Nutmeg—beets, Brussels sprouts, carrots, cabbage, cauliflower, greens, green beans, onions, spinach, sweet potatoes, winter squash, sauces

Oregano—baked beans, broccoli, cabbage, cauliflower, green beans, lima beans, onions, peas, potatoes, spinach, tomatoes, turnips, beef, pork, veal, poultry, fish, pizza, chili con carne, Italian sauces, stews

Paprika—salad dressings, shellfish, fish, gravies, eggs

Parsley Flakes—all vegetables, soups, sauces, salads, stews, potatoes, eggs

Pepper—most vegetables, meats, salads

Poppy Seeds—salads, noodles

Rosemary—mushrooms, peas, potatoes, spinach, tomatoes, vegetable salads, beef, lamb, pork, veal, poultry, stews, cheese, eggs

Saffron—rice

Sage—eggplant, onions, peas, tomato dishes, salads, pork, veal, poultry, ham, cheese

Savory—baked beans, beets, cabbage, carrots, cauliflower, lima beans, potatoes, rice, squash, egg dishes, roasts, ground-meat dishes

Sesame Seed—asparagus, green beans, potatoes, tomatoes, spinach

Tarragon—asparagus, beets, cabbage, carrots, cauliflower, mushrooms, tomatoes, salads, macaroni-and-vegetable combinations, beef, poultry, pork

Thyme—artichokes, beets, carrots, eggplant, green beans, mushrooms, peas, tomatoes, pork, veal, poultry, cheese and fish dishes, stuffings

Turmeric—mustards and curries, chicken

APPETIZERS AND SNACKS

Although we normally serve fruit for appetizers when we entertain, the low-fat dips in this section make for interesting contrasts when you are looking for something different.

Check out the spreads in the Sandwich Makings section of this chapter for additional appetizer and snack ideas.

GARBANZO BEAN DIP

1 large can (20 ounces) garbanzo beans (chickpeas), drained and rinsed
3 tablespoons tahini (sesame seed paste)

¼ cup lemon juice
3 garlic cloves, crushed
1 scallion, minced
dash salt
parsley sprigs

1. Combine all ingredients except parsley in a blender or food processor. Blend into a thick paste.
2. Transfer to a serving bowl and chill for at least one hour.
3. Garnish with parsley and serve with whole-grain crackers, fat-free tortilla chips, or raw vegetables.

20 SERVINGS (2 TABLESPOONS EACH)

PER SERVING: *62 calories, 2 grams fat, 0 saturated fat, 0 cholesterol, 13 mg. sodium, 2 grams fiber*

SPINACH ARTICHOKE BAKE

A long walk in the park and a craving for a local restaurant's spinach artichoke dip inspired the quick creation of this recipe. Jamie shared the first version with her neighbors along with hot French bread. It was an instant hit!

2 cans (14 ounces each) artichoke hearts, drained and diced
1 package (10 ounces) frozen chopped spinach, thawed
1 can (10¾ ounces) reduced-fat cream of celery soup

½ cup reduced-fat mayonnaise
½ teaspoon garlic powder
¼ teaspoon fresh-ground black pepper
4 ounces Parmesan cheese, grated

1. Squeeze excess moisture from thawed spinach.
2. Combine with diced artichoke hearts in medium bowl.
3. Stir in cream soup, mayonnaise, garlic powder, pepper, and grated Parmesan.
4. Turn into a shallow 2-quart casserole that has been coated with nonstick cooking spray. Bake at 350 degrees for 35–40 minutes or until browned around edges and bubbly.
5. Serve with French bread or fat-free tortilla chips.

12 SERVINGS

PER SERVING: *101 calories, 3 grams fat, 2 grams saturated fat, 8 mg. cholesterol, 565 mg. sodium, 2 grams fiber*

TOFU SPINACH DIP

2 cups baby spinach, washed

1 package (12 ounces) extra-firm silken tofu

2 scallions, chopped

2 tablespoons fresh parsley, chopped

1 garlic clove, crushed

1½ tablespoons lemon juice

½ teaspoon salt

½ teaspoon ground mustard powder

½ teaspoon thyme

¼ teaspoon ground cumin

¼ teaspoon crushed red pepper

fresh-ground black pepper to taste

1. Remove coarser stems from spinach and then, in a microwave-safe bowl, cook spinach on high, covered, for 2–3 minutes until it is wilted.
2. With a slotted spoon, remove spinach from microwave bowl to a food processor. (Reserve liquid for another use.)
3. Add remainder of ingredients and process until smooth.
4. Chill. Serve as a dip with fresh carrot, bell pepper, and celery sticks.

MAKES ABOUT 2 CUPS OF DIP

PER SERVING (¼ CUP): *66 calories, 4 grams fat, 1 gram saturated fat, 0 mg. cholesterol, 158 mg. sodium, 1 gram fiber*

SEASONINGS

Taste buds adapt to the taste of salt and sugar so that the more you use, the less sensitive to the flavor you become. The converse is also true—that is, the less you use, the more sensitive you become. About 15 percent of the population is "salt sensitive," which means, if you belong to this group, that your blood pressure may become elevated in response to the overconsumption of salt. By and large, Americans eat eight to ten times more salt than our bodies need to stay healthy. Most health professionals, including myself, think we need to cut back. I don't think you need to cut salt down to the barest minimum unless your physician has determined that it's necessary. Start by using less salt in cooking, adding just a small amount during food preparation in order to help bring out the other food flavors. If you find the food needs more salt, add it at the table. Most people find they use much less salt when they add little or none during cooking and then just sprinkle a bit on the finished product after tasting it. In this way, the salt hits your taste buds as soon as the food enters your mouth. When a recipe says "salt to taste," go lightly. Try about one-eighth of a teaspoon in a recipe for four. In this way you will be adding only about 250 milligrams of salt to the entire recipe, which is less than 65 milligrams per serving.

Experiment with using other herbs and spices rather than relying primarily on salt for flavor. Try the seasoning mixtures presented here for starters. They are proven favorites. You might also try one or more of the many commercially available salt-free blends. They have distinctive combinations of herbs. If you are not trying to severely restrict your salt intake, add a dash and it will help bring out the herb flavors. Use plain onion and garlic powder, not blended garlic and onion salt, which are high in sodium. Many people find that the use of hot spices does, in time, reduce the preference for salt as well as for sweet things. When you use hot spices, the thermic effect of food is increased, which means you get the added benefit of burning a few extra calories while eating and digesting your meals.

HERB SALT

This is a popular blend of dried herbs with just enough salt to let your taste buds know it's there as it embellishes the other herb flavors. It contains only about 285 milligrams of sodium per teaspoon, compared to approximately 2200 in a teaspoon of plain salt.

½ teaspoon basil   *¼ teaspoon celery seed*
¼ teaspoon thyme   *¼ teaspoon parsley*
¼ teaspoon dill weed   *¼ teaspoon salt*

Combine all ingredients except salt and grind with a mortar and pestle. Add salt, mix, and store in a small herb jar.

MAKES ABOUT 1 ³/₄ TEASPOONS

Except for the sodium mentioned, the mixture contains trace amounts of other nutrients too small to be meaningful in the amounts used.

INDIAN SPICE BLEND

Indians make many different spice blends (called *garam masalas*) by combining a selection of different hot or pungent spices to suit their personal tastes and the food for which they are intended. Ginger, coriander, cardamom, cayenne, cinnamon, chilies, mustard seed, turmeric, cumin, black (and other color) pepper, poppy seeds, fenugreek, fennel, mace, and cloves are among the spices found in traditional *garam masalas*. In addition to imparting different flavors, these spices hit different taste buds and make for full-flavored dishes. I have a variety of such blends on my shelf, and keep one like this on hand whenever a recipe simply calls for curry powder. It will also add an authentic Indian flavor to baked beans or a chili. Try it with Basic Better Beans, or in place of the spices called for in dishes like our Curried Vegetables.

8 teaspoons ground cumin *2 teaspoons cayenne*
4 teaspoons ground ginger *4 teaspoons turmeric*
2 teaspoons ground coriander *2 teaspoons black pepper*

Combine all ingredients and store in an airtight spice jar.

MAKES ABOUT 7 TABLESPOONS

In the amounts normally used, this mixture contains only trace amounts of various nutrients.

SAUCES

In addition to these three basic sauces, you will find a number of others associated with different recipes in this book that you can use, in some of your own favorite recipes, to replace higher-fat sauces.

BARBECUE SAUCE

This tasty sauce, stored in an airtight container, will keep for about a week and a half in the refrigerator.

1 can (12 ounces) no-salt-added tomato paste
½ cup dry red wine (or substitute water)
1½ cups water or stock
2 tablespoons red wine vinegar
2 teaspoons lemon juice
½ medium onion, chopped fine
½ medium bell pepper, chopped fine
1 tablespoon Worcestershire sauce

2 tablespoons brown sugar
1 tablespoon honey
2 teaspoons Liquid Smoke
1 teaspoon garlic powder
1 tablespoon chili powder
1 tablespoon dry mustard
crushed red pepper to taste
dash of Tabasco
2 tablespoons fresh parsley, minced
¼ teaspoon celery seed
½ teaspoon salt (optional)

1. Combine all ingredients except parsley and celery seed in a large kettle or saucepan.
2. Bring to a low boil, then reduce heat and simmer about 20 minutes.
3. Add the parsley and celery seed (and salt, if desired), and simmer for another 5 minutes or so.

MAKES ABOUT 1 QUART

PER 2-TABLESPOON SERVING: *16 calories, 0 fat, 0 saturated fat, 0 cholesterol, 5 mg. sodium, 0 fiber*

LIGHT BÉCHAMEL (WHITE SAUCE)

This is a low-fat sauce for making creamed vegetables. It can also be used in place of tomato purée to convert the Red Clam Sauce recipe to a white sauce.

¼ cup vegetable or chicken
  stock
¼ cup flour or 2 tablespoons
  cornstarch
2 cups nonfat or 1% milk
½ cup nonfat dry milk

1 bay leaf
½ teaspoon thyme
½ teaspoon ground white pepper
1 teaspoon vegetable seasoning
  (optional)

1. Heat stock in a saucepan over moderate heat.
2. Gradually add the flour or cornstarch and blend with wire whisk
   or wooden spoon.
3. Simmer on very low heat until heated through but not browned.
4. Remove from heat and add remaining ingredients.
5. Return to heat and simmer, stirring constantly, until thickened.

MAKES 2½ CUPS

PER ¼ CUP (USING FLOUR): 42 calories, 0 fat, 0 saturated fat, 1
mg. cholesterol, 63 mg. sodium (without vegetable seasoning), 0 fiber

ONION GRAVY

This is a nice gravy for grain dishes and many vegetables, especially
those in the cabbage family.

1 teaspoon sesame oil (or olive
  oil)
2 teaspoons water
1 onion, chopped
⅛ teaspoon garlic powder

¼ teaspoon ground ginger
¼ teaspoon salt
1 tablespoon soy sauce
1 cup water (divided)
1 tablespoon cornstarch

1. In a small saucepan combine the oil and 2 teaspoons water.
2. Add the onion and sauté, partially covered, over medium heat,
   stirring often, until onions are translucent and are just barely
   starting to brown.
3. Add the spices and soy sauce.
4. Add water, reserving 2 tablespoons.
5. Cook, covered, until the onions are tender.
6. Combine the cornstarch with the reserved water and blend.
7. Add to the onions and cook until the gravy thickens.

MAKES ABOUT 1 1/2 CUPS GRAVY

PER 1/4 CUP SERVING: *21 calories, 1 gram fat, 0 saturated fat, 0 cholesterol, 260 mg. sodium, 0 fiber*

SOUPS

It's a fact: People who include soup with their meals find it easier to lose weight and maintain their losses! I strongly encourage you to try it to prove it to yourself. Clear soups are generally lower in fat than cream soups, but you can make low-fat "cream" soups by substituting skim or low-fat milk for cream or whole milk, adding some nonfat dry milk, flour, or cornstarch to make the soup richer and thicker.

Save water used for steaming or microwaving vegetables to use as vegetable stock for soups or other recipes. Freeze it, with a label, so that you will know what it is and can consider with what recipes that particular stock will add good flavor. I occasionally use Morga Vegetable Broth for soup and other recipes. It adds a pleasant mixed vegetable flavor at the expense of 710 mg. of sodium per teaspoon, so it needs to be used sparingly. You can easily adapt your own favorite soup recipes by cutting fat and experimenting with seasonings.

*CHILLED CELERY SOUP

1 medium onion, chopped
1 tablespoon olive oil
3 cups vegetable bouillon
3 cups chopped celery
1 bay leaf
1/2 teaspoon caraway seed
1/2 teaspoon salt
fresh-ground pepper to taste
1 cup nonfat or 1% milk
2 tablespoons lemon juice

1. In a large saucepan, sauté onion in olive oil, partially covered, until onion is translucent.
2. Add bouillon, bay leaf, and caraway seeds and bring to a boil.
3. Reduce heat and simmer, covered, until celery is very tender, about 30 minutes.

4. Meanwhile, combine milk with lemon juice and chill.
5. When celery is tender, remove bay leaf and allow vegetables to cool.
6. When cool enough to handle, remove vegetables with a slotted spoon and purée them in a blender or food processor.
7. Return vegetables to broth, add milk/lemon juice mixture, and mix until smooth.
8. Add salt and pepper to taste and chill at least 1 hour before serving.

4 SERVINGS

PER SERVING: *80 calories, 4 grams fat, 0.5 gram saturated fat, 1 mg. cholesterol, 422 mg. cholesterol, 2 grams fiber*

COLD PUMPKIN SOUP

1 tablespoon olive oil + 1 table-
  spoon water
1 onion, chopped
2 garlic cloves, minced
2 teaspoons grated fresh ginger
1 leek, sliced
4 cups vegetable bouillon
2 cups canned pumpkin

½ teaspoon ground nutmeg
1 teaspoon salt
cayenne pepper to taste
fresh-ground black pepper to
  taste
1 cup nonfat or 1% milk
4 scallions, chopped

1. In a large skillet, over medium heat, sauté onion, garlic, ginger, and leek in oil/water mixture until onions are translucent.
2. Add vegetable bouillon and bring to a boil. Then lower heat, cover, and simmer until onion and leek are soft (about 15 minutes).
3. With a slotted spoon, transfer vegetables to a food processor or blender and purée.
4. Return puréed vegetables to the broth and stir in pumpkin until smooth. Add nutmeg, salt, and cayenne and black peppers to taste. Simmer 10–15 minutes longer.
5. Add milk and blend well.
6. Chill at least 1 hour before serving.
7. Sprinkle each portion with chopped scallions.

8 SERVINGS

PER SERVING: *62 calories, 2 grams fat, 0 saturated fat, 1 mg. cholesterol, 327 mg. sodium, 2 grams fiber*

*CREAM OF BROCCOLI SOUP

*1½ pounds fresh broccoli,
  chopped
2 cups water
¾ cup celery, chopped
½ cup onion, chopped
2 tablespoons olive oil
2 tablespoons flour*

*2½ cups vegetable bouillon
¾ teaspoon salt
⅛ teaspoon fresh-ground pepper
dash of ground nutmeg
¾ cup evaporated nonfat milk*

1. In a large pot, heat 2 cups water to boiling. Add broccoli, celery, and onion. Cook until vegetables are tender, about 10 minutes.
2. Transfer vegetables along with cooking water to a food processor or blender and process until smooth. Set aside.
3. Meanwhile, heat oil in same pot where vegetables were cooked. Gradually add flour, stirring until smooth.
4. Remove from heat and stir in 2½ cups bouillon. Return to heat and cook to boiling, stirring constantly. Cook and stir one additional minute after mixture comes to a boil.
5. Reduce heat. Stir in broccoli mixture and seasonings. Heat just to boiling. Stir in evaporated milk, heat slightly (do not boil), and serve.

6 SERVINGS

PER SERVING: *114 calories, 5 grams fat, 1 gram saturated fat, 1 mg. cholesterol, 385 mg. sodium, 4 grams fiber*

*CREAM OF PORTABELLA SOUP

12 ounces Portabella mushrooms
1 small onion, chopped
1 garlic clove, minced
1 tablespoon olive oil
1½ cups vegetable bouillon

6 tablespoons nonfat or 1%
  milk
2 tablespoons 2% cottage cheese
½ teaspoon salt
fresh-ground pepper to taste
chopped scallions (optional)

1. Wash mushrooms and pat them dry. Quarter and slice thinly.
2. In a large saucepan cook onion, garlic, and mushrooms in olive oil over medium heat. Stir frequently and cook until liquid has evaporated.
3. Meanwhile, in a small processor or blender, process milk and cottage cheese until completely smooth. Refrigerate.
4. Add bouillon to ingredients in the saucepan.
5. Cover and simmer over low heat for about 5 minutes. Let cool.
6. With a slotted spoon, transfer half of the vegetables to a food processor or blender and purée until smooth.
7. Return vegetables to saucepan and stir until blended.
8. Add milk/cottage cheese mixture to saucepan and stir until blended.
9. Add salt and pepper to taste and heat, but do not boil.
10. Serve and sprinkle each serving with chopped scallions, if desired.

4 SERVINGS

PER SERVING: 81 calories, 4 grams fat, 0.5 gram saturated fat, 1 mg. cholesterol, 364 mg. sodium, 3 grams fiber

Note: Other kinds of mushrooms may be used instead of the Portabellas, but be aware that most mushrooms have more moisture and so may need a longer cooking time in Step 2.

CREAMY CARROT-PARSNIP SOUP

I was never very fond of parsnips until, after being given a batch, my wife Enid was inspired by a much higher-fat version to come up with this recipe. I think it will surprise you just as it did our guests when we did a tasting.

3 medium parsnips, washed and cut in chunks
6 medium carrots, washed and cut in chunks
2 small onions, sliced
2 garlic cloves, minced
1 tablespoon olive oil + 1 tablespoon water
1 teaspoon salt

fresh-ground pepper to taste
1 teaspoon fresh grated ginger
½ teaspoon dried dillweed
2 tablespoons fresh parsley, chopped
4 cups broth or bouillon
1 cup nonfat or 1% milk
1 teaspoon honey (optional)

1. In a large pot, sauté onions and garlic in oil/water mixture.
2. Add all other ingredients except for milk and honey.
3. Bring to a boil.
4. Turn down heat, cover, and simmer until vegetables are tender.
5. With a slotted spoon, transfer vegetables to a food processor or blender and purée until smooth.
6. Return puréed vegetables to the broth and stir until smooth.
7. Add milk, and honey, if desired, and stir.
8. Heat (but do not boil) and serve.

10 SERVINGS

PER SERVING: *89 calories, 2 grams fat, 0 saturated fat, 0 cholesterol, 390 mg. sodium, 4 grams fiber*

*CURRIED SQUASH/CAULIFLOWER SOUP

This unusual soup may seem like a strange concoction, but give it a try. It's been a great success with our tasters and at dinner parties. Freezing will not harm the flavor, and when we make it for ourselves we store half in the freezer for future occasions.

2 tablespoons olive oil	1 teaspoon salt
1 head cauliflower, coarsely chopped	2 teaspoons turmeric
	1 teaspoon ground coriander
1 large onion, chopped	1 teaspoon chili powder
4 cups vegetable bouillon, divided	1 teaspoon ground ginger
	1 teaspoon thyme
2 cups cooked butternut or acorn squash, puréed	½ teaspoon ground cumin
	fresh-ground pepper to taste

1. Put the oil in a 6-quart pot. Add the cauliflower and braise over low heat, partially covered, for about 5 minutes.
2. With a slotted spoon, lift the cauliflower into a bowl and set aside.
3. Add the onion to the pot and braise until translucent.
4. Add 2 cups of the bouillon and simmer, covered, for 15 minutes.
5. Lift the onion out with a slotted spoon and purée in a food processor or blender.
6. Return the onion to the broth.
7. Add the remaining bouillon and the cauliflower, squash, and spices.
8. Simmer, covered, for about 30 minutes or until the cauliflower is tender.

6 SERVINGS

PER SERVING: *124 calories, 6 grams fat, 1 gram saturated fat, 0 cholesterol, 352 mg. sodium, 4 grams fiber*

*FRESH PEA SOUP

1 small onion, chopped	8 cups vegetable bouillon
1 tablespoon olive oil	1 bay leaf
1 medium-size potato, cut in chunks	6 large lettuce leaves, shredded
	1 teaspoon thyme
3 10-ounce packages frozen fresh peas	½ teaspoon salt
	fresh-ground pepper to taste

1. In a large stockpot sauté onion in olive oil until translucent.
2. Add all other ingredients except salt and pepper and bring to a boil.
3. Lower heat, cover, and simmer until potatoes are tender.
4. Remove bay leaf and let cool.
5. Put a colander in a large bowl and pour in soup, draining vegetables.
6. Return drained broth to pot. Purée vegetables in batches in a food processor.
7. Return puréed vegetables to the broth, blend well, add salt and pepper to taste, heat, and serve.

8 SERVINGS

PER SERVING: *116 calories, 2 grams fat, 0 saturated fat, 0 cholesterol, 428 mg. sodium, 6 grams fiber*

*FRESH VEGETABLE SOUP

This recipe was contributed several years ago by a former first lady of Tennessee, Betty Dunn, wife of Governor Winfield Dunn. It's been popular with readers and weight-management group participants ever since. It will keep in the refrigerator for up to a week, but we're betting it won't stay around that long!

1 tablespoon olive oil
2 quarts chicken or vegetable broth
3 garlic cloves, minced
2 tablespoons chopped celery leaves
1 large stalk celery, chopped
1 teaspoon oregano
1 green bell pepper, chopped
2 carrots, thinly sliced
3 red potatoes, sliced, with peel
2 yellow squash, coarsely chopped

2 zucchinis, sliced
2 cups fresh tomatoes, chopped, or a 16-ounce can stewed tomatoes
1 tablespoon basil
⅛ teaspoon cayenne pepper
Tabasco to taste
1 cup cooked spaghetti or macaroni
Parmesan cheese, grated (optional)

1. Combine all ingredients except spaghetti and Parmesan cheese in a large soup kettle.
2. Bring to a boil, reduce heat, and simmer covered for about 50 minutes.
3. Add the spaghetti and simmer 10 minutes more.
4. Serve sprinkled with Parmesan cheese, if desired.

12 SERVINGS

PER SERVING: *95 calories, 2 grams fat, 0.5 gram saturated fat, 1 mg. cholesterol, 530 mg. sodium, 2 grams fiber*

*MINESTRONE

1 medium onion, chopped
1 stalk celery, chopped
2 medium carrots, chopped
1 cup fresh or frozen green beans
1 medium zucchini, chopped
1 package (10 ounces) frozen chopped spinach

1 can (28 ounces) tomatoes
½ cup uncooked macaroni
1 can (15 ounces) navy beans, with juice
¼ teaspoon basil
¼ teaspoon oregano
¼ teaspoon cayenne pepper
6 cups water

1. Combine all ingredients in a large pot.
2. Bring to a boil, reduce heat and simmer for about 30 minutes or until vegetables are tender.
3. Add additional water if needed, to make desired consistency.

12 SERVINGS

PER SERVING: *137 calories, 1 gram fat, 0 saturated fat, 0 cholesterol, 207 mg. sodium, 8 grams fiber*

*WHITE CHILI

Although we are classifying this chili as soup, it is certainly a meal all by itself, and a tasty one at that.

4 boneless, skinless chicken
  breast halves
2½ cups water
1 tablespoon olive oil
1 onion, chopped
1 garlic clove, minced
2 (9 ounces each) packages
  frozen white corn
2 (4 ounces each) cans diced
  green chilies

2 teaspoons ground cumin
½ teaspoon salt
juice of 1 lime
2 cans (15 ounces each) Great
  Northern beans, drained
salsa
1 cup crushed fat-free tortilla
  chips

1. In a saucepan, cover the chicken breasts with 2½ cups of water and bring to a boil. Reduce heat, cover, and simmer about 25–30 minutes.
2. Drain (reserve stock for later) and set chicken aside.
3. In the bottom of a large pot, sauté the onion and garlic in the olive oil until tender.
4. Add the corn, chilies, cumin, salt, lime juice, and beans.
5. Cut the chicken into ½-inch pieces and add to pot.
6. Add ¼–½ cup reserved stock to make desired consistency.
7. Continue cooking until thoroughly heated and flavors are blended.
8. Serve with salsa and top with crushed tortilla chips.

6 SERVINGS

PER SERVING: *365 calories, 4 grams fat, 1 gram saturated fat, 46 mg. cholesterol, 293 mg. sodium, 12 grams fiber*

SALADS AND SALAD DRESSINGS

Nutritionists recommend that about half the vegetables we eat each day should be raw because they generally retain more of their nutritional value in their uncooked state. But not all salads or all ingredients in a multi-ingredient salad need be raw. Both raw salads and cooked salads served cold are excellent ways to increase the amount of plant foods in your diet and to reduce the amount of fat. We now know that in some cases, particularly for foods in the cabbage family, certain healthful phytochemicals may become more available to the body after cooking.

But watch out for the salad bar when eating out! Many of the pre-mixed pasta, potato, bean, and vegetable salads at restaurant salad bars are loaded with high-fat dressings. So are the fish and ham salads. If you are attempting to eat a more healthful diet, be careful after making low-fat vegetable and fruit choices when you get to the salad dressings. By using several tablespoonfuls of a high-fat salad dressing at 8 or 9 grams of fat per tablespoon, you can end up adding 30 to 40 grams of fat and several hundred calories to an otherwise healthful meal.

We have greatly increased the number of salads in our daily menus in the past several years, using delicately flavored vinegar, olive oil, lemon juice, and many different seasonings found in Mediterranean cuisine. The dressings used in any particular salad in this section can be used in many different recipes. When you find one that you like in one salad, let your instinct and imagination tell you whether it might work well with other salad foods.

The Honey Mustard and Tarragon Dijon Dressings are good stand-by recipes for just about any mixed vegetable salad.

BULGUR SALAD OUR WAY

This salad is hearty and satisfying enough to serve as a main course (in larger-size servings). For freshest flavor, it's important to add the tomatoes just before serving.

1¼ cups water
1 cup bulgur, dry
¼ teaspoon salt
2 scallions, chopped
1 garlic clove, crushed
⅓ cup daikon radish, diced
½ large red bell pepper, diced
¼ cup packed fresh parsley,
    chopped
1 stalk celery, chopped

2 tablespoons olive oil
1 tablespoon lemon juice
1 teaspoon brown rice vinegar
¼ teaspoon ground cumin
½ teaspoon ground coriander
1 teaspoon chili powder
½ teaspoon salt
pepper to taste
3–4 Roma (red Italian) toma-
    toes, chopped

1. In a small saucepan, bring water to a boil.
2. Add bulgur and salt. Stir, cover, and remove from heat. Set aside for 20–30 minutes.
3. Combine all other ingredients except tomatoes in a medium-size bowl.
4. When bulgur is ready, toss with a fork and add to other ingredients in bowl.
5. Chill at least 1 hour before serving.
6. When ready to serve, add tomatoes and toss to combine.

6 SERVINGS

PER SERVING: *137 calories, 5 grams fat, 1 gram saturated fat, 0 cholesterol, 311 mg. sodium, 5 grams fiber*

COLLARD POTATO SALAD WITH MUSTARD DRESSING

The collards in this zesty salad are one of the best vegetable sources of calcium.

2 pounds small potatoes, washed
1 pound collards, washed
2 tablespoons Dijon mustard
2 tablespoons brown rice vinegar
4 tablespoons olive oil
fresh-ground black pepper to taste

1 garlic clove, crushed
1 teaspoon fresh ginger, grated
2 scallions, chopped
2 tablespoons fresh parsley, chopped
½ teaspoon salt
¼ teaspoon crushed red pepper (optional)

1. Put potatoes in a large pot with enough water to cover. Bring to a boil, then reduce heat and simmer about 20 minutes until just tender.
2. Transfer potatoes to a colander, using a slotted spoon, and let cool, reserving potato water.
3. Remove tough stems from collards and discard. Cut leaves into 1-inch pieces and place in potato water. Cook for about 10 minutes.

4. In a small bowl, combine remaining ingredients and whisk until blended.
5. Cut potatoes into chunks and place in large bowl.
6. When collards are cooked, drain them in a colander and cool with running water.
7. Remove collards from colander and press dry in a clean towel. Put in bowl with potatoes, separating the collard pieces.
8. Add dressing and toss to coat. Chill until ready to serve.

10 SERVINGS

PER SERVING: *124 calories, 5 grams fat, 0.5 gram saturated fat, 0 cholesterol, 329 mg. sodium, 3 grams fiber*

CRABMEAT SALAD

This is one of our favorite pita-pocket salad filings. We like it with sliced tomatoes.

2 cans crabmeat (4 ounces each)
3 ounces daikon radish, peeled and chopped
½ large yellow bell pepper, chopped
2 scallions, chopped
¼ cup black olives, chopped
⅛ teaspoon garlic powder
¼ teaspoon ground coriander
¼ teaspoon celery seed
¼ teaspoon dillweed
½ teaspoon salt
fresh-ground pepper to taste
2 tablespoons reduced-calorie mayonnaise
2 teaspoons Dijon mustard
1 tablespoon brown rice vinegar

1. Drain crabmeat; place in a colander and rinse. Set aside.
2. Combine all other ingredients in a large bowl.
3. Press out excess moisture from crabmeat and add to mixture in bowl.
4. Mix well and chill for about 1 hour before serving.

4 SERVINGS

PER SERVING: *107 calories, 4 grams fat, 0 saturated fat, 52 mg. cholesterol, 657 mg. sodium, 1 gram fiber*

CUCUMBER SALAD

2 large cucumbers
¼ teaspoon salt
⅓ cup brown rice vinegar
¼ cup water
2 teaspoons sugar

1 garlic clove, crushed
1 teaspoon dill seed
fresh-ground pepper to taste
2 large tomatoes
8 black olives

1. Trim the ends of the cucumber; then score them lengthwise with a fork and slice very thin.
2. Place cucumbers in a colander, sprinkle with salt, and set aside to drain for about 1 hour.
3. In a small saucepan bring vinegar, water, sugar, garlic, and spices to a boil and cook, stirring until sugar is dissolved. Set aside to cool.
4. Rinse cucumbers and squeeze out excess moisture.
5. In a bowl, combine cucumbers with vinegar mixture and chill for at least 1 hour.
6. To serve, cut tomatoes in half. Then prepare each half by making shallow cuts in the tomato flesh. Fan tomato out.
7. With a slotted spoon, place ¼ of the cucumber mixture on each tomato half and garnish with black olives.

4 SERVINGS

PER SERVING: *76 calories, 2 grams fat, 0 saturated fat, 0 cholesterol, 231 mg. sodium, 2 grams fiber*

ENDIVE SLAW

3 or 4 endive bulbs, sliced thin
1 red bell pepper, diced
2 tablespoons fresh parsley,
　chopped
2 tablespoons brown rice vine-
　gar

1 tablespoon olive oil
1 garlic clove, crushed
½ teaspoon tarragon
¼ teaspoon salt
fresh-ground pepper to taste

1. Combine endive, bell pepper, and parsley.
2. In another bowl, whisk the remainder of the ingredients.
3. Pour over the endive mixture.
4. Chill for at least 1 hour before serving.

4 SERVINGS

PER SERVING: *51 calories, 4 grams fat, 0 saturated fat, 0 choles-*
terol, 148 mg. sodium, 2 grams fiber

HAROLD'S GARBANZO SALAD

My brother, Harold Klein, lives in the little town of West Winfield, New York. We don't get to see him often, but he has always been a good cook. A love of good food and much pleasure in its preparation seem to run in our family, and he often shares recipes with us. During one telephone call on a dark and dreary rainy day in Nashville, he shared this recipe while talking with my wife, Enid. It is very pungent and satisfying. Perked us right up!

1 can (16 ounces) garbanzos
　(chickpeas)
¼ red onion, chopped
½ cup chopped roasted bell
　peppers
1 can (2 ounces) anchovies,
　drained well
2 garlic cloves, crushed

¼ cup fresh parsley, chopped
½ teaspoon oregano
¼ teaspoon salt
1 tablespoon olive oil
1 tablespoon lemon juice
1 teaspoon brown rice vinegar
fresh-ground pepper to taste

1. Drain and rinse the garbanzos. Place in a large bowl and mash coarsely.
2. Add the onion and roasted peppers.
3. Chop the anchovies and add along with the remainder of the ingredients.
4. Mix well and chill before serving.

4 SERVINGS

PER SERVING: *212 calories, 6 grams fat, 1 gram saturated fat, 12 mg. cholesterol, 1068 mg. sodium, 5 grams fiber*

HONEY MUSTARD SALAD DRESSING

½ cup plain nonfat yogurt
¼ cup fat-free or reduced-calorie mayonnaise
1 tablespoon olive oil
¼ cup honey

2 tablespoons Dijon mustard
2 tablespoons prepared yellow mustard
1 tablespoon cider vinegar

1. Combine all ingredients in an airtight container, mixing well.
2. Cover and chill for at least 1 to 2 hours.

MAKES 1 ½ CUPS

PER 2-TABLESPOON SERVING: *52 calories, 2 grams fat, 0.5 gram saturated fat, 1 mg. cholesterol, 58 mg. sodium, 0 fiber*

MAIN COURSE GREEK SALAD

This is a personal favorite that, with a big bowl of chopped greens, can make a whole meal. Try it along with some whole-grain pita bread.

20 Greek or other black olives,
  pitted and halved
2½ teaspoons capers
1 bunch radishes, chopped
  (about 10)
1 bunch chives (about ¼ cup)
1 peeled cucumber, scored with
  fork tines, then halved,

seeded, and cut in chunks
4 fresh Italian plum tomatoes,
  cut in chunks
2 ounces feta cheese, crumbled
1 tablespoon olive oil
juice of ½ fresh lemon
1 teaspoon dried oregano
fresh-ground pepper to taste

1. Combine all ingredients except the oil, lemon juice, oregano, and pepper in a large bowl.
2. Whisk the last four ingredients and pour over the salad. Toss to coat, then chill. Serve with mixed salad greens if desired.

6 SERVINGS

PER SERVING (WITHOUT SALAD GREENS): *90 calories, 7 grams fat, 2 grams saturated fat, 8 mg. cholesterol, 756 mg. sodium, 1 gram fiber*

RED CABBAGE AND PARSLEY SLAW

2 cups red cabbage, shredded
2 cups packed parsley leaves,
  chopped
4 scallions, chopped
2 tablespoons brown rice vine-
  gar
1 tablespoon olive oil

1 garlic clove, crushed
¼ teaspoon celery seed
¼ teaspoon salt
fresh-ground pepper to taste
4 large lettuce leaves
12 large black olives

1. Combine cabbage, parsley, and scallions.
2. In another bowl, combine vinegar, oil, garlic, celery seed, salt, and pepper.
3. Pour the sauce over the cabbage mixture and chill at least 1 hour.
4. When ready to serve, line each of 4 salad plates with a lettuce leaf.
5. Divide the slaw evenly among the plates and garnish each with 3 black olives.

4 SERVINGS

PER SERVING (INCLUDING LETTUCE AND OLIVES): *82 calories, 6 grams fat, 1 gram saturated fat, 0 cholesterol, 279 mg. sodium, 2 grams fiber*

POTATO AND GREEN BEAN SALAD WITH CITRUS DRESSING

1½ pounds red potatoes, cut in bite-sized chunks
½ cup water
¾ pound green beans, trimmed
2 scallions, chopped
2 garlic cloves, crushed
1 small bell pepper, diced
24 pitted black olives, halved
½ cup packed fresh parsley, chopped

1 tablespoon olive oil
2 tablespoons fresh lemon juice
2 tablespoons fresh orange juice
1 teaspoon brown rice vinegar
½ teaspoon salt
¼ teaspoon crushed red pepper
fresh-ground black pepper to taste

1. Place potatoes and water in a microwave-safe bowl; cover and cook on high for about 12 minutes or until the potatoes are tender.
2. Transfer potatoes with a slotted spoon to a large mixing bowl. Set aside.
3. Cut green beans diagonally into 1½-inch pieces.
4. Put green beans in the same microwave bowl used to cook the potatoes. Add more water, if necessary, and cook on high about 7 minutes or until tender.
5. Remove beans from cooking liquid with a slotted spoon and add to the potatoes.
6. Stir in scallions, garlic, bell pepper, olives, and parsley.
7. In a small bowl, whisk together the remainder of the ingredients and pour over the potato/green bean mixture.
8. Toss to mix and chill until ready to serve.

8 SERVINGS

PER SERVING: *116 calories, 4 grams fat, 0 saturated fat, 0 choles-terol, 263 mg. sodium, 3 grams fiber*

*SWEET 'N' SAVORY CHICKEN SALAD

½ cup plain, nonfat yogurt
1 tablespoon lemon juice
¾ teaspoon dried tarragon,
  crushed
2 cups cooked chicken breast,
  cut in chunks
1 can (20 ounces) pineapple
  chunks, unsweetened,
  drained

1 can (10½ ounces) mandarin
  oranges, unsweetened,
  drained
1 can (4 ounces) water chest-
  nuts, drained
1 small cucumber, diced
1 scallion, finely chopped
  lettuce leaves

1. Mix together the yogurt, lemon juice, and tarragon to make a dressing.
2. In a large bowl, combine the remaining ingredients, except the lettuce leaves.
3. Pour the dressing over the chicken salad and toss lightly.
4. Serve on lettuce leaves of your choice.

MAKES 6 CUPS

PER 1-CUP SERVING: *195 calories, 2 grams fat, 0.5 gram satu-rated fat, 40 mg. cholesterol, 57 mg. sodium, 3 grams fiber*

TARRAGON DIJON DRESSING

1 tablespoon olive oil
5 tablespoons red wine vinegar
2 tablespoons lemon juice
6 tablespoons water
1 teaspoon Dijon mustard
1¼ teaspoon tarragon, crushed
1 garlic clove, crushed

2 tablespoons shallots or scal-
  lions, finely minced
1 tablespoon honey
¼ teaspoon paprika
salt and fresh-ground pepper to
  taste

1. Combine all ingredients in an airtight container, mixing well.
2. Store covered in refrigerator.

MAKES 1 CUP

PER SERVING (2 TABLESPOONS): *27 calories, 2 grams fat, 0 saturated fat, 0 cholesterol, 9 mg. sodium (without salt to taste), 0 fiber*

*TUNA WITH CHICKPEAS

This is a satisfying main dish dinner salad, originating in Greece. It's great as a leftover dish at lunch.

1 can (15 ounces) chickpeas, drained
2 cans (6 ounces each) tuna packed in water, drained
4 scallions, chopped
1 stalk celery, chopped
2 tablespoons olive oil
2 garlic cloves, crushed
1 tablespoon lemon juice

grated rind of ½ lemon
3 tablespoons fresh parsley, chopped (plus additional leaves for garnish, optional)
1 teaspoon dried dillweed
½ teaspoon salt
fresh-ground pepper to taste
¼ teaspoon dried mustard

1. Drain chickpeas, rinse, then coarsely mash in a medium-size bowl.
2. Add tuna and combine.
3. Stir in the scallions and celery.
4. In another bowl, combine all other ingredients and whisk to blend.
5. Stir dressing into tuna mixture.
6. Cover and chill several hours before serving. Garnish with parsley leaves if desired.

4 SERVINGS

PER SERVING: *263 calories, 9 grams fat, 1 gram saturated fat, 26 mg. cholesterol, 817 mg. sodium, 6 grams fiber*

BREADS AND MUFFINS

Except for vitamin B_{12}, bread made from whole wheat contains a similar vitamin and mineral profile as beef (beef has more B_{12}). A slice of whole-grain bread contains about 1 gram of fat (naturally occurring as part of the grain) and 2 grams of fiber, which is removed in the processing of the grain for white bread. Almost all of the recipes that follow call for a combination of all-purpose and whole-wheat flour, since breads and muffins made exclusively with whole-wheat flour tend to have a heavy consistency. While the average commercial muffin may contain between 5 and 10 grams of fat, some baked in local bakeries and for restaurants may contain more than 25 grams! Try some of the recipes included here for low-fat alternatives. Many of them flavored with fruit and spices make for great snacks; no butter or margarine needed to improve palatability.

*APRICOT MUFFINS

1 cup boiling water
1½ cups (approximately ½ pound) dried apricots, cut in small pieces
2 cups all-purpose flour
1 cup whole-wheat flour
1 cup sugar
1 tablespoon baking powder
1 teaspoon baking soda
½ teaspoon salt
2 eggs, beaten, or ½ cup egg substitute
¼ cup canola oil
1 cup orange juice

1. In a bowl, pour the boiling water over the dried apricot pieces. Set aside to cool.
2. In a large bowl, combine the flours, sugar, baking powder, baking soda, and salt.
3. Stir the eggs, oil, and orange juice into the apricot mixture.
4. Make a well in the center of the dry ingredients and add the liquid apricot mixture, stirring enough to moisten (do not overmix).
5. Spray muffin tins with nonstick cooking spray or line with muffin cups. Fill each ⅔ full with batter.
6. Bake for 20–25 minutes in a preheated 375-degree oven.

MAKES 24 MEDIUM MUFFINS

PER MUFFIN: *138 calories, 3 grams fat, 0.5 gram saturated fat, 18 mg. cholesterol, 126 mg. sodium, 2 grams fiber*

*CARROT PINEAPPLE BREAD

Reminiscent of carrot cake, this is wonderful as a dessert bread, a snack with coffee, or a special breakfast bread; or serve it with fruit salad and cottage cheese for lunch.

1¼ cup applesauce
1¾ cup sugar
2 tablespoons canola oil
2 teaspoons vanilla extract
4 eggs or 1 cup egg substitute
1½ cups whole-wheat flour
1½ cups all-purpose flour
1 tablespoon baking powder

1 teaspoon baking soda
1 teaspoon salt
1 tablespoon ground cinna-mon
2½ cups shredded raw carrots
1 can (8 ounces) crushed pineapple with juice

1. Combine the applesauce, sugar, oil, and vanilla in a large mixing bowl.
2. Beat by hand or with an electric mixer until well blended.
3. Beat in eggs, one at a time.
4. In a separate bowl, combine the flours, baking powder, soda, salt, and cinnamon; whisk thoroughly.
5. Add to the applesauce mixture, stirring just until combined.
6. Fold in carrots and pineapple.
7. Divide the batter between two loaf pans that have been coated with cooking spray, smoothing tops with a spatula.
8. Bake in a preheated 350-degree oven for 50 minutes or until the bread shrinks slightly from the side of the pan. Allow to cool in pans for 15 minutes, then remove to cool on a wire rack.

24 SERVINGS (2 LOAVES)

PER SERVING: *150 calories, 2 grams fat, 0 saturated fat, 35 mg. cholesterol, 112 mg. sodium, 2 grams fiber*

*CORN BREAD

2 cups self-rising cornmeal
½ cup light sour cream
1 can (15 ounces) cream-style
  corn

¾ cup buttermilk
¼ cup egg substitute or 1 egg,
  lightly beaten

1. Combine all ingredients in a medium mixing bowl, stirring just until blended.
2. Pour the batter into an 8-inch baking pan that has been coated with cooking spray.
3. Bake in a preheated 375-degree oven 25–30 minutes, or until the top is lightly browned and the corn bread pulls slightly from the edge of the pan.

9 SERVINGS

PER SERVING: *173 calories, 3 grams fat, 1 gram saturated fat, 0 cholesterol, 586 mg. sodium, 2 grams fiber*

*DATE-BRAN BREAD

1 cup all-purpose flour
1 cup whole-wheat flour
1½ cups all-bran cereal
2 teaspoons baking powder
½ teaspoon baking soda
1 teaspoon salt
½ cup molasses

1½ cups nonfat or 1% milk
1 egg, lightly beaten, or ¼ cup
  egg substitute
¼ cup applesauce
1 cup finely chopped pitted
  dates

1. In a large mixing bowl, whisk together the flours, bran, baking powder, soda, and salt.
2. In another bowl, combine the molasses, milk, egg, and applesauce.
3. Add to the dry ingredients. Stir just until combined (do not overmix).
4. Pour into a loaf pan that has been coated with cooking spray. Bake in a preheated 350-degree oven for about 1 hour or until the loaf shrinks slightly from the side of the pan.

5. Cool in pan 15 minutes and then remove to cool completely on a wire rack.

16 SERVINGS

PER SERVING: *146 calories, 1 gram fat, 0 saturated fat, 14 mg. cholesterol, 330 mg. sodium, 5 grams fiber*

*LIGHT WHEAT BISCUITS

Living in the South makes it a must to include a biscuit variation. Serve with a fruit preserve or honey.

1½ cups self-rising flour   *⅓ cup stick margarine or butter*
½–¾ cup whole-wheat flour   *¾ cup buttermilk*

1. Combine flours. Cut in butter with two knives or pastry blender to form coarse crumbs.
2. Stir in the buttermilk with a fork, mixing only to moisten (do not overmix).
3. Transfer dough to lightly floured surface. Knead gently for 1 minute.
4. Roll to approximately ½-inch thickness. Cut into 10 biscuits with a biscuit cutter or moistened drinking glass.
5. Bake on an ungreased cookie sheet for 8–10 minutes in a pre-heated 475-degree oven.

MAKES 10 BISCUITS

PER BISCUIT: *148 calories, 7 grams fat, 1 gram saturated fat, 1 mg. cholesterol, 328 mg. sodium, 1 gram fiber*

*OATMEAL MOLASSES BREAD

2 cups boiling water
1½ cups old-fashioned or
  quick-cooking oatmeal
¼ teaspoon sugar
1½ packages active dry yeast
⅓ cup warm water

1 tablespoon butter, softened
1½ teaspoons salt
½ cup dark molasses
1½ cups whole-wheat flour
3 cups all-purpose flour, or
  more as needed

1. In a large bowl, pour the boiling water over the oatmeal and let stand for 1 hour.
2. In a small bowl, sprinkle sugar and yeast over ⅓ cup lukewarm water, stir to dissolve, and let stand until foamy, about 10 minutes.
3. Stir the yeast mixture into the oatmeal along with the butter, salt, and molasses.
4. Gradually add the whole-wheat flour and 2½ cups of the all-purpose flour, beating well.
5. Turn the dough out onto a floured surface and knead, adding a little more all-purpose flour as needed to form a soft but slightly sticky dough.
6. Form the dough into a ball, place in a buttered bowl, and turn to coat with the butter. Cover with plastic wrap and a kitchen towel and let rise in a warm place for about 1 hour, or until doubled in size.
7. Punch down dough, knead for 3–5 minutes, and form into 2 loaves. Place in loaf pans that have been coated with cooking spray.
8. Cover and let rise for 45 minutes, or until doubled.
9. Bake in a preheated 375-degree oven for 1 hour, or until loaves are browned and sound hollow when tapped.
10. Remove from pans and cool on wire rack.

32 SERVINGS (2 LOAVES)

PER SERVING: 98 calories, 1 gram fat, 0 saturated fat, 0 cholesterol, 105 mg. sodium, 2 grams fiber

*QUICK MUSTARD-RYE BREAD

This bread makes any sandwich special!

3–4 cups all-purpose flour, divided
1½ teaspoons salt
3 packages active dry yeast
2 cups water

¼ cup Dijon mustard
⅓ cup brown sugar
3 tablespoons butter or margarine
2 cups rye flour

1. Combine 2 cups of the all-purpose flour, salt, and yeast in an electric mixer bowl. Set aside.
2. In a saucepan or in the microwave, heat water, mustard, brown sugar, and butter until warm (110–115 degrees).
3. Add to dry ingredients and mix for 3 minutes on medium speed.
4. Add the 2 cups rye flour and 1 to 2 cups of the all-purpose flour, mixing by hand, until it forms a soft dough.
5. Transfer to a floured surface and knead for 5 minutes.
6. Shape into a ball, place in a bowl that has been coated with nonstick cooking spray, turn once to coat, and loosely cover with plastic wrap and a cloth towel.
7. Let rise 15 minutes. Punch down dough and divide in half.
8. Shape each half into a round loaf. Place on a cookie sheet that has been sprayed with cooking spray, press down lightly, cover, and let rise another 15 minutes.
9. Make diagonal cuts across each loaf and bake for 25–35 minutes in a preheated 375-degree oven.
10. Remove from cookie sheets and cool on a wire rack.

MAKES 2 LOAVES, 14 SLICES PER LOAF

PER SLICE: *100 calories, 2 grams fat, 1 gram saturated fat, 2 mg. cholesterol, 159 mg. sodium, 2 grams fiber*

*REFRIGERATOR BRAN MUFFINS

A great way to have fresh, hot muffins any time. The batter, stored in the refrigerator and tightly covered, will keep for at least a week.

3 cups all-purpose flour

2 cups whole-wheat flour

1 teaspoon salt

4 teaspoons ground cinna-
mon

5 teaspoons baking soda

3 cups sugar

2 cups rolled oats

1 box (15 ounces) raisin bran
cereal

1 pound raisins

1 jar (22 ounces) applesauce

¼ cup canola oil

4 eggs, lightly beaten, or 1 cup
egg substitute

4 cups (1 quart) buttermilk

1. In a very large mixing bowl, whisk together the flour, salt, cinnamon, soda, sugar, and rolled oats.
2. Add the bran cereal and raisins and stir to combine.
3. In a separate bowl, combine the applesauce, oil, eggs, and buttermilk and mix thoroughly.
4. Add to the dry ingredients; stir well.
5. Transfer to a large airtight storage container and refrigerate.
6. Prepare muffins as needed by filling paper-lined or cooking
spray–coated muffin cups ⅔ full.
7. Bake in a preheated 400-degree oven for 15–20 minutes, or until
the muffins are lightly browned and springy to the touch.

72 MUFFINS

PER MUFFIN: *130 calories, 2 grams fat, 0 saturated fat, 12 mg.
cholesterol, 138 mg. sodium, 3 grams fiber*

SPICED BANANA BREAD

This is a favorite combination of spices and ripe bananas. We almost
always make a double recipe and either freeze the second loaf or
give it to a friend.

2 bananas, mashed

½ cup sugar

¼ cup egg substitute

1 teaspoon vanilla

¼ cup canola oil

2 tablespoons plain nonfat yogurt

1¼ cups whole-wheat flour

⅓ cup soy flour

1 teaspoon baking soda

1 teaspoon cinnamon

½ teaspoon ground ginger

½ teaspoon nutmeg

¼ teaspoon salt

½ cup raisins

¼ cup nuts, coarsely chopped

1. Combine mashed bananas, sugar, egg substitute, vanilla, and oil. Stir until smooth.
2. Add yogurt and mix well.
3. In another bowl, sift the whole-wheat and soy flours with the baking soda, spices, and salt.
4. Gradually add the flour mixture to the banana mixture and blend just until dry ingredients are moistened.
5. Stir in raisins and nuts.
6. Coat a loaf pan with cooking spray and spoon the banana bread mixture into it.
7. Bake in a preheated 350-degree oven for 40–45 minutes until a toothpick inserted in the center comes out clean.

16 SERVINGS

PER SERVING: *142 calories, 5 grams fat, 0.5 gram saturated fat, 0 cholesterol, 124 mg. sodium, 2 grams fiber*

*ZUCCHINI MUFFINS

This recipe offers lots of opportunities for variation—substitute grated carrots for the zucchini, for example, or try chopped fresh or dried fruit instead.

½ cup whole-wheat flour
½ cup all-purpose flour
2 teaspoons baking powder
½ teaspoon salt
½ cup sugar

1 egg white
½ cup nonfat or 1% milk
1 tablespoon butter, melted
½ cup grated zucchini

1. Combine the flours, baking powder, salt, and sugar.
2. In a small bowl, using a wire whisk, beat the egg white just until foamy.
3. Add beaten egg white to milk along with melted butter.
4. Drain excess moisture from zucchini and then add it along with the liquid ingredients to the flour mixture, stirring just enough to moisten.
5. Spray muffin tin with cooking spray or line with muffin cups. Fill each ¾ full.

6. Bake in a preheated 375-degree oven for 15–20 minutes or until lightly browned.

MAKES 8 MEDIUM MUFFINS

PER MUFFIN: *124 calories, 2 grams fat, 1 gram saturated fat, 2 mg. cholesterol, 247 mg. sodium, 1 gram fiber*

BREAKFAST FOODS

Many people who are trying to lose weight skip breakfast with the idea that it helps cut down the total calories eaten in a day. Most of the time, it doesn't. Skipping breakfast can lead to overconsumption later in the day because you may build up a "hidden hunger." By skipping breakfast (or any other meal) you can greatly deplete your glycogen stores, which can generate strong hunger signals and lead to overeating at a future meal. Here are some recipes that you can use to vary standard breakfast routines. Remember, if it appeals to you, there is nothing wrong with enjoying leftovers from yesterday's evening meal for breakfast.

*BRAN CAKES

¼ cup egg substitute	*1½ cups all-purpose flour*
2 cups nonfat or 1% milk	*1 tablespoon baking powder*
¾ cup All-Bran, Bran Buds, or	*¼ teaspoon salt*
Fiber One cereal	*2 tablespoons sugar*

1. Mix the egg substitute with the milk and then stir into the cereal. Let stand 5 minutes.
2. Stir together the flour, baking powder, salt, and sugar in medium mixing bowl.
3. Add the cereal mixture, stirring just to combine, and let stand 5 minutes.
4. Drop the batter, using ¼ cup for each pancake, onto a griddle preheated to medium and coated with cooking spray. Cook, turning once, until golden brown on both sides.

MAKES 12 PANCAKES

PER SERVING (2 PANCAKES): *195 calories, 1 gram fat, 0 saturated fat, 0 cholesterol, 85 mg. sodium, 5+ grams fiber*

*FRENCH TOAST

This is good served with fresh fruit, applesauce, or a sprinkle of powdered sugar to go with the cinnamon. Of course, it's hard to beat a tablespoon or two of real maple syrup, but it doesn't need any butter.

¼ cup egg substitute
2 tablespoons nonfat or 1% milk

¼ teaspoon cinnamon
2 slices whole-grain bread

1. Whisk together the egg substitute, milk, and cinnamon. Dip the bread in the mixture, coating both sides.
2. Spray a skillet with nonstick cooking spray and heat over medium heat.
3. Fry the bread in the pan, turning once, until golden brown on both sides.

1 SERVING

PER SERVING: *210 calories, 4 grams fat, 0.5 gram saturated fat, 2 mg. cholesterol, 395 mg. sodium, 4 grams fiber*

*FRUIT TOPPING

Try instead of syrup as a topping for pancakes, waffles, or French toast.

1 cup fresh or unsweetened frozen berries or other fruit
¼ cup unsweetened apple juice

1½ teaspoons cornstarch
Dash nutmeg, cinnamon, and/or ground ginger

1. Place the fruit in a saucepan.
2. Combine the apple juice and cornstarch and pour over the fruit.
3. Heat over medium-low heat, stirring occasionally, until thickened.
4. Add spices to taste as desired. Serve hot.

MAKES ABOUT 1 CUP

PER ¼-CUP SERVING: *31 calories, 0 fat, 0 saturated fat, 0 cho-*
lesterol, 1 mg. sodium, 2 grams fiber

*FRUITY BREAKFAST BARLEY

1 cup orange juice   *1 cup quick-cooking barley*
¼ cup dried apricots, chopped   *1 tablespoon honey*
dash of ground cloves

1. In a medium saucepan, combine the orange juice, apricots, and
   cloves with 1½ cups of water. Bring to a boil.
2. Stir in the barley. Cover and simmer 12–15 minutes or until the
   barley is tender.
3. Stir in the honey. Serve with nonfat milk, if desired.

4 SERVINGS

PER SERVING: *165 calories, 0 fat, 0 saturated fat, 0 cholesterol, 54*
mg. sodium, 5 grams fiber

*MIXED-GRAIN CEREAL

A wholesome hot cereal that combines oats, barley, and bulgur
grains.

1 cup regular rolled oats   *1 cup raisins*
1 cup quick-cooking barley   *½ cup millet*
1 cup cracked wheat (bulgur)

1. Combine all ingredients in an airtight storage container.
2. To make 2 servings: In a saucepan, bring 1⅓ cups water to a boil. Stir in ¾ cup of the cereal mixture.
3. Cover, reduce heat, and simmer for 12–15 minutes or until the cereal has the desired consistency.
4. Serve with nonfat milk and honey.

12 SERVINGS

PER SERVING: *208 calories, 1 gram fat, 0 saturated fat, 0 cholesterol, 46 mg. sodium, 6 grams fiber*

OATMEAL PANCAKES

1 cup rolled oats
1 cup buttermilk
1 large egg, slightly beaten, or
   ¼ cup egg substitute

¼ cup all-purpose flour
1½ teaspoon sugar
½ teaspoon baking powder
½ teaspoon baking soda

1. Pour the buttermilk over the oats in a medium bowl and let stand for 5 minutes.
2. Stir in the egg.
3. In a separate bowl, whisk together the flour, sugar, baking powder, and baking soda.
4. Add to the buttermilk mixture and stir just until combined. The batter should be lumpy.
5. Coat a griddle with cooking spray and heat over moderate heat until a drop of water dances on the surface. Drop the batter by ¼ cupfuls onto the griddle and cook the pancakes until bubbles form over the surface; turn and brown the other side.
6. Serve with fruit topping or syrup.

4 SERVINGS (2 PANCAKES)

PER SERVING: *312 calories, 6.3 grams fat, 2 grams saturated fat, 110 mg. cholesterol, 321 mg. sodium, 5 grams fiber*

*WHOLE-WHEAT PANCAKES

An excellent basic pancake batter recipe. This will keep in the refrigerator for a few days; if, after storing, the mixture becomes very thick, add more buttermilk and stir before using.

1 cup whole-wheat flour
1 cup all-purpose flour
½ teaspoon salt
1 tablespoon baking powder
1 teaspoon baking soda

1 whole egg and 2 egg whites,
   lightly beaten (or ½ cup egg
   substitute)
2 tablespoons applesauce
2½ cups buttermilk

1. In a bowl or wide-mouthed pitcher, whisk together the flours, salt, baking powder, and baking soda.
2. Add the eggs, applesauce, and buttermilk and stir just until blended. The batter should be lumpy.
3. Drop by ¼ cupfuls onto a hot griddle that has been sprayed with cooking spray. When the edges begin to brown and bubbles appear across the surface, turn and lightly brown the other side.
4. Serve with fruit topping or syrup.

6 SERVINGS (2 PANCAKES)

PER SERVING: *190 calories, 2 grams fat, 1 gram saturated fat, 38 mg. cholesterol, 656 mg. sodium, 3 grams fiber*

SANDWICH MAKINGS

These sandwich makings can help you cut back on the amount of meat and saturated fat you may be eating. You may find that the Soycuts make a good substitute for a meat sandwich.

*CREAMY CRAB SPREAD

1 can (6 ounces) crabmeat
1 package (12 ounces) silken
  tofu extra-firm
2 scallions, chopped
1 garlic clove, crushed
1 stalk celery, chopped
2 tablespoons fresh parsley,
  chopped
½ red bell pepper, diced
1 tablespoon reduced-calorie
  mayonnaise

2 teaspoons prepared mustard
½ teaspoon dried dillweed
½ teaspoon thyme
½ teaspoon salt
1 teaspoon paprika
pinch cayenne
fresh-ground pepper to taste
3 whole-wheat pita breads,
  halved

1. Combine all ingredients except for the pita bread.
2. Chill until ready to serve.
3. Serve on pita or other bread.

6 SERVINGS

PER SERVING (WITH ½ WHOLE-WHEAT PITA): *182 calories, 6 grams fat, 1 gram saturated fat, 26 mg. cholesterol, 451 mg. sodium, 4 grams fiber*

*HERBED PINTO BEAN SPREAD

1 can (16 ounces) pinto or kidney beans
1 tablespoon olive oil
2 scallions, chopped
1 teaspoon capers
½ teaspoon marjoram

½ teaspoon basil
½ teaspoon thyme
⅛ teaspoon garlic powder
¼ teaspoon crushed red pepper
¼ teaspoon salt and fresh-
  ground pepper to taste

1. Drain and rinse the pinto or kidney beans.
2. Mash the beans coarsely.
3. Add all other ingredients and mix until well blended.
4. Chill until ready to serve.
5. Serve on whole-wheat toast or pita bread.

4 SERVINGS

PER SERVING: *129 calories, 4 grams fat, 0 saturated fat, 0 choles-terol, 391 mg. sodium, 6 grams fiber*

*SALMON-HERB SPREAD

1 cup plain nonfat yogurt
1 can (15 ounces) salmon
  packed in water, drained
2 tablespoons green onions,
  finely chopped
1 tablespoon fresh parsley,
  minced

1 tablespoon reduced-calorie
  mayonnaise
¼ teaspoon dried dillweed
¼ teaspoon thyme
⅛ teaspoon salt

1. Put yogurt in a strainer that has been lined with a large coffee fil-ter or, better, several layers of cheesecloth. Allow to drain over a bowl for at least 1 hour.
2. Meanwhile, combine remaining ingredients in a bowl.
3. Fold in yogurt. Store in an airtight container. Serve chilled.

MAKES 1½ CUPS

PER ¼-CUP SERVING: *137 calories, 6 grams fat, 1 gram satu-rated fat, 32 mg. cholesterol, 468 mg. sodium, 0 fiber*

Note: You can substitute 8 ounces of softened fat-free cream cheese for the yogurt.

*VEGGIE SANDWICH SPREAD

This flavorful spread is great on bagels, whole-grain breads, or pita. Serve with soup and fruit to round out an easy meal.

½ cup diced raw vegetables (try
  a combination of carrots,
  green onions, broccoli,
  mushrooms, bell peppers,

  and zucchini)
1 cup light ricotta cheese
2 teaspoons Dijon or spicy mus-tard

1. Blend the combination of finely diced vegetables with ricotta and mustard.
2. Keep refrigerated (use original ricotta container for leftovers).

6 SERVINGS

PER ¼-CUP SERVING: *45 calories, 1 gram fat, 0 saturated fat, 2 mg. cholesterol, 165 mg. sodium, 1 gram fiber*

SOYCUTS FOR SANDWICHES

This is not a spread, but it has become one of my favorite spicy substitutes for salami or other meat used as a cold cut for sandwiches. Experiment with your own seasonings after you try this recipe. While the recipe uses a large amount of soy sauce, you will find that almost half will remain in the pan and dry up in the cooking. Thus the sodium count is not as high as you might expect.

If you like, you can press some of the liquid out of the tofu before applying the seasoning by placing it on a large dish before you slice it, and then covering it with about three of the same-size dishes (inverted with serving side down on the tofu) as you prepare the seasonings. This procedure will squeeze a tablespoon or two of liquid out of the tofu and allow for greater absorption of the seasonings. But it is not necessary.

I use soycuts on sandwiches with sliced tomato. I also like to use a small amount of nayonnaise, a mayonnaise-like dressing with one-quarter the fat and great flavor made from soy and polyunsaturated (not hydrogenated) oil. You can find this at most health food stores.

2 ounces soy sauce
1 teaspoon steak sauce
½ teaspoon ground ginger
¼ teaspoon garlic powder
10 twists of fresh-ground black pepper

¼ teaspoon onion powder
¼ teaspoon turmeric
pinch of cinnamon
pinch of cloves
1 pound firm tofu

1. Mix all the seasonings together in a small bowl, making sure the powders have dissolved in the liquid.

2. Using a sharp chef's knife, slice the tofu lengthwise into 8 equal pieces (it's easiest to get equal slices if you start first by cutting the block of tofu in halves, then quarters, and then in eighths).
3. Place the slices of tofu on a foil-lined baking sheet, lifting the edges of the foil to prevent liquid from flowing out.
4. Spread about a teaspoon of the seasoning on each slice of the tofu, then turn the tofu over and cover the other side.
5. Bake in a 350-degree oven for 30 minutes. At this point, the soy-cuts are done, but soft to the touch. If you find you like your soy-cuts drier, turn the oven down to 250 degrees and let the tofu sit there for up to another hour. They will now be quite dry and have a meatier texture (which is the way I like them).
6. Wrap in foil and chill in the refrigerator. They will keep for several days.

MAKES 8 SLICES

PER SLICE: *50 calories, 3 grams fat, 0 saturated fat, 0 cholesterol, 258 mg. sodium, 1 gram fiber*

MEATLESS MAIN COURSES/VEGETARIAN ENTRÉES

Because the daily consumption of red meat increases your risk for certain cancers and heart disease, health experts strongly recommend that you begin to cut back. You don't need to worry that you will fail to get enough protein when you do this; if you have been eating the typical American diet, you have probably been consuming twice as much protein as you need each day. When you obtain your protein from meat, you also end up eating more total fat, saturated fat, cholesterol, and dangerous chemical residues (which are concentrated in the animal's fat cells) than when you obtain protein from plant foods.

Because plant foods tend to be deficient in one or another of the essential amino acids, it was thought for many years that legumes, grains, and seeds needed to be eaten at the same meal in order for you to obtain the same quality of protein that's found in foods of animal origin. By combining different plant foods, the amino acid missing in one would be supplied by the other. This is now known to be incorrect. The body is able to extract, retain, and combine the various amino acids found in the protein of different plant foods even if these foods are consumed at different times during the day.

If you have been accustomed to eating red meat every day, start out by planning just one day without. At first you might make it a day that includes fish or poultry, but aim for one completely meatless day a week. For the past five years we have been trying out different meatless main courses, and the eighteen recipes in this section are among the best.

Look also in the Vegetable and Grain Side Dishes section later in this chapter for additional recipes that you can use on your meatless day. We often combine two, three, or even more of these in a single meal.

Cooking Whole Grains

To cook whole grains such as brown rice, you need about twice as much liquid (water or stock) as grain—in other words, about two cups of liquid to one cup of grain. Although there are rather complex ways of preparing, for example, a risotto, using wine, oil, and seasonings to lightly sauté the rice before adding any water, this isn't really necessary as your basic procedure. Simply bring your liquid to a boil, add the rinsed grain, bring to a boil again, cover, reduce heat, and let simmer for about forty minutes. Stirring is unnecessary. Especially when cooked in stock, no added fat is needed to make whole grains taste good, but if your grains come out too sticky, add a teaspoon or two of olive oil to the liquid before adding the rice. Add the rice and, in this case, give it a stir so that the oil will coat each grain. You can also add herbs, spices, or minced vegetables such as garlic, scallions, dried bell peppers, or carrots if you want more flavor.

*ASPARAGUS-NUT STIR-FRY

*1 tablespoon olive oil + 1 table-
   spoon water*
*1 pound asparagus, sliced di-
   agonally into 1-inch pieces*
1 leek, thinly sliced
1 teaspoon grated fresh ginger
3 garlic cloves, minced
½ cup chopped walnuts
5 ounces water
1 tablespoon cornstarch

1 tablespoon soy sauce
*1 tablespoon miso (fermented
   soybean paste)*
¼ teaspoon salt
fresh-ground pepper to taste
*¼ teaspoon crushed red pepper
   (optional)*
*2 teaspoons sesame seeds,
   toasted*
cooked rice or pasta

1. In a large skillet, heat olive oil + water.
2. Add leek and ginger and cook, stirring, about 2 minutes. Lower
   heat.
3. Stir in asparagus, garlic, and nuts and cook, stirring, 5 more minutes.
4. Combine the cornstarch, soy sauce, and miso with a small
   amount of the 5 ounces of water. Then add this mixture and the
   remainder of the water to the skillet. Stir.
5. Add salt and pepper to taste and crushed red pepper if desired.
6. Cover and continue cooking over low heat until asparagus is tender.
7. Serve over cooked rice or pasta and top with sesame seeds.

4 SERVINGS

PER SERVING (WITHOUT RICE OR NOODLES): *194 calories, 13
grams fat, 1 gram saturated fat, 0 cholesterol, 567 mg. sodium, 4
grams fiber*

*BASIC BETTER BEANS

The use of stock instead of water for cooking, and whole onions
stuck with whole cloves, make beans even more flavorful. Serve
with cooked grain for a main course.

2 cups dried beans, or lentils
  (your choice)
4 cups chicken or vegetable
  stock
2 large onions

6 whole cloves
2 tablespoons olive oil
salt and fresh-ground pepper to
  taste

1. Soak the beans in water, enough to cover, along with the onions that have been stuck with the cloves, overnight in the refrigerator.
2. Remove the onions and cloves with a slotted spoon. Discard the cloves.
3. Drain and rinse beans.
4. In a pot, pour stock over soaked beans and cook until beans are just tender (about 2 hours).
5. Chop the onions and sauté in the olive oil until translucent.
6. Place all ingredients (except cloves) in a large casserole dish and bake for 1 hour at 325 degrees.

8 SERVINGS

PER SERVING: *181 calories, 5 grams fat, 0.5 gram saturated fat, 0 cholesterol, 438 mg. sodium, 6 grams fiber*

COLLARDS, TOFU, CHEESE CASSEROLE

1 pound collards, washed and
  chopped
¼ cup water
½ cup egg substitute
1 cup 2% cottage cheese
8 ounces tofu
⅓ cup whole-wheat flour
¼ cup feta cheese

¼ teaspoon thyme
¼ teaspoon salt
¼ teaspoon crushed red pepper
fresh-ground black pepper to
  taste
2 tablespoons grated Parmesan
  cheese

1. Place collards and water in a microwave-safe bowl. Cover and microwave on high for about 12–15 minutes until collards are tender.
2. In another large bowl, mix all other ingredients except for Parmesan cheese.

3. Drain cooked collards and add to bowl mixture. Stir together.
4. Pack collard mixture into a casserole dish that has been coated with cooking spray.
5. Sprinkle Parmesan cheese on top.
6. Bake in a 350-degree oven for about 45 minutes.

8 SERVINGS

PER SERVING: *106 calories, 4 grams fat, 2 grams saturated fat, 8 mg. cholesterol, 439 mg. sodium, 3 grams fiber*

CURRIED VEGETABLES

This is a full-bodied meatless curry. If you don't feel like taking the trouble to measure out the spices called for, just substitute 3 teaspoons of Indian Spice Blend (see Seasonings section in this chapter) for the spices (from ginger through black pepper) called for in this recipe.

2 tablespoons olive oil
1 small onion, coarsely chopped
10 whole raw cashews
6 ounces nonfat or 1% milk, divided
¼ cup 2% cottage cheese
2 tablespoons catsup
1 medium tomato, diced
flowerets from small head cauliflower
1 cup frozen peas, thawed
1 medium carrot, cut in julienne strips
¼ cup packed parsley, chopped

½ cup vegetable bouillon
¼ cup raisins
½ teaspoon salt
¼ teaspoon garlic powder
¼ teaspoon ground ginger
½ teaspoon ground cumin
1 teaspoon ground coriander
1 teaspoon cinnamon
⅛ teaspoon ground cardamom
Pinch of ground cloves
⅛ teaspoon cayenne
fresh-ground black pepper to taste
3 cups cooked brown rice

1. In a skillet, heat olive oil and sauté onions and cashews over medium heat until onion begins to brown.
2. In a blender or food processor, combine the onion/cashew mix-

ture with 4 ounces of the 1% milk and the catsup. Process until smooth. Remove from blender and set aside.

3. In the same blender or food processor, process the remaining 2 ounces of milk with the cottage cheese until smooth. Combine with first milk mixture and set aside.

4. Put chopped tomato in the skillet, cover, and cook over low heat for 1 minute.

5. Add all remaining vegetables, including the parsley, and stir-fry for 3 minutes over low heat.

6. Add bouillon, raisins, and all the spices. Bring to a boil; then lower heat, cover, and simmer for about 12 minutes until the vegetables are just tender.

7. Add the milk mixture and stir well over low heat until sauce is smooth and heated through.

8. Serve over cooked brown rice.

6 SERVINGS

PER SERVING (WITH ½ CUP BROWN RICE): *268 calories, 7 grams fat, 1 gram saturated fat, 1 mg. cholesterol, 372 mg. sodium, 7 grams fiber*

*EASY BEAN BURRITOS FOR TWO

*4 large flour tortillas, prefer-
ably whole wheat*
*1 can (15 ounces) refried
beans*
2 cups lettuce, chopped
1 cup tomatoes, chopped
¼ cup onion, chopped
2 tablespoons jalapeño peppers,

*chopped (some people like to
use gloves when chopping)*
*¼ cup shredded sharp cheddar
cheese*
*½ cup plain nonfat yogurt or
sour cream*
½ cup salsa or taco sauce

1. Warm tortillas according to package directions and heat refried beans.

2. Spread each tortilla with ¼ can refried beans.

3. Top with vegetables and shredded cheese. Add a dollop of non-fat yogurt or sour cream. Serve with salsa or taco sauce.

2 SERVINGS

PER SERVING: *248 calories, 6 grams fat, 3 grams saturated fat, 9 mg. cholesterol, 696 mg. sodium, 8 grams fiber*

*EGGPLANT PARMESAN

An oven-baked, low-fat version of traditional Eggplant Parmesan, which is usually quite high in fat and calories because the eggplant is breaded and fried in oil—and eggplant absorbs a lot of oil!

1 large or 2 small eggplants	*½ cup bread crumbs*
2 egg whites or ½ cup egg substitute	*2 tablespoons grated Parmesan cheese*
2 tablespoons nonfat or 1% milk	*2 cups meatless spaghetti sauce*
¼ cup wheat germ	*¾ cup shredded reduced-fat mozzarella cheese*

1. Peel the eggplant and cut into ½-inch-thick slices.
2. Beat together the egg and milk in a shallow bowl.
3. In another bowl, combine the wheat germ, bread crumbs, and Parmesan cheese.
4. Dip the eggplant slices in the egg mixture, coating well. Dip into the bread crumb mixture and place on a baking sheet that has been lined with foil and sprayed with cooking spray.
5. Bake for 15 minutes in a preheated 350-degree oven, turn slices over, and bake another 10 minutes.
6. Line the bottom of a casserole dish (that has been coated with cooking spray) with eggplant slices.
7. Top with half of the tomato sauce, then with half of the shredded cheese. Repeat the layers.
8. Cover and bake for about 25 minutes, then uncover and bake an additional 15 minutes.
9. Serve with pasta and additional tomato sauce if desired.

4 SERVINGS

PER SERVING: *235 calories, 7 grams fat, 3 grams saturated fat, 13 mg. cholesterol, 583 mg. sodium, 7 grams fiber*

*HEARTY VEGETARIAN CHILI

1 pound pinto beans
6 cups water
6 cups vegetable bouillon
2 large onions, chopped
4 garlic cloves, minced
2 bay leaves
2 tablespoons olive oil
1 pound frozen tempeh,
   thawed and crumbled
1½ teaspoons oregano

2 teaspoons ground cumin
1 teaspoon sage
1 teaspoon thyme
1 teaspoon salt
¼ teaspoon ground cloves
¼ teaspoon cayenne
2 cans (4 ounces each)
   chopped green chilies
1 jar (16 ounces) salsa

1. Wash beans and soak overnight in the 6 cups of water.
2. The next day, drain and rinse the beans. Place in a large kettle with the 6 cups of vegetable bouillon, ½ of the onions, ½ of the garlic, and both bay leaves.
3. Cover and bring to a boil; then lower heat and let simmer until beans are tender (2½–3 hours). Stir occasionally.
4. Meanwhile, in a skillet, sauté the remaining onions and garlic with the tempeh in 2 tablespoons of oil. Stir often and cook over low heat, partially covered, until the onions are tender.
5. Add all the spices and cook 1 minute longer, stirring constantly.
6. Add the green chilies and stir. Set aside.
7. When the beans are tender, add the onion/tempeh/spice mixture. Bring to a boil; then lower heat, cover, and simmer for 1 hour.
8. Place in a serving bowl and pour the salsa over the top.

10 SERVINGS

PER SERVING: *301 calories, 7 grams fat, 1 gram saturated fat, 0 cholesterol, 641 mg. sodium, 16 grams fiber*

*MEATLESS MEATLOAF

The high-gluten whole-wheat flour that we buy in a health food store and use in this recipe gives our loaf a very firm texture. If you like a softer texture, use a fifty-fifty mixture of breadcrumbs and flour.

3 cups textured vegetable protein granules
2¼ cups boiling water
8 ounces tomato sauce
1 medium onion, chopped
1 tablespoon olive oil
¾ cups high-gluten whole-
  wheat flour (or half flour,
  half breadcrumbs)

2 tablespoons soy sauce
1 tablespoon Worcestershire
  sauce
¼ teaspoon fresh-ground black
  pepper
1 teaspoon each garlic powder,
  basil, oregano, and marjoram
½ cup fresh parsley, minced

1. Place the soy granules in a large mixing bowl, add the boiling water and tomato sauce, mix well, and let stand for 10 minutes.
2. Place the chopped onion and oil in a microwave-safe dish and microwave on high until soft (about 3 minutes), or sauté until soft on the stove in a small skillet.
3. Add onions and all remaining ingredients to the rehydrated soy granules and mix well.
4. Put the mixture in loaf pan (9 × 5 × 2½ inches) or a suitably sized casserole that has been coated with nonstick spray. Press down firmly with a large spoon or spatula, smoothing the top.
5. Bake at 350 degrees for 45 minutes, or until firm (if it begins to brown too deeply before it is done, cover with foil).
6. Remove from oven, let stand 10 minutes, run a knife around the edges, and turn loaf out on a platter to serve.

8 SERVINGS

PER SERVING: *225 calories, 3 grams fat, 0 saturated fat, 0 choles-terol, 452 mg. sodium, 12 grams fiber*

*NO-FRY FALAFEL

This is an inspired alternative to traditional deep-fried Middle East-ern falafel. Serve in whole-wheat pita pockets with shredded lettuce and tahini mixed with nonfat plain yogurt and some lemon juice.

1 cup mashed potatoes (leftover
  or instant)
3 cans (15 ounces each) garbanzo beans, drained and
  mashed
2 tablespoons regular or
  toasted tahini (sesame paste)
2 tablespoons plain nonfat yogurt
¾ cup bread crumbs, prefer-

ably whole wheat
⅔ cup red onion, finely
  chopped
2 garlic cloves, minced
1 tablespoon ground cumin
2 teaspoons paprika
¼ teaspoon cayenne pepper
½ teaspoon salt
¼ cup fresh cilantro, minced

1. In a large bowl, combine the potatoes, mashed beans, tahini, yogurt, and bread crumbs.
2. Add the onion, garlic, cumin, paprika, cayenne, salt, and cilantro.
   Mix well.
3. Shape into 6 patties and arrange on an aluminum foil–lined
   cookie sheet that has been coated with cooking spray.
4. Bake for 10 minutes at 450 degrees, turn, and continue baking
   until browned.

6 SERVINGS

PER SERVING (WITH ONE 6-INCH WHOLE-WHEAT PITA): *375
calories, 6 grams fat, 1 gram saturated fat, 0 cholesterol, 932 mg.
sodium, 14 grams fiber*

*POLENTA WITH SPAGHETTI SQUASH

1 spaghetti squash, roasted (to
  roast squash, prick with a
  fork, set on baking sheet,
  and bake for 1 hour at 375
  degrees; this can be done the
  day before)
1 cup cornmeal
4 cups vegetable bouillon, divided
1 teaspoon salt
1 can (28 ounces) tomato
  sauce

1 onion, chopped
2 garlic cloves, minced
1 bell pepper, diced
1 tablespoon olive oil
½ teaspoon chili powder
½ teaspoon ground cumin
⅛ teaspoon cayenne
½ teaspoon cilantro
1 teaspoon basil
1 chopped jalapeño pepper (optional)
4 tablespoons goat cheese

1. In the top of a double boiler, combine cornmeal with ½ cup of the vegetable bouillon and salt. When smooth, add remainder of bouillon and stir well.
2. In the bottom of the double boiler, bring about 2 inches of water to a boil. Then, lower heat, place cornmeal mixture on top, and cover.
3. Cook over low heat, stirring very frequently, until cornmeal (polenta) gets thick (about 25 minutes).
4. Oil an 8 × 11½ × 2–inch casserole and put polenta in it. Smooth it over the bottom and refrigerate.
5. Put olive oil in a small skillet. Add onion, garlic, and bell pepper. Sauté over low heat, partially covered, until pepper is soft.
6. Add tomato sauce and spices and let simmer about 5 minutes.
7. Cut roasted squash in half and scoop out the seeds. Discard seeds.
8. Scoop out squash from shells and mash.
9. Spread squash over refrigerated polenta.
10. Spread tomato mixture over this and dot with goat cheese.
11. Bake at 350 degrees for about 40 minutes until bubbly.

8 SERVINGS

PER SERVING: *162 calories, 4 grams fat, 2 grams saturated fat, 6 mg. cholesterol, 952 mg. sodium, 4 grams fiber*

*SASSY SALSA BEANS

2 cups dried navy beans, washed

2 cups water

2 teaspoons vegetable bouillon powder

1 can (28 ounces) tomato sauce

1 teaspoon dried garlic flakes

3 tablespoons medium-hot salsa

extra water as needed

1. In a large saucepan, combine beans, 2 cups water, bouillon powder, tomato sauce, garlic flakes, and salsa.
2. Bring to a boil; cover, lower heat, and simmer for 1 hour. Stir often and add extra water as needed to be sure beans are always covered with sauce.

3. After one hour, place in a casserole. Cover with casserole lid or foil and bake in a 300-degree oven for 2 hours until beans are tender and sauce reaches desired consistency.

8 SERVINGS

PER SERVING: *206 calories, 1 gram fat, 0 saturated fat, 0 choles-terol, 630 mg. sodium, 14 grams fiber*

*SHEPHERD'S PIE

This vegetarian version retains the hearty, satisfying character of a traditional Shepherd's Pie. The combination of miso, soy sauce, and ginger give it a unique, full flavor. Our tasters could not believe a vegetarian Shepherd's Pie could be this satisfying.

¾ pound green beans, trimmed and cut diagonally in 1-inch pieces
½ cup water
2 medium carrots, sliced
1 large onion, chopped
2 garlic cloves, minced
1 teaspoon grated fresh ginger
2 tablespoons olive oil, divided
1 large zucchini, diced
1 tablespoon miso (fermented soybean paste)
1 tablespoon soy sauce
3 tablespoons whole-wheat flour
1 cup or more water for sauce
4 medium potatoes, cubed
water to cover
½ teaspoon salt
½ teaspoon thyme
fresh-ground pepper to taste
paprika

1. In a microwave-safe bowl, place green beans and ½ cup water. Cover and cook on high for 5 minutes.
2. Add carrots, and microwave on high an additional 8–10 minutes until vegetables are tender.
3. With a slotted spoon, transfer beans and carrots to a bowl and set aside.
4. Measure cooking water and add 1 cup or more water to make a total of 1½ cups water. Set aside.
5. In a skillet, sauté the onion, garlic, and ginger in 1 tablespoon of the olive oil until onion is translucent and just starting to brown (about 5 minutes).

6. Add zucchini and sauté 5 minutes more until zucchini is tender. Add the green beans and carrots and stir.
7. Using a small amount of the 1½ cups of water you have set aside, dissolve the miso along with the soy sauce.
8. Add the flour to this miso mixture and stir until smooth.
9. Add this mixture to the skillet along with the remainder of the reserved water.
10. Cook, stirring, until the sauce begins to thicken.
11. Place in a 3-quart casserole and set aside.
12. Cook the potatoes, covered, in a saucepan with water to cover.
13. When fork tender, drain, add the remaining 1 tablespoon of olive oil, the salt, thyme, and pepper. Mash well and add as much of the cooking water as you need to get a smooth, creamy consistency. (Save any remaining cooking water for soups, stews, etc.)
14. Spread the potatoes over the vegetables in the casserole and sprinkle with paprika.
15. Bake at 350 degrees for 30 minutes until bubbly.

6 SERVINGS

PER SERVING: *182 calories, 5 grams fat, 1 gram saturated fat, 0 cholesterol, 488 mg. sodium, 6 grams fiber*

STUFFED EGGPLANT

2 small eggplants (about 14 ounces each)
1 tablespoon olive oil + 1 table- spoon water
1 onion, chopped
2 garlic cloves, minced
1 small bell pepper, diced
1 teaspoon grated fresh ginger
1 tablespoon miso (fermented soybean paste) + 1 table-
spoon water
1 tablespoon soy sauce
½ teaspoon ground coriander
¼ teaspoon ground cumin
½ teaspoon crushed red pepper
1 tablespoon dried parsley
¼ cup walnuts, chopped
¼ cup feta cheese, crumbled
fresh-ground pepper to taste

1. Cut eggplants in half and scoop out the flesh, leaving ¼-inch rim. Set shells aside.

2. Cut eggplant flesh into bite-sized chunks and set aside.
3. In a large skillet, sauté onion, garlic, bell pepper, and ginger in the oil/water mixture, partially covered, until tender.
4. Add eggplant chunks, miso/water mixture, soy sauce, spices, and nuts. Cover and simmer until eggplant is tender (about 5 minutes).
5. Add feta cheese and salt and pepper to taste. Cook 1 minute longer. Let cool.
6. Stuff eggplant shells.
7. Place on a baking sheet and bake at 350 degrees for 30–40 minutes until hot.

4 SERVINGS

PER SERVING: *184 calories, 10 grams fat, 2 grams saturated fat, 8 mg. cholesterol, 526 mg. sodium, 6 grams fiber*

*TEMPEH BARBECUE ON MASHED POTATOES

Barbecue

1 medium onion, diced
1 garlic clove, minced
1 teaspoon grated fresh ginger
1 tablespoon olive oil
1 package (8 ounces) tempeh, defrosted and crumbled
2 tablespoons soy sauce

½ cup ketchup
½ teaspoon thyme
½ teaspoon crushed red pepper (optional)
1 teaspoon prepared Dijon mustard

1. In a large saucepan, sauté onion, garlic, ginger, tempeh, and soy sauce in olive oil over medium heat, stirring occasionally, until onion is tender (about 10 minutes).
2. Add remaining ingredients and simmer, uncovered, about 10 minutes longer, stirring often. Cover and keep mixture warm.

Mashed potatoes

2 medium potatoes, cut in chunks
water to cover
1 tablespoon olive oil

1 teaspoon soy sauce
fresh-ground pepper to taste
reserved potato water as needed

1. In a large saucepan, place potatoes with water to cover.
2. Bring to a boil; then lower heat, cover, and simmer until potatoes are tender.
3. Drain potatoes reserving the water.
4. Add oil and soy sauce and pepper to taste.
5. Mash potatoes, adding reserved potato water as needed to make it a desirable consistency.
6. Serve tempeh barbecue over the mashed potatoes.

4 SERVINGS

PER SERVING: *291 calories, 11 grams fat, 2 grams saturated fat, 0 cholesterol, 1004 mg. sodium, 6 grams fiber*

TEX-MEX BULGUR

1 tablespoon olive oil
1 onion, chopped
1 red or yellow bell pepper, diced
1 medium carrot, grated
¼ cup fresh parsley, chopped
1 teaspoon chili powder
½ teaspoon salt
1 teaspoon sage
½ teaspoon ground cumin

¼ teaspoon crushed red pepper
black pepper to taste
1 large garlic clove, minced
2 cups vegetable bouillon
1 cup bulgur
1 can (16 ounces) kidney beans, drained
1 cup kernel corn, drained
¼ cup shredded cheddar cheese

1. In a large skillet, heat oil slightly over medium heat.
2. Stir in onion, bell pepper, and grated carrot. Cook, partially covered, for about 5 minutes, stirring often.
3. Stir in parsley, chili powder, salt, sage, cumin, crushed red pepper, black pepper, and garlic.
4. Add bouillon and bring to a boil. Stir in bulgur, beans, and corn. Then lower heat, cover, and simmer about 15 minutes.
5. Remove from heat and let stand, covered, until all liquid is absorbed (about 5 minutes).
6. Place in a large serving bowl, sprinkle with cheese, and serve.

8 SERVINGS

PER SERVING: *169 calories, 4 grams fat, 1 gram saturated fat, 4 mg. cholesterol, 426 mg. sodium, 7 grams fiber*

*VEGETABLE TOFU BAKE

1 bag ready-to-use baby
  spinach (10 ounces)
1 leek, tough green section removed
2 carrots, shredded
1 tablespoon olive oil
1 pound firm tofu, drained
  and cubed
½ cup pine nuts, toasted
1 cup egg substitute

2 tablespoons tahini
2 tablespoons soy sauce
1 teaspoon dried tarragon
¼ teaspoon nutmeg
¼ teaspoon garlic powder
½ teaspoon salt
fresh-ground pepper to taste
4 tablespoons stuffing mix
salsa

1. Coat an 8 × 11½ × 2–inch baking dish with cooking spray. Set aside.
2. Remove tough stems from spinach.
3. Wash leek and cut into 1-inch pieces.
4. In a food processor, process the spinach and the leek until finely chopped.
5. Put oil in a skillet and add the spinach, leek, and shredded carrots. Cook about 2 minutes; remove to a large bowl and set aside.
6. Put tofu and toasted pine nuts in the food processor and process until smooth.
7. Add egg substitute, tahini, soy sauce, spices, salt, and pepper. Process to mix.
8. Combine with vegetables in the large bowl.
9. Pour all into baking dish. Sprinkle with stuffing mix.
10. Bake at 350 degrees for about 30 minutes until set.
11. Cut into squares and serve with salsa on the side.

8 SERVINGS

PER SERVING (WITH 2 TABLESPOONS SALSA): *204 calories, 11 grams fat, 2 grams saturated fat, 0 cholesterol, 690 mg. sodium, 4 grams fiber*

*ZUCCHINI NUT SKILLET

*2 large zucchinis, cut in bite-
    sized chunks*
1 small onion, chopped
1 garlic clove, minced
1 teaspoon grated fresh ginger
*1 tablespoon olive oil + 1 table-
    spoon water*
*1 tablespoon miso (fermented
    soybean paste)*
1 tablespoon soy sauce

1 tablespoon dried parsley
½ teaspoon ground coriander
¼ teaspoon ground cumin
⅓ cup walnuts, chopped
*¼ cup shredded Parmesan
    cheese*
fresh-ground pepper to taste
*3 cups cooked brown rice or
    other grain*

1. In a skillet, sauté onion, garlic, and ginger in the oil/water mixture until onions are translucent.
2. In a small bowl, mix the miso with the soy sauce until well
   blended.
3. Add the miso/soy sauce mixture to the skillet.
4. Add the zucchini and spices. Lower heat and cover.
5. Let simmer about 8 minutes until the zucchini is tender.
6. Add cheese and let cook 1 minute longer.
7. Add pepper.
8. Serve over cooked rice or other cooked grain.

6 SERVINGS

PER SERVING (WITH ½ CUP BROWN RICE): *214 calories, 9
grams fat, 2 grams saturated fat, 3 mg. cholesterol, 362 mg. sodium,
4 grams fiber*

ZUCCHINI PIE

1 small onion, chopped
2 garlic cloves, minced
1 tablespoon olive oil
1½ pounds zucchini, diced
*½ cup whole kernel corn,
    drained*
1 tablespoon nutritional yeast

1 teaspoon paprika
½ teaspoon thyme
½ teaspoon oregano
1 teaspoon salt, divided
*fresh-ground black pepper to
    taste*
½ cup 2% cottage cheese

1 cup egg substitute
1 cup skim milk
½ cup whole-wheat flour

¾ cup shredded wheat, crumbled

2 tablespoons Parmesan cheese

1. Coat an 8 × 8 × 2–inch baking dish with cooking spray.
2. In a skillet, sauté onion and garlic in oil until onion is tender (about 3 minutes).
3. Add zucchini and cook about 10–12 minutes more, until zucchini is just tender.
4. Add corn, yeast, spices, and ½ teaspoon of the salt. Cook 1 minute more, stirring often. Place in baking dish and set aside.
5. In blender or food processor, process cottage cheese until smooth and creamy.
6. Add egg substitute, milk, flour, remaining ½ teaspoon salt, and shredded wheat and process until smooth.
7. Pour this mixture over the vegetables in the baking dish.
8. Sprinkle with Parmesan cheese and bake at 400 degrees about 25 minutes until bubbly around the edges and browned on top.
9. Let stand 5 minutes before serving.

6 SERVINGS

PER SERVING: *171 calories, 4 grams fat, 1 gram saturated fat, 4 mg. cholesterol, 625 mg. sodium, 4 grams fiber*

PASTA

High in carbohydrates and low in fat, pasta has become almost as common as hearty bread in my own diet. I usually mix whole-grain and regular semolina fifty-fifty because, while whole-grain pasta contains more fiber, it tends to have a pasty texture; the combination with semolina prevents this. Don't overcook your pasta—cook it *al dente* and then mix it with the sauce. Many different grains are now being used to make pasta, including rice, corn, Jerusalem artichoke, and soy, among others, but none of them except perhaps the Jerusalem artichoke make as good a pasta as wheat.

An average serving of 1 cup of cooked pasta contains about 2 grams of fat. Pastas with added egg (for example, egg noodles) will contain about 50 milligrams of cholesterol per serving.

*BROCCOLI PESTO

Flowerets from 2 stalks broccoli
   (about 4 cups)
½ cup vegetable bouillon
4 garlic cloves, chopped
½ cup pine nuts (or walnuts)
¼ cup packed fresh parsley
2 tablespoons olive oil
1 teaspoon lemon juice

½ teaspoon ground coriander
½ teaspoon salt (or more to
   taste)
fresh-ground black pepper to
   taste
¼ teaspoon crushed red pepper
12 ounces thin spaghetti

1. Place broccoli and vegetable bouillon in a microwave-safe covered container and microwave on high for 5 minutes. Let cool.
2. In a food processor, process garlic and pine nuts until finely chopped.
3. Add oil, lemon juice, and spices. Process until smooth.
4. Add broccoli and bouillon. Process until smooth.
5. Cook spaghetti according to directions on package. Drain in colander and return to pot.
6. Add pesto and toss to distribute evenly.
7. Heat briefly and serve.

6 SERVINGS

PER SERVING: *332 calories, 11 grams fat, 2 grams saturated fat, 0 cholesterol, 217 mg. sodium, 3 grams fiber*

CANNELLONI

This recipe takes a bit of extra time, which I think you will find well worthwhile. It's an illustration of how to use cheese in moderation to produce a very tasty dish that remains relatively low in fat. By the way, it was a "winner" at a local charity pasta event against much higher-fat competition!

Sauce

1 garlic clove, crushed
1 tablespoon olive oil
3 tablespoons water
¼ cup all-purpose flour
1½ teaspoons instant chicken
bouillon
⅛ teaspoon white pepper
2 cups evaporated skim milk
¼ cup farmers or grated sap-
sago cheese

Filling

3 tablespoons sliced green
onions
2 teaspoons olive oil plus 2 teaspoons water
1 package (10 ounces) frozen
chopped spinach, thawed
and drained
1 cup finely chopped cooked
chicken breast
¼ cup grated farmers or sap-
sago cheese
1 egg, beaten, or ¼ cup egg
substitute
2 tablespoons nonfat or 1%
milk
¾ teaspoon liquid Italian seasoning
¼ teaspoon pepper

Other ingredients

6 cannelloni (or manicotti) shells

1. To make the sauce, sauté the garlic in the olive oil and water in a medium saucepan over moderate heat.
2. Stir in the flour, bouillon, and pepper.
3. Remove from heat and gradually stir in milk.
4. Return to heat and bring to a boil, stirring constantly. Boil and stir for 1 minute.
5. Reduce heat to low. Stir in the cheese until melted. Remove from heat and set aside.
6. Parboil the pasta shells according to package directions. Rinse and drain.
7. While shells are cooking, make the filling. In a small skillet, sauté the onion in the olive oil/water just until tender.
8. Combine remaining ingredients in a bowl, add onion, and mix well.
9. Fill shells with mixture and arrange in a shallow 2-quart casserole dish that has been coated with cooking spray.
10. Spoon sauce over filled cannelloni.
11. Bake for 20 minutes at 350 degrees, then broil for 5 minutes or until sauce is bubbly and golden. Serve immediately.

4 SERVINGS

PER SERVING (1 ½ SHELL WITH SAUCE): *478 calories, 11 grams fat, 3 grams saturated fat, 95 mg. cholesterol, 889 mg. sodium, 4 grams fiber*

*CHICKEN AND VEGETABLES ALFREDO

8 ounces uncooked linguine
2 cups broccoli, chopped
2 cups carrots, thinly sliced
1 cup mushrooms, sliced
1 chicken bouillon cube
½ cup onion, chopped
2 cloves garlic, minced
3 tablespoons flour
¼ teaspoon fresh-ground pep-

per
1 can (12 ounces) evaporated skim milk
1½ cups cubed cooked chicken breast
1 container (8 ounces) reduced-fat sour cream
⅓ cup grated Parmesan cheese

1. Cook linguine according to package directions. Drain and set aside.
2. Meanwhile, in a medium saucepan combine the broccoli, carrots, mushrooms, and enough water to cover the vegetables.
3. Bring to a boil, reduce the heat, and cook about 5 minutes until just tender. Drain, reserving ¼ cup of the liquid. Set the vegetables aside.
4. Spray a large nonstick skillet with cooking spray. Dissolve the chicken bouillon in the reserved liquid over medium-high heat.
5. Add the onion and garlic, and cook until onion is tender.
6. Stir in the flour and pepper. Gradually stir in the evaporated milk.
7. Cook until the sauce boils and thickens, stirring constantly.
8. Stir in the vegetables, chicken, sour cream, and ¼ cup of the Parmesan cheese.
9. Heat thoroughly without boiling. Add hot linguine, tossing to mix. Sprinkle with remaining Parmesan cheese before serving.

6 SERVINGS

PER SERVING: *345 calories, 4 grams fat, 2 grams saturated fat, 36 mg. cholesterol, 442 mg. sodium, 5 grams fiber*

*ONCE-A-WEEK PASTA

When you look in your refrigerator at the end of the week you are likely to find a few vegetables that have just passed their prime for use in salads or in recipes where the freshest yield the flavor and texture you desire. Almost every vegetable, even after it's begun to grow a bit limp with age, can be added to a garlic-and-oil base for an excellent pasta sauce. Start by sautéing plenty of garlic in an olive oil/water mixture (1–2 tablespoons oil + 1 tablespoon water for every four servings of the final dish), then add the vegetables from your crisper in order of the amount of time it takes to cook. For example, if you have broccoli, celery, and carrots, they would go in the pot before mushrooms and spinach leaves. The tougher, more fibrous vegetables should be chopped into small pieces. As the cooking proceeds, you can add ¼ to ½ cup of chicken or vegetable bouillon to create enough sauce for the amount of pasta you plan to prepare. Vegetables are 80 to 90 percent water, and as they cook down, your sauce will expand with healthful, tasty vegetable juices.

Once-a-Week Pasta is always a new experience, which is what makes this dish so much fun to prepare and serve. Here is an example of a pasta dish that I prepared one Saturday evening with the remnants of our salad vegetables and other leftover vegetables. It's the kind of recipe where you just line up ingredients and mince, chop, or slice one item at a time and add to the sauce as you go along. Since the sauce can simmer for quite a time to its advantage, I usually wait to start my pasta until I'm near the end of my preparations for the sauce.

3 tablespoons olive oil + 2 tablespoons water
12 garlic cloves, minced
4 stalks broccoli, about an inch of the toughest lower stem removed, and the rest chopped in small pieces
2 leeks, sliced thin
¼ white onion, chopped
2 stalks celery, chopped
1 large green bell pepper, diced
½ large red bell pepper, diced
1 small piece napa cabbage

(the heart), chopped
3 large mushrooms, sliced
1 ounce fresh spinach
¼ to ½ cup chicken or vegetable bouillon (optional)
3 or 4 dried hot red peppers (optional, but they add zip!)
fresh-ground black pepper to taste
4 tablespoons shredded or grated Parmesan cheese
1 pound favorite pasta, cooked

1. Heat the oil and water in a 3-quart or larger saucepan, add the minced garlic, and sauté over low heat until translucent.
2. Add the chopped broccoli to the garlic and oil, cover, and begin simmering over low heat.
3. Prepare, one at a time (my projected order of cooking required time), leeks, onion, celery, green pepper and red bell pepper, napa cabbage, mushrooms, and spinach. Add to the sauce, stir, cover the pot, and simmer in between additions. (Toward the end of these preparations, I put the water on to heat for my pasta.)
4. If the sauce does not appear to have enough liquid, add the bouillon.
5. Add the dried red peppers (optional), black pepper, and Parmesan cheese and stir. Continue simmering until pasta is ready.
6. Drain the pasta, pour the sauce into a spacious casserole dish, and add the pasta to the sauce. Mix and top with extra Parmesan if desired. If necessary, place in a warm oven (under 200 degrees) until serving time. Let each person add salt to taste at the table.

8 GENEROUS SERVINGS

PER SERVING (WITH PASTA): *315 calories, 7 grams fat, 1 gram saturated fat, 3 mg. cholesterol, 157 mg. sodium, 6 grams fiber*

Note: I have also used carrots, zucchini, yellow summer squash, tomatoes, cauliflower, cucumbers, various greens and cabbages, garbanzo beans, lettuce, and herbs such as parsley and basil in my Once-a-Week Pasta sauce. Also, if you like, substitute tomato sauce or tomato juice for the bouillon.

REAL ITALIAN TOMATO SAUCE

Here is our favorite basic marinara sauce. This sauce can be used for any recipe calling for tomato sauce, from pasta to eggplant to fish. You can store this in an airtight container in the refrigerator for several days, or freeze for later use. If you want to cut down on sodium, look for no-salt-added canned tomato products.

1 tablespoon olive oil
1 medium onion, cut in
  chunks
8 ounces fresh mushrooms,
  sliced or quartered
1 to 3 tablespoons dried basil
  (three times more if you use
  fresh!)
2 large garlic cloves, minced
1 large bay leaf
1 can (28 ounces) tomatoes
1 can (10 ¾ ounces) tomato
  purée
1 can (6 ounces) tomato paste
salt and fresh-ground black
  pepper to taste

1. Heat a large kettle over medium heat. Put in the oil, onion, mush-rooms, basil, and garlic. Cover, and reduce heat to medium low. Stir frequently—you may need to add a tablespoon or two of water to keep it from sticking.
2. When the onions are translucent, add the remaining ingredients, except the salt and pepper. Bring to a boil on high heat, then reduce to simmer and let cook for an hour or so, stirring occasionally to break up the whole tomatoes.
3. Add salt and pepper to taste.

MAKES ABOUT 6 CUPS

PER CUP: *110 calories, 3 grams fat, 0 saturated fat, 0 cholesterol, 326 mg. sodium, 4 grams fiber*

*RED CLAM SAUCE

When you use canned clams in a recipe, it's a good idea to add them last and cook only for a short time to preserve their tenderness.

2 cups chopped onions
12 ounces mushrooms, sliced
6 garlic cloves, crushed
2 tablespoons olive oil
½ teaspoon salt
¼ cup red wine (optional)
¼ teaspoon fresh-ground black
  pepper
⅛ teaspoon cayenne pepper
1 can (10½ ounces) tomato
  purée
4 cans (6½ ounces each)
  clams, minced, drained; re-serve liquid

1. In a 3-quart saucepan, sauté onion, mushrooms, and garlic in the olive oil over medium-high heat for about 5 minutes, or until onions are translucent.
2. Add remaining ingredients except for drained clams (include liquid from clams) and cook, covered, for 40 minutes.
3. Add clams and cook for an additional 5 minutes.
4. Serve over favorite pasta.

MAKES ABOUT 8 CUPS

PER CUP: *124 calories, 5 grams fat, 1 gram saturated fat, 63 mg. cholesterol, 185 mg. sodium, 2 grams fiber*

*SPAGHETTI SAUCE WITH TEMPEH AND BROCCOLI

2 stalks broccoli, diced
½ cup water
1 tablespoon olive oil
8 ounces tempeh, thawed and crumbled
1 small onion, chopped
2 garlic cloves, minced
1 teaspoon grated fresh ginger
1 tablespoon soy sauce

3 cups tomato sauce
1 teaspoon basil
1 teaspoon sage
1 teaspoon thyme
¼ teaspoon crushed red pepper (optional)
¼ teaspoon salt
fresh-ground pepper to taste
12 ounces spaghetti, uncooked

1. Place the broccoli and water in a microwave-safe covered bowl and microwave on high for 5 minutes.
2. In a large skillet, sauté the tempeh, onion, garlic, and ginger in the olive oil over low heat, partially covered, until onion is translucent. Stir frequently.
3. Add the soy sauce, broccoli with the water, tomato sauce, and spices. Bring to a boil; then lower heat, cover, and simmer about 15 minutes more.
4. Meanwhile, cook the spaghetti and drain. Keep warm.
5. When sauce is done, combine with the spaghetti and serve.

8 SERVINGS

PER SERVING (WITH 1 CUP COOKED SPAGHETTI): *277 calories, 5 grams fat, 1 gram saturated fat, 0 cholesterol, 845 mg. sodium, 6 grams fiber*

*SPINACH LASAGNA

This recipe has always been a favorite with Jamie's weight-management participants. It's great for dinner parties—leftovers are delicious!

½ pound lasagna noodles
1 medium onion, chopped
2 garlic cloves, minced
1 teaspoon olive oil
16 ounces "light" ricotta or 2% cottage cheese
¼ cup grated Parmesan cheese
1 ½ pounds fresh spinach, washed and chopped, or 1 package (10 ounces) frozen chopped spinach, thawed

and drained
2 egg whites, beaten, or ¼ cup egg substitute
¼ teaspoon fresh-ground pepper
2–3 tablespoons fresh parsley, chopped
6 cups meatless spaghetti sauce
8 ounces reduced-fat mozzarella cheese, grated

1. Spray a 13 × 9–inch casserole dish with cooking spray. Preheat the oven to 300 degrees.
2. Sauté the onion and garlic in olive oil in a nonstick skillet, adding water as needed to prevent sticking.
3. Combine the ricotta, Parmesan, spinach, egg whites, pepper, parsley, and sautéed onion and garlic, mixing well.
4. Spread ¼ of the tomato sauce (1½ cups) over the bottom of the prepared casserole dish.
5. Arrange ⅓ of the noodles (uncooked) over the sauce, top with ⅓ of the ricotta/spinach mixture, sprinkle with ⅓ of the mozzarella, and top with more tomato sauce.
6. Repeat layers twice more, ending with the sauce.
7. Cover with aluminum foil, crimping edges tightly. Bake for 1½ hours, remove foil, and bake another 10 minutes.

12 SERVINGS

PER SERVING: *230 calories, 6 grams fat, 3 grams saturated fat, 13 mg. cholesterol, 633 mg. sodium, 4 grams fiber*

Note: Lessen cooking time to about 45 minutes by precooking lasagna noodles. This recipe can be turned into a nine-vegetable lasagna by incorporating other vegetables into the sauce (mushrooms, zucchini, yellow squash, red, yellow, and green peppers, plus the onions, spinach, and tomatoes . . . !).

*SUPER-EASY ANGEL HAIR WITH FETA AND SPINACH

This dish has become a favorite in Jamie's neighborhood for a quick yet special dinner after work. It takes less than ten minutes to prepare and tastes like a pasta dish you'd get at an upscale restaurant.

8 ounces angel hair pasta, un- cooked

1 package (10 ounces) creamed spinach (Green Giant or any brand marked "low-fat sauce")

6 ounces flavored feta cheese, crumbled (garlic-herb or tomato-basil are good)

pepper and garlic powder to taste

1. In a large pot, cook pasta according to package directions. Angel hair varieties can take as little as 2 minutes' boiling time.
2. Meanwhile, cook spinach in microwave according to package directions.
3. Drain pasta, return to pot, and stir in creamed spinach and seasonings.
4. Toss with feta and serve.

4 SERVINGS

PER SERVING: *334 calories, 12 grams fat, 7 grams saturated fat, 38 mg. cholesterol, 1042 mg. sodium, 2 grams fiber*

Note: For an even more special dish, add diced fresh tomatoes or a few sliced black olives.

POULTRY

Many persons who have been successful in weight management report reducing their consumption of red meat in favor of chicken and fish. A cooked half breast of chicken, about 3 ounces of white meat *without skin,* averages around 140 calories. Fat contributes only about 20 percent of its nutrient weight (about 3 grams, or 27 calories). Compare this to a *small* rib-eye steak of around 3½ ounces cooked, which could contain as much as 440 calories, with 360 of those calories (40 grams) coming from fat. Even the leanest meats tend to contain about twice the fat of a chicken breast. You can see that, as a rule, chicken is the choice to make.

White meat of chicken contains about 25 percent less fat than dark meat. When whole chickens are used, the nutritional analyses assume half white meat and half dark. When a recipe calls for chicken breasts, split breasts are assumed; that is, 4 chicken breasts means 4 half-breasts.

The fat content of turkey is similar to that of chicken. Ground turkey is an excellent "extender" for ground beef, or it can be used in place of ground beef in most recipes. But beware of prepackaged ground turkey—it can contain just as much fat as the fattest ground beef for hamburgers. Ask for extra-lean, or for ground turkey that is less than 10 percent fat (preferably 5 percent) by weight.

*BAKED CHICKEN WITH TARRAGON AND FENNEL

4 skinless chicken breast halves
1 teaspoon tarragon
¼ teaspoon fennel seeds, crushed

⅛ teaspoon ground cardamom
salt and fresh-ground pepper to taste

1. Place chicken breasts on foil-lined baking pan. Sprinkle with seasonings.
2. Cover loosely with foil to help retain moisture.
3. Bake at 350 degrees for 45 to 50 minutes, until cooked through.

4 SERVINGS

PER SERVING: *165 calories, 3 grams fat, 1 gram saturated fat, 84 mg. cholesterol, 207 mg. sodium, 0 fiber*

*BARBECUED CHICKEN

You can use this recipe with our Barbecue Sauce (in the Sauces section) or your own variation. Or substitute a store-bought brand if you wish.

3½ pounds chicken pieces   *1 cup barbecue sauce*

1. Rinse under cold running water and skin the chicken pieces.
2. Place the pieces "skin" side down in a large, shallow baking pan (you may wish to line the pan with foil for easy cleaning)
3. Baste the chicken pieces liberally with barbecue sauce, and place in the oven.
4. Bake at 350 degrees for 20 minutes, basting halfway through.
5. Turn chicken over and bake another 25 to 30 minutes, or until chicken is tender, basting occasionally.

6 SERVINGS

PER SERVING: *174 calories, 5 grams fat, 2 grams saturated fat, 78 mg. cholesterol, 86 mg. sodium, 1 gram fiber*

*CHICKEN PICANTE

½ cup medium chunky taco sauce
¼ cup Dijon mustard
6 tablespoons plain low-fat yogurt
2 tablespoons fresh lime juice

6 boneless, skinless chicken breast halves
1 teaspoon olive oil
1 lime, cut into 6 slices
fresh cilantro, chopped (optional)

1. In a large bowl, make a marinade by mixing taco sauce, mustard, yogurt, and lime juice.
2. Add the chicken, turning to coat.

3. Cover and refrigerate at least 30 minutes.
4. Coat a large skillet with cooking spray and heat olive oil over medium heat.
5. Remove the chicken from the marinade and place in skillet. Cook 5 minutes on each side.
6. Add the marinade to the skillet and cook about 5 minutes more, until a fork can be inserted in the chicken with ease and the liquid is slightly reduced.
7. Remove the chicken. Raise the heat to high and boil the marinade for 1 minute. Pour over chicken.
8. Garnish with lime slices and cilantro.

6 SERVINGS

PER SERVING: *165 calories, 3 grams fat, 1 gram saturated fat, 69 mg. cholesterol, 271 mg. sodium, 1 gram fiber*

*OVEN-FRIED CHICKEN

¾ cup wheat germ
1 teaspoon paprika
2 teaspoons dried parsley
1 teaspoon dried minced onion
¼ teaspoon garlic powder
¼ teaspoon salt

¾ teaspoon sage
6 skinless chicken breasts (bone in or boneless)
½ cup buttermilk
butter-flavored cooking spray

1. In a bowl, mix the wheat germ with the paprika, parsley, onion, garlic, salt, and sage.
2. Dip the chicken pieces in the buttermilk, then roll in the wheat germ mixture.
3. Arrange in 13 × 9–inch baking pan that has been sprayed with cooking spray. Sprinkle with any remaining wheat germ mixture.
4. Spray each piece with cooking spray.
5. Bake, uncovered, at 375 degrees for 45 minutes to 1 hour.

6 SERVINGS

PER SERVING: *191 calories, 3 grams fat, 1 gram saturated fat, 69 mg. cholesterol, 187 mg. sodium, 2 grams fiber*

*OVEN-STEWED CHICKEN AND VEGETABLES

This is a rich meal in a casserole, and easy to prepare.

4 skinless chicken breasts
2 large potatoes, halved length-
    wise and sliced ½-inch thick
2 large carrots, in ½-inch slices
1 large onion, in thick slices
4 stalks celery, thinly sliced
1 green bell pepper, in ½-inch
    slices

2 cans (15 ounces each)
    tomato sauce
2 cups chicken broth
½ teaspoon garlic powder
½ teaspoon thyme
½ teaspoon marjoram
fresh-ground pepper to taste

1. Wash the chicken breasts under cold running water and place on the bottom of a 5-quart casserole dish.
2. Spread the vegetables around on top of the chicken breasts.
3. Pour in the tomato sauce and chicken broth until the vegetables are just about covered (do not quite cover; you want the water contained in the vegetables to be released in the casserole).
4. Sprinkle the seasonings over the mixture and blend carefully into the liquids and vegetables on the surface.
5. Cover and bake in a 350-degree oven for about 1½–2 hours, stirring and mixing the ingredients ever half-hour or so.

4 SERVINGS

PER SERVING: *392 calories, 5 grams fat, 1 gram saturated fat, 88 mg. cholesterol, 1468 mg. sodium, 8 grams fiber*

*SAVORY TURKEY LOAF

The National Turkey Federation provided the inspiration for this recipe. My wife, Enid, was intrigued by the idea of combining turkey and spinach, and then went on to create her own mixture of seasonings.

1 pound lean ground turkey

1 package (10 ounces) frozen chopped spinach, thawed and drained

½ cup your favorite brand dry poultry stuffing

1 small onion, chopped

1 garlic clove, crushed

2½ tablespoons Dijon mustard

¼ cup fresh parsley, chopped

¼ teaspoon dried thyme

1 tablespoon catsup

¼ cup shredded part-skim mozzarella

1 jar (2 ounces) chopped pimentos, drained

1. In a large bowl, combine all but the last three ingredients.
2. Shape into a loaf, about 4 × 6 inches in size, and place in a 9-inch pie pan that has been coated with cooking spray.
3. Bake in a 350-degree oven for about 55 minutes or until browned.
4. Spread with catsup and sprinkle on the cheese and pimentos.
5. Bake about 5 minutes longer, until cheese is melted.

4 SERVINGS

PER SERVING: *298 calories, 12 grams fat, 4 grams saturated fat, 94 mg. cholesterol, 825 mg. sodium, 3 grams fiber*

FISH

While it's possible to use fish in complex recipes, most types can be prepared quickly, easily, and in low-fat ways: poaching, broiling, steaming, baking, and grilling. Watch cooking times carefully to avoid overcooking.

Many varieties of fish contain those important "Omega 3" fatty acids that can reduce the risk of heart disease. One of these, eicosapentanoic acid (EPA), has been shown to lower serum cholesterol and triglycerides and to increase high-density lipoproteins (HDL). Lower total cholesterol and higher HDL levels are both associated with a reduced risk of cardiovascular disease. EPA also lessens the risk of blood clots and stroke by causing some changes in the red blood cells and platelets in the bloodstream that are responsible for clotting.

The best sources of Omega 3 fatty acids are cold-water fish: salmon, mackerel, pollack (bluefish), albacore tuna, and herring.

Moderate amounts can be found in halibut, red snapper, swordfish, and shellfish, while cod, monkfish, and orange roughy have a little less. Although the varieties of fish richest in Omega 3 fatty acids contain more fat than others, they are still generally lower in fat than red meat. While flounder and sole, for example, may be very low in fat and merit frequent inclusion in your diet, the added health benefits and reasonable fat contents of the fattier fish listed above also recommend their use on a regular basis.

*BAKED FISH FILLETS

This is one of the simplest ways to prepare fish and one of the most satisfying.

1½ pounds lean fish fillets
  (sole, flounder, perch)
1 tablespoon olive oil
1 teaspoon lemon juice

salt and fresh-ground pepper to
  taste
garlic and onion powder to
  taste (optional)

1. Preheat oven to 475 degrees.
2. Pour the oil and lemon juice onto a foil-lined baking pan.
3. Swish the fish around in the liquid on both sides.
4. Sprinkle with salt and pepper, and garlic and onion powder if desired.
5. Bake 8 to 10 minutes uncovered on a rack just above the middle of your oven.
6. Be sure to test at 8 minutes and frequently thereafter. Fish is done when it flakes easily with a fork and is still moist.

4 SERVINGS

PER SERVING: *229 calories, 5 grams fat, 1 gram saturated fat, 115 mg. cholesterol, 180 mg. sodium, 0 fiber*

Variation: Make the same recipe with a fattier fish, such as salmon. Salmon fillets may take 10 to 12 minutes, as will fish steaks an inch in thickness. Until you know your oven and can gauge cooking time, check frequently for doneness. Salmon is done when there is still a little streak of pinkness in the center, and the fish is moist and flakes easily with a fork.

*DIJON SWORDFISH

This marinade is also delicious with chicken.

2 tablespoons Dijon mustard	¾ cup fresh basil, shredded (or
½ cup white wine	2 tablespoons dried)
¼ cup lemon juice	6 swordfish steaks, 1 inch thick
¼ cup olive oil	(about 6 ounces each)
1 garlic clove, minced	

1. In a bowl, combine the mustard, wine, lemon juice, and olive oil with a wire whisk. Add the garlic and basil.
2. Arrange the swordfish in a shallow baking pan.
3. Pour the marinade over the fish, turning to coat both sides. Refrigerate for 1 hour, turning once.
4. Place steaks on broiling rack and broil 7 inches from heat for 5 to 6 minutes per side.

6 SERVINGS

PER SERVING: *232 calories, 8 grams fat, 2 grams saturated fat, 64 mg. cholesterol, 214 mg. sodium, 0 fiber*

*DIKKIE'S ROASTED SALMON WITH HERBS AND PEPPER

2 tablespoons lemon juice	peppercorns
2 teaspoons olive oil	¼ cup fresh dill, chopped
5 garlic cloves, minced	¼ cup fresh parsley, chopped
1 tablespoon crushed black	2 pounds salmon fillets

1. In a small bowl, combine lemon juice, oil, and garlic.
2. In another bowl, combine peppercorns, dill, and parsley.

3. Line a 15 × 10–inch jelly roll pan with aluminum foil and coat lightly with cooking spray.
4. Place salmon fillets in pan and spoon the lemon juice/oil/garlic mixture over the tops.
5. Sprinkle on the peppercorn/herb mixture and press in gently.
6. Preheat oven to 475 degrees and bake salmon for about 12–15 minutes until fish flakes easily or temperature on thermometer placed in salmon reads 145 degrees.

4 SERVINGS

PER SERVING: *298 calories, 14 grams fat, 2 grams saturated fat, 107 mg. cholesterol, 88 mg. sodium, 0 fiber*

HALIBUT WITH LEMON
ARTICHOKE SAUCE

If you have never had a lemon artichoke sauce with a white-fleshed fish, you are in for a treat and a surprise. Halibut and a lemon artichoke sauce were made for each other, but the sauce also goes well with cod and orange roughy.

2 pounds halibut steaks
1 tablespoon olive oil
3 garlic cloves, minced
1 medium onion, chopped
1 can (14 ounces) artichokes
(net weight), drained; reserve liquid
teaspoon lemon juice
¼ teaspoon salt
fresh-ground pepper to taste

1. Preheat oven to 475 degrees.
2. In small skillet, lightly sauté garlic and onions in oil on medium-low heat until translucent and just turning lightly brown.
3. Add artichokes, lemon juice, and 1 tablespoon artichoke liquid; warm on low heat, adding a little more artichoke liquid as needed.
4. Lightly brush fish steaks with oil on both sides, and bake on baking sheet for 10–12 minutes, or until they flake easily. Do not overcook; flesh should be soft to touch and not dry.
5. When fish is done, place on serving platter and cover with sauce.
6. Add salt and pepper to taste when served.

4 SERVINGS

PER SERVING: *324 calories, 8 grams fat, 2 grams saturated fat, 70 mg. cholesterol, 554 mg. sodium, 2 grams fiber*

*ROYAL INDIAN SALMON

This recipe is an all-time favorite, delicately flavored, and easy to prepare. I include it here again because so many people have written complimentary notes to me about it. I want to make sure new readers have a chance to try it.

*4 salmon steaks, 1 inch thick
(about 6 ounces each)
¼ cup low-sodium chicken or
vegetable bouillon
2 tablespoons lemon juice
½ teaspoon fennel seeds,*

*crushed
¼ teaspoon ground cumin
¼ teaspoon ground coriander
dash of salt and fresh-ground
pepper to taste*

1. Place the steaks in a shallow pan. Pour the bouillon and the lemon juice over the steaks. Add the seasonings.
2. Marinate, covered, in the refrigerator for at least 2 hours, turning the steaks occasionally.
3. To cook, place the steaks on a foil-covered broiling pan. Spoon 2 teaspoons of the marinade on top of each steak.
4. Place under broiler not too close to the source of the heat for 8–10 minutes, or until slightly brown on the edges. Turn steaks over, spoon on remaining marinade, and broil for an additional 8–10 minutes. (The internal temperature of the fish should reach 145 degrees.)

4 SERVINGS

PER SERVING: *285 calories, 8 grams fat, 2 grams saturated fat, 120 mg. cholesterol, 225 mg. sodium, 0 fiber*

*ORANGE ROUGHY WITH SPINACH

Orange roughy is a medium-fatty fish that can be prepared as specified in Baked Fish Fillets, the first recipe in the Fish/Seafood section. It also lends itself to a rich-tasting Florentine combination. You can use any lean to medium-fatty fillets in this recipe.

1½ pounds orange roughy fillets (2 fillets)
8 ounces fresh spinach
2 teaspoons olive oil
2 tablespoons soy sauce
2 teaspoons Worcestershire sauce

1 medium onion, thinly sliced
1 medium tomato, thinly sliced
2 tablespoons grated Parmesan cheese
fresh-ground black pepper to taste

1. Preheat oven to 375 degrees.
2. Line a 3-inch-deep baking pan with half the spinach.
3. Place fish on top.
4. Combine olive oil with soy sauce and Worcestershire and drizzle over the fish.
5. Partially cook the onion (5 minutes on high in the microwave).
6. Spread the onion and tomato slices over the fish.
7. Sprinkle with the Parmesan cheese and pepper. Spread remaining spinach on top.
8. Cover lightly with foil and bake 20–25 minutes or until fish flakes easily with a fork.

4 SERVINGS

PER SERVING: *218 calories, 5 grams fat, 1 gram saturated fat, 47 mg. cholesterol, 786 mg. sodium, 2 grams fiber*

OVEN-FRIED CATFISH

Fried catfish is very popular in the South. Created as a lower-fat alternative, we think fried-fish lovers will approve. You can substitute any lean or medium-fatty fish.

2 tablespoons nonfat or 1%
 milk
¼ cup egg substitute or 2 egg
 whites
½ cup yellow cornmeal
¼ teaspoon paprika

¼ teaspoon salt
¼ teaspoon onion or garlic
 powder
1 pound catfish fillets
½ teaspoon olive oil

1. In a shallow bowl, beat the milk and egg substitute together.
2. In another shallow bowl, combine the cornmeal and seasonings.
3. Dip each fish fillet in the egg substitute and then coat thoroughly with the cornmeal.
4. Coat a shallow baking dish with cooking spray and then add the olive oil, turning the dish to distribute the oil evenly.
5. Place the fish in a single layer in the baking dish.
6. Bake in a 500-degree oven for about 12 minutes or until fish flakes easily with a fork.

4 SERVINGS

PER SERVING: *203 calories, 6 grams fat, 1 gram saturated fat, 66 mg. cholesterol, 242 mg. sodium, 2 grams fiber*

*SALMON LOAF

1 can (16 ounces) salmon,
 drained
2 scallions, chopped
1 garlic clove, minced
1 stalk celery, chopped fine
¼ cup fresh parsley, chopped
1 cup oats
2 teaspoons dry mustard

1 tablespoon fresh lemon juice
¾ cup nonfat or 1% milk
1 tablespoon soy sauce
¼ cup egg substitute (or 2 egg
 whites)
fresh-ground pepper to taste
paprika

1. Coat a loaf pan or similar casserole dish with cooking spray.
2. In a large bowl, combine all ingredients except paprika.
3. Turn into prepared loaf pan or casserole and sprinkle with paprika.
4. Bake at 350 degrees for 35 minutes or until a crust forms.

8 SERVINGS

PER SERVING: *147 calories, 5 grams fat, 1 gram saturated fat, 25 mg. cholesterol, 468 mg. sodium, 1 gram fiber*

*TUNA TERIYAKI

The teriyaki-style sauce can be used for other fatty fish, such as salmon. If you have the time, try mincing 3 cloves of fresh garlic, 2 or 3 green onions, and an inch of fresh ginger (peeled) in place of the powdered form. Fresh garlic, onions, and ginger give it a much different, richer flavor than the powders. We make the extra effort for company. A good rule for baking fish at 475 degrees is to allow about 10 minutes per inch of thickness. Seven or 8 minutes will be enough for thinner salmon fillets. If broiling or grilling thick steaks— about 2 inches thick—allow 7 minutes per side, turning once.

It's not always possible to obtain tuna steaks that are exactly an inch thick, so adjust the baking time according to thickness, as indicated in the directions below.

2 pounds tuna steaks (about 1 inch thick, blue or yellow fin)
1 tablespoon olive oil
2 tablespoons soy sauce
1 teaspoon steak sauce

1 teaspoon lemon juice
½ teaspoon onion powder
½ teaspoon garlic powder
½ teaspoon ground ginger
¼ teaspoon fresh-ground black pepper

1. Preheat oven to 475 degrees.
2. Place all ingredients except for the tuna on a foil-lined baking sheet and mix them together with a spoon.
3. Swish the fish around in the mix until well coated on both sides with the seasonings.
4. Bake 8–12 minutes (10 minutes per inch of thickness) or until the fish flakes easily but remains soft to the touch. Do not overcook.

4 SERVINGS

PER SERVING: *349 calories, 14 grams fat, 3 grams saturated fat, 83 mg. cholesterol, 607 mg. sodium, 0 fiber*

MEAT

Beef

Compared with poultry and most seafood, beef is high in saturated fat. More and more health professionals are encouraging Americans to cut back on meat consumption, since eating meat, even just once a week, appears to be associated with an increased risk of heart disease and certain cancers. The risk is greater if your cholesterol level is above normal and there is a history of heart disease or cancer in your family. (Part of the problem associated with the consumption of meat, and with poultry and fish as well, is that the contaminants—including herbicides, pesticides, hormones, and antibiotics—that they have eaten are concentrated and stored in their fat cells. When you eat them, you consume far more of these undesirable elements than when you eat plant foods.)

If you do eat beef, I strongly encourage you to limit yourself to the low-fat cuts: top and bottom round, eye of round, sirloin tip, flank steak, London broil, tenderloin (including filet mignon, chateaubriand, fillet steak, and tournedos), and, of course, extra-lean hamburger. However, markets vary in the fat content they put into "lean" or "extra-lean" hamburger. "Extra-lean" may contain anywhere from 5 to 15 percent total fat. Sometimes you will find the percentage marked on the package. If it is not listed, ask. You can also ask the butcher to grind you some that's less than 10 percent fat, preferably 5 percent.

Whatever cut of beef you use, examine it carefully and trim all visible fat. Experiment with using beef as a condiment combined with lots of vegetables, as in Asian cooking.

*STEAK MARINADE

These two marinades for flank steak, London broil, or any other lean cut of beefsteak can be used for tasty oven or pan broiling or for outdoor grilling. The wine and soy sauce, like other acidic liquids, have a tenderizing effect. Marinate in a large covered bowl or plastic bag for at least two hours in the refrigerator, turning once or twice to be sure all of the meat has been well covered. (Sometimes recipes call for basting with a marinade, which is acceptable if the food continues to cook until it is brought up to the correct temperature. In all other cases, in order to prevent foodborne illness, be sure to dispose of the marinade after using; *do not allow cooked meat to come in contact with uncooked marinade.*)

The amounts are sufficient for 2 pounds of meat.

Basic marinade

2 teaspoons of olive oil
½ cup dry red wine (you can use white wine for light-colored meats)
¼ teaspoon Herb Salt (see Sea-

sonings section of this book)
1 bay leaf
1 teaspoon chives
1 small onion, minced

Asian marinade

2 teaspoons olive oil
¼ cup soy sauce
¼ cup dry red wine
4 garlic cloves, minced
4 scallions, minced

6 whole peppercorns
⅛ teaspoon ground coriander
1-inch cube fresh ginger, peeled and grated or minced

Olive oil contains approximately 35 calories and a little over 4 grams of fat per teaspoon. However, very little remains on the meat after it is removed from the marinade and cooked. The other ingredients provide negligible calories, including the wine, since the alcohol will evaporate and the sugar content is low. Soy sauce is high in sodium, but it is difficult to predict how much will penetrate or adhere to the meat. My guess is that the sodium content per serving—for example, assuming a serving size of 4½ ounces of flank steak—would be moderate, perhaps 300 milligrams.

*BAKED FLANK STEAK

1½ pounds flank steak
1 tablespoon olive oil
1 cup hot water
1 bay leaf
1 large garlic clove, crushed
1 teaspoon salt

4 tablespoons minced celery
¼ teaspoon fresh-ground black pepper
2 teaspoons lemon juice
1 medium carrot, diced
¼ medium bell pepper, diced

1. Trim away any visible fat from the steak. Sear the steak in the oil over medium to medium-high heat. Place the steak in a casserole dish.
2. For extra flavoring, pour the water into the skillet you seared the meat in, and stir. Pour this over the meat, then add all the other ingredients.
3. Cook, uncovered, at 350 degrees for 30 minutes, or longer if you prefer your meat well done.

Light Gravy (optional): Heat 1 tablespoon vegetable oil, and stir in 2 tablespoons whole-wheat flour. Take a cup of liquid from the meat and stir into the roux. Stir until thickened, and serve over the meat

MAKES 4 SERVINGS, 4 ½ OUNCES EACH, PLUS SAUCE, BUT WITHOUT OPTIONAL GRAVY

PER SERVING: *273 calories, 12 grams fat, 2 grams saturated fat, 88 mg. cholesterol, 630 mg. sodium, 1 gram fiber (gravy adds 30 calories and 3 grams of fat; nutrient values of the meat liquid and other ingredients are included in the original analysis)*

*POT ROAST

2 pounds eye of round (or other lean beef), cut in 2-inch cubes
2 cups sliced onions
4 garlic cloves, chopped
1 bell pepper, sliced
4 large stalks celery, cut in 2-inch pieces
6 medium carrots, cut in 2-inch pieces
3 large potatoes (about 2 pounds), cut in eighths

1 can (28 ounces) whole tomatoes
1 can (15 ounces) tomato sauce
1 tablespoon soy sauce
1 teaspoon Worcestershire sauce
1 cup beef stock
1 tablespoon dried basil
fresh-ground black pepper to taste

1. Place meat, onions, garlic, bell pepper, celery, carrots, and potatoes in large roasting pan.

2. Cover with canned tomatoes, tomato sauce, soy sauce, Worcestershire, and stock. Sprinkle with basil and pepper.

3. Bake covered at 350 degrees for 45 minutes. Reduce heat to 250 degrees and bake for 3 hours or until meat is very tender to the fork. Baste occasionally.

6 SERVINGS

PER SERVING *(4 ounces cooked beef with assorted vegetables): 473 calories, 8 grams fat, 3 grams saturated fat, 78 mg. cholesterol, 667 mg. sodium, 8 grams fiber*

Pork

As with beef, some cuts of pork are lean. Tenderloin, butt, blade, and sirloin each run about 30 to 35 percent fat, with from about 9 to 12 grams of fat per 3½-ounce serving. Combined with vegetable side dishes, fresh salad, and whole-grain bread, or used in an Asian-style main dish, pork will not contribute an excessive amount of fat to your diet. Taken packaged right from the meat counter, however, even these lean cuts may still have considerable fat remaining, so be sure to trim them well.

Compared with the cuts of pork I have mentioned, bacon may contain over twice the fat and calories, and much more sodium. Try substituting lean ham or Canadian bacon (half the fat of regular bacon) in your own recipes that call for bacon. Many people have found "turkey bacon" to be a satisfactory replacement. It is only 5 percent fat (a little over 1 gram per ounce).

*FRAGRANT PORK ROAST

This is tender, moist, and redolent of the herbs that flavor it. It smells wonderful while it roasts.

1 pound pork tenderloin
1 stalk leafy celery, sliced
½ small onion, sliced
1 garlic clove, slivered
1 rosemary sprig, or ¼ teaspoon dried

3 sage leaves, or ¼ teaspoon dried
1 sprig thyme, or ¼ teaspoon dried
1 teaspoon Dijon mustard
fresh-ground pepper to taste

1. Preheat oven to 325 degrees.
2. Place the pork tenderloin on a piece of aluminum foil that is a few inches longer than the length of the meat. Separate the tenderloin into 2 lengthwise sections. (This has probably already been done by the butcher; if not, simply cut it right down the middle.)
3. In a small bowl, combine the celery, onion, garlic, rosemary, sage, and thyme; mix well.
4. Spread the flat side of both halves with mustard. Place one half flat side up, sprinkle with pepper, and top with an even layer of the vegetable mixture. Press the flat side of the remaining tenderloin half against the first so that the roast is assembled with vegetables and herbs sandwiched between the two halves.
5. Wrap foil snugly around the roast and fold ends over tightly to seal.
6. Bake for 1½–2 hours. Remove foil and let stand 5 minutes before serving.

4 SERVINGS

PER SERVING: *192 calories, 5 grams fat, 2 grams saturated fat, 90 mg. cholesterol, 89 mg. sodium, 0 fiber*

*PORK TENDERLOIN WITH ORANGE MARMALADE

1 pork tenderloin (1 pound)
1½ tablespoons grainy, course prepared mustard
1 garlic clove, minced
¼ teaspoon fresh rosemary, finely chopped

pinch fresh-ground black pepper
¼ cup low-sugar orange marmalade
½ cup water
¼ cup chicken stock

1. Make a cut lengthwise down the center about halfway through the pork tenderloin.
2. In a small bowl, mix together mustard, garlic, rosemary, and pepper. Spread mixture along the cut surface of the tenderloin.
3. Reshape and tie in several places. Place on rack above roasting pan.

4. Brush with 2 tablespoons marmalade. Add water to pan.
5. Bake in a 400-degree oven for 40–45 minutes or until internal temperature of meat reaches 160 degrees.
6. Mix together remaining marmalade and chicken stock in a small saucepan. Simmer 2–3 minutes until thickened. Spoon sauce over sliced tenderloin and serve immediately.

4 SERVINGS

PER SERVING: *160 calories, 3 grams fat, 1 gram saturated fat, 74 mg. cholesterol, 175 mg. sodium, 0 fiber*

VEGETABLE AND GRAIN SIDE DISHES

Fresh raw or steamed vegetables are a low-fat complement to any meal. Cooked in a microwave, vegetables retain their nutrients perhaps better than through any other way of cooking. Check your microwave manual for the simple instructions for cooking vegetables.

Leave edible skins on most vegetables and fruits, such as apples, carrots, and potatoes. The skins contain healthful nutrients and fiber, but wash them well to remove contaminants. (There are a number of products on the market, such as *Clean Greens!,* that may aid in the removal of contaminants. Check at your supermarket or health food store.)

Frozen vegetables are good to have on hand in a pinch, and because of the quick way in which they are processed, they are as nourishing as fresh. Many people find that canned vegetables have been overcooked, oversalted, or preserved with ingredients you may prefer to avoid, so read labels carefully.

Because of the role that hundreds of different phytochemicals may play in strengthening our immune systems and preventing cancer and heart disease, and because the various colors of different vegetables indicate the presence of different phytochemicals, health experts suggest that we eat vegetables of different colors every day. Red, green, and yellow are basic, but good advice is to "eat a rainbow" every day. For people who have difficulty digesting milk and milk products, and who are therefore in danger of having low intakes of calcium, remember that many leafy greens, such as collards, are good sources of calcium. And they contain no fat!

*ASPARAGUS WITH MUSTARD SAUCE

2 pounds asparagus	⅛ teaspoon salt
½ cup water	1 ½ teaspoons mustard seeds
1 tablespoon Dijon mustard	1 teaspoon olive oil
1 tablespoon lemon juice	

1. Wash asparagus; snap off and discard tough ends. Cut asparagus diagonally into 1-inch pieces.
2. Put asparagus and ½ cup water in a microwave-safe bowl and cover. Microwave on high for about 10 minutes, stirring every 3 minutes, until asparagus is just tender. Drain and set aside.
3. In a small bowl, combine mustard, lemon juice, and salt. Set aside.
4. In a large skillet, over medium heat, toast the mustard seeds in the olive oil, stirring constantly, for 1 minute.
5. Add asparagus and mustard mixture to the skillet. Cook about 2 minutes until heated through.

8 SERVINGS

PER SERVING: *37 calories, 1 gram fat, 0 saturated fat, 0 cholesterol, 86 mg. sodium, 3 grams fiber*

*BAKED BEETS AND POTATOES

This is another of our discoveries about foods that go remarkably well with each other. It's great in chunks, but try it mashed smooth in a blender or food processor.

2 large beets, thinly sliced (about 10–12 oz.)	½ teaspoon sage
	½ teaspoon thyme
2 large potatoes, thinly sliced (about 1–1½ pounds)	½ teaspoon salt
	1 tablespoon chopped fresh parsley
1 large onion, thinly sliced	
2 tablespoons olive oil	1 garlic clove, minced
1 tablespoon lemon juice	fresh-ground pepper to taste
1 tablespoon water	

1. Coat a 2 ½-quart casserole with nonstick cooking spray.
2. In a large bowl, combine all ingredients.
3. Place in casserole and cover.
4. Bake at 350 degrees 45 minutes to 1 hour until beets are tender.
5. Uncover for the last 10 minutes if you like a drier top.

6 SERVINGS

PER SERVING: *152 calories, 5 grams fat, 1 gram saturated fat, 0 cholesterol, 240 mg. sodium, 3 grams fiber*

*BESSIE'S LIMA BEAN CASSEROLE

1 pound dried lima beans
6 cups water
1 tablespoon olive oil + 1 table-
 spoon water
6 large carrots, cut in bite-
 sized chunks
½ bunch of celery (5–6 stalks),
 chopped

1 bunch fresh dill (¾ ounce),
 chopped
2 bunches scallions, chopped
2 ½-3 cups vegetable bouillon
2 cups tomato sauce
1 teaspoon salt, or to taste
fresh-ground pepper to taste
1 tablespoon olive oil

1. In a large ceramic, glass, or stainless steel bowl, soak limas in 6 cups water overnight.
2. The next day, drain and rinse the limas and set aside.
3. In a large pot, heat the olive oil + water and add the carrots, celery, dill, and scallions. Lower heat and sauté, partially covered, for 5 minutes, stirring frequently.
4. Add limas and vegetable bouillon and bring to a boil. Then, lower heat, cover, and let simmer about 45 minutes until beans are just tender.
5. Drain off any excess liquid and save for use in soups, stews, and the like.
6. Combine beans and vegetables with the tomato sauce, salt, and ground pepper.
7. Place in a large casserole, drizzle the 1 tablespoon of olive oil over the top, and bake in a 300-degree oven for 1 hour.

10 SERVINGS

PER SERVING: *117 calories, 3 grams fat, 1 gram saturated fat, 0 cholesterol, 580 mg. sodium, 6 grams fiber*

*BRAISED CABBAGE AND LEEKS

1 small cabbage (about 1 ½
  lbs.)
1 large leek
1 tablespoon olive oil
2 tablespoons marsala wine
⅓ cup water
½ teaspoon tarragon

¼ teaspoon celery seed
¼ teaspoon salt
1 tablespoon soy sauce
1 teaspoon paprika
fresh-ground black pepper to
  taste

1. Slice the cabbage in half and remove the core. Thinly slice the cabbage and shred or grate the core.
2. Slice the leek thinly.
3. In a large skillet, place the oil, marsala, and water and heat briefly over medium heat.
4. Add the cabbage, leek, tarragon, celery seed, and salt. Cover and cook, stirring occasionally, for about 10 minutes, until the cabbage is just tender.
5. Add the soy sauce, paprika, and black pepper and stir to combine.

8 SERVINGS

PER SERVING: *48 calories, 2 grams fat, 0 saturated fat, 0 cholesterol, 219 mg. sodium, 3 grams fiber*

BRAISED KOHLRABI

1 tablespoon olive oil
1¼ pounds kohlrabi, peeled
  and cut into ¼-inch julienne
  strips
1 small onion, chopped

1 teaspoon grated fresh ginger
1 cup vegetable bouillon
1 bay leaf
½ teaspoon salt
fresh-ground pepper to taste

1. In a small saucepan, sauté the kohlrabi, onion, and ginger over medium heat, stirring often, until they are just barely turning brown.
2. Add the remainder of the ingredients and bring to a boil.
3. Then, lower heat and simmer, partially covered, for about 15–20 minutes or until the kohlrabi is just tender.
4. Remove bay leaf and serve.

4 SERVINGS

PER SERVING: *79 calories, 4 grams fat, 0 saturated fat, 0 choles-terol, 325 mg. sodium, 6 grams fiber*

BRAISED SWISS CHARD

1 bunch swiss chard (about 8 leaves)
½ cup water
1 medium onion, chopped
1 garlic clove, minced

1 tablespoon olive oil
½ teaspoon balsamic vinegar
¼ teaspoon salt
fresh-ground pepper to taste

1. Remove the center rib from each chard leaf and cut it on the diagonal into 1 ½-inch pieces.
2. Place in a microwave-safe bowl and add ½ cup water. Cover and microwave on high for 4 minutes.
3. Meanwhile, stack the leaves and cut them lengthwise down the middle. Then, cut crosswise into 1 ½-inch strips.
4. When the stems have cooked for 4 minutes, add the leaves and cook on high for an additional 4–6 minutes until tender.
5. In a skillet, sauté the onions and garlic in the oil until the onions are tender.
6. When the chard is tender, add it and the cooking liquid to the skillet and toss to combine.
7. Add the salt, pepper, and balsamic vinegar and stir to combine. Serve.

4 SERVINGS

PER SERVING: *60 calories, 4 grams fat, 0.5 grams saturated fat, 0 cholesterol, 351 mg. sodium, 2 grams fiber*

*CAULIFLOWER SAUTÉ

1 cauliflower, cut in bite-sized chunks
½ cup water + extra water if necessary
½ teaspoon vegetable bouillon powder
1 tablespoon olive oil
1 large leek, cleaned and sliced

4 ounces mushrooms, sliced
½ red bell pepper, sliced thin
½ teaspoon chili powder
½ teaspoon salt
¼ teaspoon ground nutmeg
fresh-ground pepper to taste
2 tablespoons Parmesan cheese (optional)

1. In a microwave-safe casserole, place cauliflower and ½ cup water. Cover and microwave on high for 6 minutes.
2. Meanwhile, in a large skillet heat the oil and sauté the leeks, mushrooms, and bell peppers, stirring frequently, until peppers are tender and leeks are starting to brown (about 3 minutes).
3. When cauliflower has been microwaved, remove it from its liquid with a slotted spoon and add it to the skillet mixture.
4. Measure the cauliflower liquid and add enough water to make ½ cup.
5. Add the liquid to the skillet along with the bouillon powder, chili powder, salt, and nutmeg. Partially cover and cook, stirring often, until cauliflower is tender and liquid has evaporated (about 6 minutes).
6. Add pepper to taste and Parmesan, if desired. Toss to combine and serve.

6 SERVINGS

PER SERVING: *66 calories, 3 grams fat, 1 gram saturated fat, 2 mg. cholesterol, 261 mg. sodium, 3 grams fiber*

Note: This is wonderful over mashed potatoes, or it can be served with any grain.

*COUSCOUS, CHICKPEAS, AND VEGETABLES

This is a big recipe and makes great leftovers. And, if you are like me (I'm normally not a fan of turnips), you won't believe how good the turnips taste in this dish.

2 cups vegetable or chicken
  bouillon, divided
1½ cups couscous, dry
1 tablespoon olive oil
1 small onion, thinly sliced
black pepper to taste
1 teaspoon salt
⅛ teaspoon cayenne (optional)
2 small carrots, thinly sliced
1 teaspoon ground cumin
¼ teaspoon cinnamon

1 small turnip, cut in match-
  stick pieces
1 small green or red bell pepper, diced
1 medium zucchini, quartered
  lengthwise and cut in ½-inch
  slices
1 can (15 ounces) chickpeas,
  drained and rinsed
2 tablespoons fresh parsley,
  chopped

1. In a small saucepan bring 1½ cups of the bouillon to a boil.
2. Add the couscous, stir, cover, and set aside.
3. Heat the oil in a 6-quart kettle and sauté the onions, covered, over low heat until they are translucent.
4. Add the remaining bouillon and the pepper, salt, and cayenne, if desired.
5. Bring to a boil and add the carrots, cumin, and cinnamon.
6. Lower heat, cover, and cook for 3 minutes.
7. Add the turnip and bell pepper.
8. Cook about 5 minutes more until the turnip is tender.
9. Add the zucchini, chickpeas, and parsley and cook until the zucchini is tender.
10. Add the cooked couscous, toss to blend, correct the seasonings, and serve.

10 SERVINGS

PER SERVING: *173 calories, 2 grams fat, 0 saturated fat, 0 cholesterol, 378 mg. sodium, 4 grams fiber*

*GLAZED ORANGE-SPICE CARROTS

2½ cups carrots, thinly sliced
water
½ cup orange juice
1½ teaspoons cornstarch

⅛ teaspoon ground ginger
⅛ teaspoon nutmeg
fresh cilantro or parsley sprigs
  (optional)

1. Steam carrots in a steamer over boiling water until just tender.
2. Meanwhile, combine orange juice, cornstarch, ginger, and nutmeg in a saucepan. Heat over medium heat until sauce begins to thicken.
3. Stir in carrots and heat through. Serve garnished with cilantro or parsley sprigs if desired.

4 SERVINGS

PER SERVING: *48 calories, 0 fat, 0 saturated fat, 0 cholesterol, 24 mg. sodium, 2 grams fiber*

*LEMON BROCCOLI RISOTTO

Broccoli mixture

1 pound broccoli, flowerets cut
  into bite-sized chunks; stems
  diced and kept separate from
  flowerets
6 cups vegetable broth or bouil-
  lon

grated rind of ½ lemon
juice of ½ lemon
1 teaspoon grated fresh ginger
½ teaspoon salt
fresh-ground pepper to taste

Rice mixture

1 small onion, chopped
2 garlic cloves, minced
2 tablespoons olive oil

1½ cups brown rice, uncooked
¼ cup grated Parmesan cheese
  (optional)

1. In a large saucepan, bring the broth to a boil.
2. Put broccoli flowerets in broth, lower heat, and simmer for 3 minutes.
3. Remove flowerets with a slotted spoon and reserve.

4. Add broccoli stems, grated lemon rind, lemon juice, ginger, salt, and pepper. Simmer for 5 minutes.
5. Meanwhile, in another saucepan, sauté onion and garlic in olive oil over medium heat until onion is softened.
6. Add rice, stirring until coated with oil.
7. Place rice mixture in a large baking dish.
8. Bring broth mixture to a boil and pour over rice.
9. Bake, uncovered, in a 350-degree oven for 45 minutes.
10. Mix in reserved broccoli flowerets and Parmesan cheese, if desired, and bake until all the liquid has been absorbed (about 15 minutes).

12 SERVINGS

PER SERVING *(including Parmesan):* 130 calories, 4 grams fat, 1 gram saturated fat, 2 mg. cholesterol, 161 mg. sodium, 2 grams fiber

*MACARONI AND CHEESE

1 tablespoon olive oil
1 tablespoon water
1 small onion, finely chopped
¼ cup whole-wheat flour
2 cups skim milk
1 cup 2% cottage cheese
2 tablespoons shredded ched-
  dar cheese
½ cup wheat germ
1 tablespoon nutritional yeast
1 teaspoon paprika

1 teaspoon dried mustard
¼ teaspoon garlic powder
1 teaspoon salt
¼ teaspoon crushed red pepper
fresh-ground black pepper to
  taste
2 cups cooked macaroni
3 tablespoons your favorite
  brand of dry commercial
  stuffing

1. Heat oil and water in a skillet; add onion and cook over medium heat until tender.
2. Add flour and stir to mix.
3. In a food processor or blender, process cottage cheese and cheddar cheese until smooth and creamy. Set aside.
4. Add milk to skillet mixture in small amounts and stir until smooth; heat, stirring, until mixture begins to thicken.

5. Stir in cheeses, wheat germ, yeast, and spices and mix until smooth.
6. Stir in macaroni and pour into a 1-quart casserole that has been coated with cooking spray.
7. Top with stuffing mix and bake in a 350-degree oven for 25–30 minutes.

8 SERVINGS

PER SERVING: *179 calories, 4 grams fat, 1 gram saturated fat, 5 mg. cholesterol, 511 mg. sodium, 2 grams fiber*

*MASHED CARROTS AND PARSNIPS

Another illustration, along with our Creamy Carrot-Parsnip Soup, of how well carrots and parsnips go together.

6 carrots, cut in chunks   *½ teaspoon rosemary*
3 parsnips, cut in chunks   *½ teaspoon thyme*
water to cover   *¼ teaspoon salt*
1 tablespoon olive oil   *fresh-ground pepper to taste*
1 tablespoon soy sauce

1. In a large saucepan, place carrots, parsnips, and water to cover.
2. Bring to a boil; then lower heat, cover, and simmer until tender.
3. Drain vegetables and add oil, soy sauce, rosemary, and thyme.
4. Mash and add salt and pepper to taste.

6 SERVINGS

PER SERVING: *118 calories, 3 grams fat, 0 saturated fat, 0 cholesterol, 302 mg. sodium, 5 grams fiber*

Note: Vegetable water can be saved in a plastic container in the refrigerator or freezer for use in soups and stews.

MEDITERRANEAN-STYLE SPINACH

This method of preparation can be used with just about any variety of greens, fresh, or frozen.

2 garlic cloves, crushed
1 tablespoon olive oil
2 packages (10 ounces each) frozen chopped spinach, defrosted and drained

¼ teaspoon salt
fresh-ground black pepper to taste
2 tablespoons feta cheese

1. In a 2-quart saucepan sauté the garlic in the olive oil until translucent.
2. Add spinach, salt, and pepper, and mix and cook, covered, for about 5–7 minutes.
3. Add feta cheese and toss to blend.

4 SERVINGS

PER SERVING: *77 calories, 5 grams fat, 1 gram saturated fat, 4 mg. cholesterol, 330 mg. sodium, 3 grams fiber*

*MIXED GREENS WITH ORANGES AND OLIVES

1 navel orange, peeled and sectioned
½ small red onion, sliced thin
1 garlic clove, crushed
1 tablespoon fresh parsley, chopped
1½ tablespoons olive oil

1 teaspoon brown rice vinegar
pinch ground cumin
¼ teaspoon salt and fresh-ground pepper to taste
5 cups mixed salad greens
12 Greek black olives

1. Cut orange sections into bite-sized chunks. Place in a large bowl.
2. Add onion, garlic, parsley, oil, vinegar, and cumin. Mix well.
3. Add mixed greens and salt and pepper to taste.
4. Toss well and divide into 4 small salad bowls.
5. Place 3 olives on each salad and serve.

4 SERVINGS

PER SERVING: *89 calories, 6 grams fat, 0.5 gram saturated fat, 0 cholesterol, 274 mg. sodium, 2 grams fiber*

*OVEN-FRIED POTATO STICKS

A lower-fat alternative to deep fat–fried French fries. You'll love them!

*4 medium potatoes
1 tablespoon olive oil
⅛ teaspoon garlic powder
⅛ teaspoon onion powder*

*1 ½ teaspoons paprika
¼ teaspoon salt
¼ teaspoon fresh-ground black
  pepper*

1. Wash the potatoes well, and slice them lengthwise into strips, leaving the skins on.
2. Line a shallow baking pan with foil, and put all the ingredients into the pan, tossing well to coat the potatoes with the oil and seasonings.
3. Bake at 425 degrees for about 35 minutes, stirring often, until the potatoes are tender. Adjust the seasonings as you desire.

4 SERVINGS

PER SERVING *(about 1 cup): 178 calories, 4 grams fat, 0 saturated fat, 0 cholesterol, 142 mg. sodium, 4 grams fiber*

*PARMESAN-DILL BRUSSELS SPROUTS

*1 pound fresh Brussels sprouts
¼ cup water
½ teaspoon salt
1 tablespoon fresh lemon juice
1 tablespoon grated Parmesan
  cheese*

*2 teaspoons olive oil (or butter,
  melted)
½ teaspoon dried dill weed
fresh-ground black pepper to
  taste*

1. Wash sprouts and remove tough outer leaves. Make a shallow cut in the bottom of the stems. If some of the sprouts are very large you may want to halve them.

2. Microwave in a shallow bowl or casserole, covered lightly, with the water and salt for 7–9 minutes on high, stirring after 4 minutes.
3. When tender, drain, place in serving dish, and toss with remaining ingredients.

4 SERVINGS

PER SERVING: *77 calories, 3 grams fat, 0 saturated fat, 0 cholesterol, 293 mg. sodium, 6 grams fiber*

POTATO CASSEROLE

2 tablespoons olive oil
2 medium onions, sliced very thin
2 garlic cloves, minced
1 teaspoon caraway seed
2 pounds potatoes, sliced very thin
1 teaspoon salt
1 cup nonfat or 1% milk
1 cup part-skim ricotta
fresh-ground black pepper to taste
paprika

1. In a large skillet, heat oil slightly and then sauté onions, garlic, and caraway over medium heat, partially covered, until onions are tender (about 10 minutes).
2. Add potatoes, salt, and pepper and cook another 2 minutes.
3. Put potato mixture into a large, flat casserole that has been coated with cooking spray.
4. In a bowl, blend milk and ricotta; pour over potatoes.
5. Sprinkle with paprika.
6. Cover with foil and bake at 350 degrees for 30 minutes. Uncover and bake 30 minutes more until the potatoes are tender.

10 SERVINGS

PER SERVING: *148 calories, 5 grams fat, 2 grams saturated fat, 8 mg. cholesterol, 282 mg. sodium, 2 grams fiber*

*POTATOES AU GRATIN

*3½ cups potatoes, peeled and
  finely chopped
½ cup 2% cottage cheese
½ cup buttermilk
1 tablespoon fresh chives,
  chopped
1 tablespoon fresh parsley,
  chopped*

*2 teaspoons cornstarch
½ teaspoon salt
¼ teaspoon fresh-ground pepper
½ cup (2 ounces) reduced-fat
  cheddar cheese
⅛ teaspoon paprika*

1. Cook the potatoes in boiling water for 8 minutes, or until just tender. Drain and set aside.
2. Combine the cottage cheese and buttermilk in a food processor or blender; process until smooth.
3. Transfer to a bowl and stir in the potatoes, chives, parsley, cornstarch, salt, and pepper.
4. Spoon into a 1 ½-quart casserole that has been coated with cooking spray and bake, uncovered, for 20 minutes at 350 degrees.
5. Sprinkle with cheese and paprika and bake an additional 5–10 minutes or until cheese is melted and bubbly.

6 SERVINGS

PER SERVING: *123 calories, 2 grams fat, 0 saturated fat, 3 mg. cholesterol, 397 mg. sodium, 2 grams fiber*

*POTATOES AND SPINACH

*1 pound small potatoes,
  scrubbed
water to cover
1 large bunch fresh spinach,
  washed
1 tablespoon olive oil*

*½ teaspoon dried garlic flakes
¼ teaspoon crushed red pepper
  (optional)
½ teaspoon salt
fresh-ground black pepper to
  taste*

1. Place potatoes in a large saucepan with water to cover.
2. Bring water to a boil; then lower heat and simmer potatoes, covered, until just tender (about 25–30 minutes).

3. While potatoes are cooking, remove and discard stems of spinach and coarsely chop the leaves.
4. When potatoes are just tender, remove from water with a slotted spoon and place in a 2½-quart casserole. Let cool.
5. Put chopped spinach in the potato water and cook until barely tender (about 3 minutes).
6. When potatoes are cool enough to handle, cut into bite-sized chunks.
7. When spinach is cooked, remove from water with a sieve or slotted spoon and add to potatoes.
8. In a small bowl combine all other ingredients and pour over potato-spinach mixture, tossing gently to coat.
9. Cover and heat in oven or microwave until hot.

6 SERVINGS

PER SERVING: *98 calories, 3 grams fat, 0 saturated fat, 0 cholesterol, 242 mg. sodium, 3 grams fiber*

*ROASTED MUSHROOMS, PEPPERS, AND ONIONS

8 ounces mushrooms, whole or halved
2 bell peppers, seeded and cut in chunks
1 large onion, cut in ½-inch rounds
1 tablespoon brown rice vinegar

2 tablespoons olive oil
2 teaspoons fresh thyme, chopped
1 teaspoon grated lemon peel
1 teaspoon grated fresh ginger
2 garlic cloves, crushed
¼ teaspoon salt
fresh-ground pepper to taste

1. Place vegetables in a medium-size bowl.
2. In a small bowl, combine remainder of ingredients.
3. Pour over vegetables and toss gently to coat.
4. Preheat oven to 450 degrees.
5. Place vegetables in a shallow pan in one layer.
6. Bake about 20 minutes, stirring occasionally, until vegetables are just tender.

4 SERVINGS

PER SERVING: *111 calories, 6 grams fat, 1 gram saturated fat, 0 cholesterol, 151 mg. sodium, 3 grams fiber*

Note: Using the same method, you can vary the vegetables (try summer squash, zucchini, leeks, carrots, fresh asparagus, or any of your choosing) as well as the seasonings (oregano and garlic make a nice combination).

*SPINACH CASSEROLE

6 tablespoons whole-wheat flour
½ teaspoon each onion powder and garlic powder
½ teaspoon salt
1 teaspoon dry mustard
dash of cayenne (optional)
1 tablespoon each fresh chopped chives, sage, and tarragon (if fresh herbs are unavailable, use 1 teaspoon each dried)

½ cup egg substitute (equivalent to 2 eggs)
2 packages (10 ounces each) frozen spinach, defrosted and drained
½ cup shredded reduced-fat cheddar cheese
1 cup plain fat-free yogurt
3 tablespoons breadcrumbs or your favorite dry commercial stuffing

1. In a large bowl, combine wheat flour, spices, herbs, and egg substitute, and beat until smooth.
2. Add spinach, cheese, and yogurt and blend.
3. Put into a casserole dish that has been coated with cooking spray, top with breadcrumbs or stuffing mix, and bake about 45 minutes at 350 degrees.

4 SERVINGS

PER SERVING: *165 calories, 2 grams fat, 1 gram saturated fat, 4 mg. cholesterol, 756 mg. sodium, 4 grams fiber*

STUFFED WINTER SQUASH

2 medium butternut or acorn
    squash
1 package (10 ounces) frozen
    baby lima beans, thawed
1 tablespoon olive oil + 1 table-
    spoon water
2 small onions, diced
2 small bell peppers, diced
2 garlic cloves, minced
1 teaspoon grated fresh ginger
¼ teaspoon crushed red pepper
    (optional)

1 ½ cups kernel corn, drained
1 teaspoon oregano
1 teaspoon thyme
½ teaspoon salt or to taste
¼ teaspoon nutmeg
fresh-ground black pepper to
    taste
4 tablespoons your favorite dry
    commercial stuffing or
    breadcrumbs

1. Cut squash in half lengthwise and scoop out seeds.
2. Place cut side down in a baking pan with a small amount of water in it.
3. Bake in a preheated oven at 350 degrees for 35–40 minutes until squash is tender when pierced with a fork.
4. Remove squash, drain, and let cool. Set aside.
5. Meanwhile, in a microwave-safe bowl, cook lima beans in ¼ cup water for about 8 minutes on high until tender. Drain and let cool.
6. Heat oil + water in a saucepan. Add onion, peppers, garlic, ginger, and crushed red pepper, if desired, and sauté 5–7 minutes until onions are translucent.
7. Add lima beans, corn, oregano, thyme, salt, nutmeg, and black pepper.
8. Cook over low heat for 5 minutes, stirring often.
9. Scoop squash from the shells, coarsely chop, and mix with vegetables in saucepan.
10. Fill squash shells with vegetables, sprinkle with stuffing mix or breadcrumbs, and bake in a 350-degree oven until slightly browned and heated through.

4 SERVINGS

PER SERVING: *293 calories, 5 grams fat, 1 gram saturated fat, 0 cholesterol, 512 mg. sodium, 13 grams fiber*

SWEET POTATO-PINEAPPLE CASSEROLE

2–3 sweet potatoes, boiled and peeled, or 1 can (40 ounces) sweet potatoes in light syrup, drained
1½ tablespoons butter
½ cup egg substitute or 2 whole eggs

1 teaspoon dried orange peel, minced
1 teaspoon cinnamon
1 teaspoon ground nutmeg
½ teaspoon salt
1 can (8 ounces) crushed pineapple

1. Mash the sweet potatoes.
2. Beat in the butter, egg substitute, orange peel, cinnamon, nutmeg, and salt.
3. Stir in the pineapple.
4. Turn into a 1½-quart casserole that has been coated with cooking spray.
5. Cover and bake in a 350-degree oven for 45 minutes.

8 SERVINGS

PER SERVING: *103 calories, 2 grams fat, 1 gram saturated fat, 6 mg. cholesterol, 200 mg. sodium, 2 grams fiber*

*TRI-COLOR PEPPER SAUTÉ

This beautiful recipe tastes as good as it looks. You can make it with just one kind of bell pepper if you like, but the three colors make it especially attractive.

6 medium bell peppers, 2 each red, yellow, and green
2 tablespoons olive oil
1 teaspoon red wine vinegar
½ teaspoon sugar
⅓ cup drained capers

4 tablespoons drained, chopped pimiento-stuffed olives
2 teaspoons dried oregano, crushed

1. Remove stems and seeds from peppers and cut into quarters.
2. Sauté, covered, in the oil until softened.
3. Mix in the remaining ingredients.

4. Simmer, covered, for about 20 minutes, or until peppers are tender but not mushy.

6 SERVINGS

PER SERVING: *90 calories, 5 grams fat, 1 gram saturated fat, 0 cholesterol, 229 mg. sodium, 3 grams fiber*

DESSERTS

When men overeat on fat, it is most often obtained from meat and meat products, while when women consume too much fat it is more often obtained from desserts and other foods that combine sugar and fat. You must take notice from people who have lost weight and successfully maintained their losses: some amount of restraint when it comes to high-fat foods, including desserts, is necessary.

If, as a rule, you follow the guidelines of the T-Factor 2000 Diet, an occasional dessert will not result in your regaining weight; nor will it interfere with losing weight, if you do not exceed your fat gram goals. However, I strongly suggest that you severely limit processed commercial desserts from your diet, both high-fat and fat-free but energy-dense varieties that can lead to overconsumption. Comparatively low-fat desserts that you can easily make yourself, such as the versions of popular desserts contained in this section, will be satisfying and helpful in weight management.

Once you begin experimenting with recipes for low-fat desserts, you will find ways to adapt many of your own favorites. The use of low-fat dairy products instead of their high-fat counterparts (skim milk instead of whole milk; half-and-half instead of cream; ricotta, Neufchâtel, or part mashed tofu instead of all cream cheese, for example) can reduce fat content considerably.

Substitute whole-wheat flour at least in part for refined white flour, for higher fiber and higher nutrient content. Use fresh and dried fruits for sweetness and reduce refined sugar. Instead of making fatty pastry crusts with lard, butter, or vegetable shortening, make crumb crusts with very little fat and honey, as in the Berry Crisp and Pumpkin Cheesecake recipes you will find in this section.

When the recipe permits, such as for cookies, cakes, and some pies, try freezing a portion so that one recipe can be used on two or more occasions. If you pack lunches, avoid high-fat commercial products by including a serving of a homemade dessert.

*BERRY CRISP

Filling
4 cups berries (any kind)

½ cup sugar

2 tablespoons cornstarch

Topping
1 cup rolled oats

3 tablespoons whole-wheat flour

1 teaspoon cinnamon

¼ teaspoon salt

¼ cup firmly packed brown sugar

3 tablespoons light olive oil

2 tablespoons orange juice

1. Coat a 7-inch casserole or a 9-inch pie pan with cooking spray.
2. Place berries, sugar, and cornstarch in a large bowl and combine.
3. Place berry mixture in casserole or pie pan.
4. Combine all topping ingredients in the same bowl that you used for the berry mixture.
5. Distribute topping evenly over berries.
6. Bake at 350 degrees for 35–40 minutes until berries are tender and juice is thickened.

8 SERVINGS

PER SERVING: *211 calories, 5 grams fat, 3 grams saturated fat, 12 mg. cholesterol, 52 mg. sodium, 4 grams fiber*

CAROB BROWNIES

4 tablespoons + ½ teaspoon light olive oil

½ cup carob powder

1 cup sugar

½ cup egg substitute

1 teaspoon vanilla

1 cup all-purpose flour

1 teaspoon baking powder

¼ teaspoon salt

¼ cup plain nonfat yogurt

½ cup walnuts, chopped

1. Preheat oven to 350 degrees.
2. Use the ½ teaspoon olive oil to lightly oil an 8-inch square baking pan.
3. In a medium-size bowl, combine the 4 tablespoons olive oil with the carob powder. Stir until smooth.
4. Stir in the sugar and mix well.
5. Add the egg substitute and vanilla and stir.
6. Add the flour, baking powder, and salt and mix.
7. Stir in the yogurt and then the walnuts.
8. Place in baking pan and bake for 30 minutes. Do not overcook. Cool on wire rack before cutting.

16 SQUARES

PER SQUARE: *144 calories, 6 grams fat, 1 gram saturated fat, 0 cholesterol, 84 mg. sodium, 2 grams fiber*

Note: This recipe works equally well with cocoa powder instead of carob.

CHESS SQUARES

These squares were inspired by my neighbor, Elizabeth Smith, who favored the whole neighborhood for many years with samples of her fantastic Chess Squares. *Nobody* could make them like Elizabeth, even though she was most generous in sharing her recipe. The original, of course, has real eggs and *lots* of margarine. Nevertheless, Elizabeth agreed that these are a tasty alternative.

1 box (16 ounces) light brown sugar
½ cup light olive oil
½ cup plain nonfat yogurt
½ cup white sugar
1 cup egg substitute

1 teaspoon vanilla
1 ⅓ cups whole-wheat flour
⅔ cup soy flour
1 ½ teaspoons baking powder
½ teaspoon salt
1 cup walnuts, chopped

1. Coat a 13 × 9–inch baking pan with cooking spray.
2. In a 2-quart saucepan, heat brown sugar in light olive oil over low heat, stirring often, for about 5 minutes. Remove from heat.

3. Add yogurt, white sugar, egg substitute, and vanilla. Mix until smooth.
4. Combine wheat and soy flours, baking powder, and salt. Stir into sugar mixture.
5. Add nuts and stir to combine.
6. Pour into prepared pan and bake in a 350-degree oven for 25–30 minutes.
7. Cool on rack before cutting.

3 2   S Q U A R E S

P E R   S E R V I N G :   *150 calories, 6 grams fat, 1 gram saturated fat, 0 cholesterol, 62 mg. sodium, 1 gram fiber*

*COCOA ZUCCHINI CAKE

This cake is moist and lightly sweet, with a satisfying, rich texture.

1 ¼ cups granulated sugar
½ cup canola oil
1 teaspoon vanilla extract
½ cup egg substitute
½ cup skim or 1% milk
1 teaspoon baking soda
1½ cups all-purpose flour

1 cup whole-wheat flour
¼ cup cocoa powder
½ teaspoon cinnamon
½ teaspoon salt
2 cups grated zucchini, un-
*   peeled (about 1½ squashes)*

1. Combine first 5 ingredients in a large bowl.
2. In another bowl, sift together the baking soda, flours, cocoa, cinnamon, and salt.
3. Add dry ingredients alternately with the zucchini to the first mixture.
4. Bake at 350 degrees for 1 hour in a Bundt pan that has been coated with cooking spray, or for 45 minutes in a 9 × 13 × 2–inch baking pan.
5. Let stand 5–10 minutes before removing from pan.

2 4   S E R V I N G S

PER SERVING: *137 calories, 5 grams fat, 1 gram saturated fat, 0 cholesterol, 90 mg. sodium, 1 gram fiber*

*DIKKIE'S CHOCOLATE CHIP MERINGUE COOKIES

This delicious cookie can be made equally well with fresh egg whites (use 2). My friend Dikkie Schoggen, whose recipe this is, says meringues made in humid weather may not turn out successfully.

4 teaspoons powdered egg whites
4 tablespoons warm water
½ cup sugar
1 teaspoon vanilla

3 tablespoons plain cocoa powder
½ cup semisweet chocolate chips

1. Preheat oven to 250 degrees.
2. Line 2 cookie sheets with foil and set aside.
3. Put the powdered egg whites and the warm water in a mixing bowl and whisk until all the powder is dissolved.
4. With an electric mixer, beat the egg whites at medium high speed until they hold stiff peaks.
5. Beat in the sugar 1 tablespoon at a time.
6. Add the vanilla.
7. Reduce the speed to low and beat in the cocoa powder.
8. Fold in the chocolate chips with a rubber spatula.
9. Drop mixture by rounded teaspoonful onto cookie sheets, spacing the cookies 1 inch apart.
10. Bake for 1 hour; then, turn oven off but let the cookies dry out there for 2 more hours.
11. Remove from cookie sheets and store in an airtight container.

ABOUT 40 COOKIES

PER SERVING: *22 calories, 1 gram fat, 0.5 gram saturated fat, 0 cholesterol, 3 mg. sodium, 0 fiber*

DIKKIE'S MANGO SORBET

*2–3 mangoes, peeled and
  puréed (about 2 cups)*
½ cup fresh orange juice

1 tablespoon fresh lime juice
2 tablespoons honey

1. Mix all ingredients until well blended.
2. Chill for at least 1 hour.
3. Pour into an ice cream freezer (such as Donvier), and process according to the manufacturer's directions.

4 SERVINGS

PER SERVING: *101 calories, 0 fat, 0 saturated fat, 0 cholesterol, 2 mg. sodium, 2 grams fiber*

*ELEGANT PEARS

This is especially good with coffee liqueur.

2 large pears
3 cups of water
*½ cup Hershey's chocolate
  syrup*

1 ounce of liqueur of choice
*1 cup vanilla ice milk or
  frozen yogurt*

1. Wash pears and cut in half.
2. Bring water to a boil in medium saucepan. Add pear halves, reduce heat, and cover. Cook until pears are soft, about 10–15 minutes.
3. While pears are cooking, combine chocolate syrup and liqueur and heat in a small saucepan or in microwave.
4. Drain pears, scoop out seeds, and wipe off excess moisture.
5. While still warm, top each pear half with ¼ cup ice milk.
6. Pour approximately 2 tablespoons of chocolate syrup mixture over pear and ice milk. Serve immediately.

4 SERVINGS

PER SERVING: *204 calories, 2 grams fat, 1 gram saturated fat, 5 mg. cholesterol, 58 mg. sodium, 4 grams fiber*

*GINGERBREAD

Adapted from Laura Ingalls Wilder's recipe. Serve this moist, sweet cake with warmed applesauce or lemon sauce.

1 cup packed brown sugar
¾ cup applesauce
1 cup molasses
2 teaspoons baking soda
1 cup boiling water
2¼ cups all-purpose flour
¾ cup whole-wheat flour
1 teaspoon ground ginger

1 teaspoon ground cinnamon
1 teaspoon ground allspice
1 teaspoon grated nutmeg
1 teaspoon ground cloves
½ teaspoon salt
2 eggs, beaten well, or ½ cup egg substitute

1. Preheat the oven to 350 degrees. Coat a 9 × 13–inch glass baking pan with cooking spray.
2. Combine the brown sugar, applesauce, and molasses in a large mixing bowl.
3. Stir the baking soda into the cup of boiling water and pour into the sugar mixture. Stir until blended.
4. In another bowl, combine the flours with the spices and salt.
5. Add to the sugar mixture with the eggs and mix well by hand.
6. Pour the batter into the prepared pan and bake for 30–40 minutes, until the gingerbread pulls slightly from the sides of the pan and springs back when touched in the center. Cool in pan or on wire rack.

16 SERVINGS

PER SERVING: *186 calories, 1 gram fat, 0 saturated fat, 13 mg. cholesterol, 189 mg. sodium, 2 grams fiber*

*PUMPKIN CHEESECAKE

This is the quintessential fall dessert but tasty anytime. You can omit the pumpkin, nutmeg, and cinnamon and have a delicious, light cheesecake that can be topped with berries or other fruit.

1½ cups graham cracker
  crumbs
2 tablespoons honey
1 tablespoon canola or light
  olive oil
2 whole eggs and 3 egg whites
  (or ¾ cup egg substitute)
8 ounces softened fat-free or
  light (Neufchâtel) cheese

12 ounces part-skim or light ricotta cheese
½ cup plain nonfat yogurt
1 can (15 ounces) pumpkin
¾ cup sugar
1 teaspoon vanilla
¼ teaspoon nutmeg'
¼ teaspoon cinnamon

1. Combine the graham cracker crumbs, honey, and oil. Mix well and press into a 9-inch pie pan.
2. In a mixing bowl, beat together the eggs and egg whites until foamy.
3. Add all other ingredients. Beat until smooth and creamy.
4. Pour into the crust and bake at 350 degrees until slightly browned and firm in the center (about 45 minutes).

10 SERVINGS

PER SERVING: *269 calories, 7 grams fat, 3 grams saturated fat, 55 mg. cholesterol, 316 mg. sodium, 2 grams fiber*

BEVERAGES

Although the research is inconsistent, I have never met an over-weight person for whom the daily use of diet drinks in place of good old water, fruit juice, or plain iced tea has been of any help in losing weight and maintaining the loss. In my experience, all they do is keep a person's taste for sweets alive. I remember an instance where a woman in one of our weight-management groups was consuming several diet drinks a day, and then finding herself out of control when she faced her favorite double chocolate cake and other sugar-sweetened *high-fat desserts*. She had a great deal of trouble losing weight. Does this sound a little like you? At least one long-term study has shown that people who drink diet drinks do *not* lose weight and keep it off as well as people who don't drink them! Please read my discussion of artificial sweeteners in Chapter 3 if you use them on a daily basis with the hope that they will help you manage your weight.

My first recommendation for no-cal beverages is WATER. Water is our most essential nutrient. We cannot live without it. If, like many people, you can't stand the taste of tap water, it may be that naturally occurring chemicals or those added in processing the water in your town have ruined the taste. Either try bottled spring water or install an activated charcoal, bacteriostatic filter for your kitchen faucet to remove chlorine and other objectionable organic matter from your water. Better yet, install a whole-house filter of this kind. You won't believe how much better your body will smell after a chlorine-free bath or shower, not to mention the air you breath while bathing. You can also try sodium-free seltzer water, either plain or with added lemon, lime, or other flavors, but with no sugar added. Check labels carefully.

I don't recommend drinking distilled water; essential minerals, including significant amounts of calcium and magnesium in many locations, will have been removed in the distilling process (they are not removed by charcoal filters).

Fruit and vegetable juices, herb teas, and combination 100 percent fruit or vegetable punches are also good substitutes for soft drinks. The calories they contain help reduce your appetite and prevent overconsumption of other foods.

Coffee and black and green tea can also serve as no-cal beverages. Add a little half-and-half or milk if desired, but count the fat grams accordingly. Both green and black tea contain powerful antioxidants that may help prevent cancer. As long as you limit yourself to no more than two cups of coffee (or perhaps three cups of tea) a day, you will probably suffer no ill effects from the caffeine. Most teas, particularly the green teas, have only about half the caffeine content of coffee. Instead of using any kind of sweetener, try adding a tablespoon of raisins to a cup of hot tea. The raisins will add a touch of raisin-flavored sweetness to the tea, and there will be a tasty little snack when you reach the bottom of the cup.

Because of increasing demand, it's now possible to obtain many varieties of decaffeinated coffee, but if you use them, buy water processed rather than those that are decaffeinated with methylene chloride. The packaging for prepackaged coffee will carry the words "water processed" if this process has been used. Methylene chloride is carcinogenic.

FRUIT SMOOTHIES

Fruit smoothies or shakes are popular as a breakfast drink or soothing snack. Here are two variations that are both delicious!

Strawberry-Kiwi-Banana Smoothie

1 cup nonfat vanilla yogurt
8 large strawberries, halved; stem removed
2 kiwi fruit, peeled and quartered

1 ripe banana, peeled and quartered
2 teaspoons of honey

Apricot Smoothie

½ cup plain nonfat yogurt
1 can (15¼ ounces) apricot halves in light syrup, drained; ¼ cup reserved

¼ cup light syrup from apricots
⅓ cup orange juice

1. In a food processor or blender, combine ingredients for either smoothie.
2. Process to a smooth consistency.
3. Refrigerate until ready to serve.

2 SERVINGS EACH

PER SERVING *(Strawberry-Kiwi-Banana Smoothie): 244 calories, 1 gram fat, 0 saturated fat, 2 mg. cholesterol, 89 mg. sodium, 5 grams fiber*

PER SERVING *(Apricot Smoothie): 198 calories, 0 fat, 0 saturated fat, 1 mg. cholesterol, 56 mg. sodium, 4 grams fiber*

HOLIDAY EGGNOG

3 cups nonfat milk
3 tablespoons sugar
3 egg yolks, lightly beaten
¾ teaspoon vanilla extract

¼ teaspoon rum flavoring or
  brandy flavoring
½ cup evaporated skim milk
½ teaspoon unflavored gelatin
grated nutmeg

1. Mix the milk, sugar, egg yolks, vanilla, and rum flavoring in a saucepan.
2. Heat over medium heat 7 to 8 minutes to just below boiling, or until the mixture starts to coat a spoon. It will thicken slightly.
3. Remove from heat and let cool. Place in refrigerator to chill completely. (This may be prepared a day in advance.)
4. Combine the evaporated milk and gelatin. Let stand 5 minutes.
5. Heat until gelatin is dissolved (about 1 minute in a microwave or in a small saucepan on the stove).
6. Using an electric mixer, beat the evaporated milk–gelatin mixture on high speed for 5 minutes, until it is whipped.
7. Fold the whipped evaporated milk into the refrigerated egg/milk mixture.
8. Ladle into punch cups, sprinkle with nutmeg, and serve.

8 SERVINGS

PER ½-CUP SERVING: *85 calories, 2 grams fat, 1 gram saturated fat, 82 mg. cholesterol, 68 mg. sodium, 0 fiber*

SPICED TEA

Pre-mixed instant teas and lemonades are usually high in sugar and additives. Here is a tangy alternative that lets you control the amount of sugar. Serve hot or over ice.

4 cups brewed black tea (4
  teabags)
2 cinnamon sticks
1 cup fresh orange juice (or
  orange-pineapple blend)
1 to 2 teaspoons of sugar (or

sugar substitute, if you desire)
1 teaspoon ground cloves
1 to 2 teaspoons lemon juice,
  or 4 slices fresh lemon

1. When brewing the tea, place cinnamon sticks in the same pan or teapot. When the tea is ready, discard the cinnamon sticks.
2. Add the remaining ingredients to the pot and serve, or chill first in a pitcher and serve over ice.

4 SERVINGS

PER SERVING: *38 calories, 0 fat, 0 saturated fat, 0 cholesterol, 9 mg. sodium, 0 fiber*

CHAPTER 9

How to Find the Slimmer, Vigorous You Hidden Inside an Overweight Body

If you are an overweight person who has never in your life culti-vated the athletic potential that lies hidden in your body, I wish I could take you from this moment to a year or two into the future. I'd like to be able to transport you to the time when you have al-ready lost the weight you'd like to lose and have been transformed into the active person I'd like to help you become. I thought about this early this morning, as I jogged around the neighborhood with my dogs. I wished once again, as I have wished many times in my career as a health psychologist trying to help overweight people, that I could take the feelings I had inside me and put them inside of you and all the fat people in this world who either hate exercise or cannot be persuaded to give it the priority it deserves in their lives. If I could, you would never be fat again.

Thirty-five years ago I was a fat man. Lugging 230 pounds around, I'd be out of breath climbing a flight of stairs. I was hypertensive and ended up with a minor coronary just a few months after taking my first job as an assistant professor of psychology at Vanderbilt Uni-versity. I was thirty-five years old.

This morning, as a much healthier, more vigorous fellow weigh-ing in at 160 pounds and in my seventy-first year, I did a four-mile tour of the neighborhood with my animal companions. We stopped a couple of times for short chats with a few of the many neighbors who have become our friends during the thirty-five years we have lived in the area. Getting to know just about all of the 205 families in the neighborhood (and every single dog and cat) has been one of the great rewards of my daily tours. Along about 4:30 or 5:00 P.M. every day, Kaycee and Bismarck, my two German shepherds, and Sheba, the Akita, come to get me and we are off again for at least a couple of miles. Walking or jogging together is as much a part of their lives as it is mine. They expect it. In fact, they demand it and they can be insistent if I'm slow to get ready.

During these past thirty-five years I have been a different person than the person I was in my first thirty-five years. In the two years after my heart attack I think I went through a personality transformation. I went from a person who had never engaged in any kind of physical activity in my life to a tennis player who began to win local tournaments and soon had a shelf full of trophies to show for it. I began to think of myself as a tennis player and it became a part of my self-concept. Thinking of myself as a tennis player, slim and physically fit, was as important to my personal identity as being a psychologist, college professor, husband, and father of two children.

As the years went on, I became interested in a number of other physical activities. I began jogging when I was fifty years old, and now that I can no longer play competitive tennis as a result of a torn rotator cuff, walking and jogging have become as essential a part of my daily life as tennis was before my injury. I am not built for running, and I rarely go very fast, but I wish I could adequately describe the exhilaration I experienced the first time I ran a quarter-mile in ninety seconds. Never in my life as a fat man who hated to walk an unnecessary block would I have believed it possible.

I was jogging at sunset on the track at David Lipscomb University, which is just about a mile from my home, with my wife and a couple of other friends. It had been a lovely fall day, cool and dry. The fall colors in the leaves on the trees across the street from the track were at their height, and intensified by the brilliance of the sunset. Everything around was bathed in a golden light.

I had been alternating my "cruising" mile-in-ten-minutes pace with my real "workout" pace of a mile in eight minutes. (As I said, I was not a fast runner.) I can't really say what made me want to challenge myself, but I was wearing a watch with a second hand and decided to see if I could round the quarter-mile track in ninety seconds rather than two minutes. It must have been the adrenaline and the endorphins, but by the time I was halfway around I was overcome with excitement—I could not believe it was me flying through space. I don't remember my feet touching the ground. I made it right on the ninetieth second, and I went mentally and emotionally sky-high. Thereafter I knew that whenever I felt like it, I could always end up with a "runner's high" by adding a few speedy intervals to my longer jogs. I also knew that I could go a lot faster than I ever thought possible.

I frequently jogged at lunchtime, or in the late afternoon when I had finished work, going several times around a one-mile loop in Nashville's Centennial Park. The loop circles a full-scale replica of the Parthenon, a small lake, and some beautiful gardens. Because it is so attractive, as well as being a measured mile, it's a favorite place for many local runners to work out. Jogging there led to making the acquaintance of two of the serious marathon runners who trained at a mile-in-5-minutes pace. They would, of course, zip by the slower runners like myself. But occasionally one of the young men would slow down "to rest" at a mere mile-in-6-minutes pace, and I would accelerate to join him for a half-mile. The first time I did this the young fellow, who was a good thirty years younger than I was, gave me a "way to go," and a pat on the back as we parted. It was a real turn-on.

A couple of years after I took up jogging, I began to do some bicycle touring, thirty or forty miles a day and sometimes even fifty or sixty miles. I've toured Yellowstone and Grand Teton National Parks on my bicycle, pedaled across the continental divides in both the Rockies and the Appalachians carrying camping gear on my back and in my wheel bags, and covered a considerable section of the beautiful Natchez Trace Parkway, sometimes racing the deer alongside the road. When we take vacations together in our home state of Tennessee, Enid and I think first of which hiking trails we'd like to cover in one of our beautiful state parks. Fat men don't do these things—but then, I am not a fat man anymore and haven't been for thirty-five years.

How can I help you discover the joy that awaits you if you become an active person? As a sedentary, overweight person, you are missing out on some great experiences that can only be known by people who lose the weight *and* get in good physical condition.

All the research on maintenance after a person has lost a significant amount of weight shows that physical activity is at least as important as adherence to a low-fat diet. But I don't think that lecturing on the physical benefits of exercise, either for weight control or car-

diovascular health, can by themselves sustain your motivation to become *and remain* an active person. The key is psychological and
emotional.

You must find some activity that contributes to your self-concept
and builds your self-esteem. Physical activity is not to be taken like
a dose of medicine. If you choose an activity that requires special
skill like tennis, you must participate in it to the point where being
good at it sends you on an ego trip. Imagine how you would think
of yourself if you were able to develop the strength and endurance
to walk, jog, swim, hike, or canoe for miles or hours at a time. Compare this with the way you think of your physical powers today.

These days I run and play with Kaycee, Bismarck, and Sheba
every morning and evening not just because it keeps me slim and
fit or helps to prevent another heart attack (which it seems to have
done these past thirty-five years). I run and play with my dogs because it's fun for all of us, it makes me feel good, and it makes them
feel good. When I think back to myself as a fat kid, 50 pounds
overweight at the age of twelve, and back to the time when I first
took up tennis and was so embarrassed with the way I looked that
I waited a year until I had lost enough weight to allow myself to un-
dress and shower in the gym with my tennis partners, I'm proud as
a peacock with what I have accomplished.

I wish I could give you at least a small taste of the experience
that's in store for you when you become an active person and raise
your level of physical fitness. But, as an old Oriental proverb states,
there are some things that you can know only by doing. This is one
of them.

Here is what you have to do.

1. First, you have to believe me! You have to believe it's possible.
I assure you that while you will like yourself better having lost
weight, the feeling will not compare with losing weight *and developing a strong, active body.*

2. I think you need to do *something* physical every day. When you
first start, you must strive to do something every day until it becomes
so much a part of you that, as with brushing your teeth, you feel un-
comfortable if you don't do it. *What you do is really less important
than doing something.*

3. People who have lost a significant amount of weight and kept
it off for years, and who truly appear to be headed toward permanent weight management, are averaging about eighty minutes of
physical activity a day! They choose to do just about anything in that

time that involves whole-body movement or employs the major muscles of the body. This includes walking, jogging, dancing, swimming, stair-stepping, bicycling (stationary and open road), treadmill, strength training—even vigorous house cleaning and yard work. Successful people are burning, on average, an extra 400 calories every day in physical activity.

4. For weight control it doesn't matter a great deal whether you move around five or ten minutes at a time, or forty-five minutes or more at a time. What counts is what works for you. But there are differences in the fitness you can achieve and in the psychological and emotional impact. I'll discuss this more fully in a moment.

5. You must set reachable goals for daily activity and a reasonable standard of performance. It has to be one that is yours alone, no one else's. If you enroll in a class or receive personal instruction in fitness, make sure that the leader's or instructor's standards are suited to your needs and abilities. (I've known a few aerobic dance leaders who keep themselves from becoming bored by using the classes to show off or to go at such a pace in order to promote their own fitness that no one else can keep up.) You should choose goals and standards that you are certain to reach, so that each day you can complete your chosen activity or activities. Depending on the kind of activity you choose, you can set a standard that involves time spent or distance covered, or perhaps the speed with which you do it, but the standard should be reachable and provide a sense of accomplishment.

6. If you choose to engage in competitive activities, your commitment will grow as your skills improve, so you should strive to become as good at the activity as time and resources allow. For example, if you ever wanted to be a tennis player, this means lessons and practice. You should choose a sport where, for you, the greatest joy is found in the game itself and is not dependent on the outcome. I have known people for whom losing a tennis match was so disturbing that they couldn't sleep well at night. This is not what we are after! In my own case, I scheduled some matches with folks who were more skilled than I was, some with folks less skilled, and some where the outcome would always be in doubt because we were so evenly matched. Over time, I won about half the time and lost the other half, and that suited my temperament just fine.

7. To experience fully the kind of gratification that results from becoming an active person may take anywhere from a couple of months to a couple of years. You must be patient and determined.

You will need to learn how to get through the change of seasons. Depending on your choice of activity and the climate where you live, you may need to learn how to deal with the heat and the cold, the rain and the snow, the dogs along your route, and the other vocational and social demands in your life. One day, having overcome all the obstacles, you will suddenly realize that you have become the person you set out to be. In addition to being fit, you will be much more self-confident and independent.

8. If you choose physical activities that are social in nature, try to find partners who are as sincere as you are. Take some initiative. Form a large enough group so that you can depend on one or more of the other members to show up at the appointed time. My wife, Enid, is part of a group of nine women who have set up times and places for walking or jogging every day of the week. They meet at three different parks on an established rotation for each day of the week, 6:30 A.M. on weekdays, and 7:00 A.M. on Saturdays and Sundays. Not all members are scheduled to meet on all days, but each member knows that there will be at least one or two others at the appointed place every weekday and a big crowd on weekends.

9. Finally, if you choose some solo activity like walking, jogging, or swimming (and I hope you do choose something you do all alone, at least as part of your total program), you may have to experiment a bit to find an approach that leads to the kind of personal satisfaction and commitment I'm speaking of. If you normally spend a great deal of time alone, then walking with friends can become an interesting social activity. There are walking groups in many cities, but you can always put notes in your neighbors' mailboxes, informing them that you are looking for walking companions. If you normally work with other people, or are under pressure when you work, then walking alone may provide you with the greatest benefits. When I have been successful in persuading people to persevere, and they have completed a year or two of walking, jogging, or swimming just about every day, they almost always tell me that it has been a period of self-discovery. Whereas they might have been bored at first, they discovered that walking alone provided them with an opportunity to talk with themselves. They found an opportunity to consider thoughts, emotions, plans, hopes, and dreams that could never have occurred otherwise. They got to know themselves, but, best of all, they grew to like themselves a great deal better than before.

That's the final component. Simply put, you will know what I'm talking about when your sense of accomplishment and self-esteem rises to the point where you can say to yourself, "The real reason I walk (jog, play tennis, dance) is that I feel like a better person for having done it."

SOME PHYSICAL AND PHYSIOLOGICAL CONSIDERATIONS

Whenever I give a lecture or workshop on weight management, someone is sure to ask, "Are there some activities that are better for weight management than others?"

I always answer, "Yes, there are." And then I go on to explain that they include any and all physical activities that give you such enduring satisfaction that you will continue doing it (or them) for the rest of your life. Everything else is really secondary. If you have been a sedentary person, you may just have to experiment, trying several different activities, until you find what you enjoy most.

Here are some general considerations.

The first rule of fitness. The golden rule for activities designed to build cardiovascular endurance and for the burning of calories for weight control, such as walking, jogging, bicycling, and swimming, is to include some periods of movement in which you go as briskly as possible *without hurting yourself.* If you hurt yourself, your activity program will go down the tubes, and I can assure you from personal experience that the pointer on your scale is likely to go up if that happens.

It's important to burn both glucose and fat in your fuel mixture. All physical activities you are likely to engage in will burn a mixture of glucose and fat in your fuel mixture. However, alternating "brisk" with "cruise" intervals in whole-body activities like walking, jogging, and swimming will add several plusses to the activity.

Recall that quick, intense physical movements burn primarily carbohydrate in the fuel mixture, while easygoing activities burn primarily fat in the fuel mixture. The brisk episodes will make sure that you burn a bit of extra glucose as well as fat in your fuel mixture. Because overloaded glucose stores can depress fat burning in your body's fuel mixture throughout the day, brisk episodes, by keeping these stores from being overloaded, encourage your body to burn an increased amount of fat drawn from your fat cells during the time you are not exercising.

While all activity tends to reduce the level of triglycerides circulating in your bloodstream and helps regulate blood glucose levels, alternating brisk and cruise intervals may promote an even greater decrease in insulin resistance and hyperinsulinemia than cruising at a steady state throughout your activity session. If you are prediabetic or suffering from NIDDM, I suggest you take this up with your physician and see if it works for you.

Brisk activity will increase cardiovascular endurance and your capacity for exercise. Brisk episodes increase cardiovascular endurance, which means that a given level of exercise intensity will become easier and easier to do as time goes on. Increased endurance also results in an increase in fat burning both during exercise and afterward. Let me give you an example from our research to show you just what this means.

In this study, conducted at the Vanderbilt Weight Management Program, the research subjects were women in their thirties and forties and approximately 60 pounds overweight on average. On the first test walk, their heart rates averaged 138 beats per minute at a three-miles-per-hour pace (twenty minutes per mile), and most of the women were tired, breathing hard, and needed to stop after twenty minutes. Walking at this level of exertion was as fast as they could go, and at this level of cardiovascular endurance, it was primarily a carbohydrate-burning activity. We estimated that on average the fuel mixture burned was about 70 percent carbohydrate and 30 percent fat and the total number of calories burned was about 100.

Over the next twelve weeks the women walked six days a week, with two objectives: Increase time to forty-five minutes, then increase speed. In order to increase speed, as their condition improved, they began to include periods of brisk walking, at a four-miles-per-hour pace (fifteen minutes per mile), throughout the workout session. By the end of the twelve weeks, all of the women were able to walk for forty-five minutes without stopping at three miles per hour, and many could maintain a four-miles-per-hour pace for a good part of the time.

We then did a second test at the three-miles-per-hour pace. Their heart rates at this pace had decreased to 112 beats per minute. This means that the heart could supply all the oxygen and nutrients that the body needed to carry out this activity with twenty-six fewer beats per minute than twelve weeks earlier. That's about a 20 percent reduction in effort. Because of their increased cardiovascular capacity, a 3-miles-per-hour pace was now their cruise speed, and the body was able to switch to burning a greater proportion of fat to carbohydrate in its fuel mixture. We estimated that the percentage of fat burned while walking at this pace increased from 30 to at least 50 percent. During the periods when they moved briskly at their four-miles-per-hour speed, they switched back to a fuel mixture similar to what it had originally been at three miles per hour in Week 1— that is, to a predominance of carbohydrate.

These results illustrate that as physical condition improves, the fat-burning potential of walking increases. This would also be true of any other whole-body movement or major-muscle utilization, such as jogging, swimming, bicycling, stair-stepping, and using a ski machine.

Because the women had been able to increase total walking each day from approximately one mile to three, the total number of both fat and carbohydrate calories burned in activity also increased significantly. On a cruise walk at a comfortable three-miles-per-hour pace, fat burning increased fivefold, from 30 calories (of the total 100 calories burned in a one-mile walk at the start of the program) to about 150 calories (of the total 300 calories burned in a three-mile walk at the end of twelve weeks). And carbohydrate burning more than doubled, from about 70 calories in a one-mile walk to 150 calories in a three-mile walk.

The value of this kind of increase in endurance and in total time spent in physical activity extends far beyond the period of activity itself. For several hours after completing an hour's walk there will be a slight increase in metabolic rate—the body may need to burn an extra fifty or so calories as it regenerates the muscle fibers that were active in exercise. In addition, as the muscles become adapted to greater use, they switch, even at rest, to burning more fat.

It's a fact: As fitness increases with daily exercise, so does the body's reliance on fat in its fuel mixture around the clock.

How should you gauge the intensity of your activity to know if you are moving toward the goal of increased cardiovascular endurance and a level of fat and carbohydrate burning in your fuel mix that will contribute to weight loss and maintenance?

I'll show you an easy and perfectly adequate way to do it on your own in a moment. But if you would like some expert help, as well as an environment that might contribute to your motivation, you might investigate joining the YMCA or YWCA. The Ys offer various fitness and exercise classes and the guidance of trained personnel. Your progress will be monitored on devices that will show you the actual physiological changes that are taking place. If a fitness club or other commercial athletic organization seems more convenient than the Y, be sure to check it out with someone who has experience there. Sometimes these organizations do not follow through on their promises, and you may not have the benefit of trained personnel in spite of their representations. Check with your local Better Business Bureau and Division of Consumer Affairs to see whether any complaints have been filed and how they have been resolved.

To do it on your own, you can make perfectly adequate progress just thinking in terms of "cruise" and "brisk" in your activity. While any continuous whole-body movement is about as good as any other for burning body fat and for combining with the T-Factor 2000 Diet for permanent weight management, walking is easiest and most convenient for most people, so I'll use that as an example.

WALKING FOR HEALTH, FITNESS, AND WEIGHT MANAGEMENT

Walking burns more calories with less perceived effort than other activities. Most of us do at least a little walking every day, and that gives us a base to build on. At a three-miles-per-hour pace you can expect to burn about 100 calories every twenty minutes. At a four-miles-per-hour pace you'll burn about 100 calories every fifteen minutes. If you don't have an area where you can measure the distance you walk in a specified length of time, such as a track or flat road on which you can measure off a mile or an exact fraction of a mile, credit yourself with a speed of three miles per hour when you take sixteen or seventeen steps every ten seconds and a pace of four miles per hour when you take about twenty-one steps every ten seconds. For many overweight persons who have had a sedentary existence, as with the women in the research I referred to above, a three-miles-per-hour pace will initially feel brisk and possibly too difficult to achieve for more than a few minutes. And, your feeling for a cruise pace and a brisk pace may not coincide exactly with either three or four miles per hour. So, I suggest you do the following.

Simply go out for a walk. Go along at the highest speed at which you could carry on a conversation with a friend and not pay attention to your breathing. That will be your initial cruise speed. Then, pick it up until you reach a pace at which you begin to feel yourself breathing hard, and at which you would have to interrupt your speech to catch your breath before you could utter another sentence. That is your brisk speed.

Now let's consider how to approach a walking program in which you set a goal of being able to walk a full forty-five minutes or an hour at a time. Remember, however, that if such a goal is not convenient or appealing, than just getting up out of your chair and doing a walk-about for five minutes every hour, or ten minutes four or five times a day, perhaps including a flight or two of stairs, will accomplish just about as much for weight control as the longer walks.

When you first start a walking program with the ultimate goal of being able to walk for forty-five or sixty minutes at a time, use the principle of gradualness and start out by aiming first for an objective of about fifteen minutes at your cruise speed. Don't even think of adding 'brisk' intervals until a full fifteen minutes at cruise feels pretty easy. In general, it's always best to *increase time before you increase your speed*. This allows your entire musculature to catch up and stay abreast of your growing cardiovascular endurance, and it will help prevent injury to your joints and leg muscles.

Take your time and build up to forty-five minutes or an hour over a period of a month or two. When that feels comfortable, it's time to do some brisk intervals: Go for one minute or about 100 steps at your brisk pace. Then relax and return to your cruise pace. Stay at your cruise pace until your breathing returns to normal. Then do another brisk interval.

When it feels comfortable to do so, increase the length of your brisk intervals. Add perhaps a minute at a time, or extra stages of 50 or 100 steps each.

You will see considerable improvement in your cardiovascular endurance within about two weeks of starting your brisk intervals. The effort will become easier and easier. If you are in a supervised fitness program, you will be able to see that your heart begins to beat much more slowly at a cruise speed of three miles per hour than at the start of your program. In addition, in a supervised program you will have been shown your personal "training" level. This is the heart rate that will result in an excellent level of cardiovascular endurance when you are able to walk at a speed that maintains it for a full twenty minutes at a time and do it about four times a week.

However, in my experience, most people who walk for health and weight maintenance prefer to use their activity as a time to escape the regimentation they find in the rest of their daily activities. You may end up being much happier and still accomplish just as much if you use a feel-good approach in building your endurance. Listen to your body, and whenever it says go faster, GO. When it says slow down, SLOW DOWN.

The walking study described earlier illustrated that as your fitness improves, you burn more fat in any given whole-body activity, such as walking. You can tell that the amount of fat being burned is increasing and the amount of carbohydrates is decreasing when, at any given pace, the feeling of effort decreases.

And now another important point: THE LONGER YOU GO, THE MORE FAT YOU BURN.

When you start out in any activity, including walking and the other activities that involve your entire body or its large muscles, the major part of the fuel mix is drawn from your glycogen pool. As you continue moving in the steady state, your body switches tanks, as it were, and begins to draw from its fat stores. The fitter you are, the sooner the switch takes place, and the longer you go, the more fat relative to glucose you will use. Thus a continuous hour of activity is likely to burn slightly more fat than walking for twelve different five-minute segments during the day or six ten-minute segments. But if brief walks are all you can manage most of the time, do them. In fact, some studies show that once people become accustomed to short segments several times a day, they are more likely to keep doing them than adhering to the forty-five- to sixty-minute daily walk regimen. Short exercise breaks from work are refreshing. Some people use them to "wash out their minds" and get a fresh grip on whatever work they have been doing. Time away from the desk in a different setting can add to creativity. If the shorter segments are more convenient on weekdays, however, try to get a couple of longer walks in on weekends so that your fitness will improve. The fitter you become, the more fat you will burn on your shorter walks.

In Table 9-1 I list approximate calories burned per fifteen minutes according to standard tables of energy expenditure. The start/stop activities like tennis or football, or those in which you keep moving most of the time but which require extreme swings in energy expenditure, like basketball, tend to burn more carbohydrate than fat, while the continuous whole-body movement exercises, like walking and cycling at a cruise pace, will tend to burn more fat than carbohydrate. The exact proportions can only be determined in the laboratory, and there will be great variability from person to person. But remember, in the end the differences are quite small, and *all activity is good activity!*

Table 9-1.

Approximate Energy Costs in Each Fifteen Minutes of Various Activities*

Activity	Calories per 15 minutes
Aerobic dancing	105
Badminton	99
Ballroom dancing, continuous	53
Basketball	141
Canoeing (recreational)	45
Cleaning house (steady movement)	63
Climbing hills (steady pace)	123
Cooking dinner	47
Cycling	
5.5 MPH, level ground	66
9.4 MPH, level ground	102
Football	135
Gardening (raking)	56
Golf, walking	87
Gymnastics	68
Horseback riding	
walking	42
trotting (English style)	113
Judo	199
Piano playing	41
Rowing (machine, fast pace)	105
Running	
11 min., 30 sec. per mile	138
10 min. per mile	174
9 min. per mile	197
8 min. per mile	213
7 min. per mile	234
6 min. per mile	260

Skiing, cross country, walking pace	146
Skiing, downhill	101
Squash	216
Swimming	
freestyle, moderate pace	143
side stroke	125
Table tennis	69
Tennis	111
Typing (electric typewriter)	27
Volleyball	51
Walking	
3 MPH, level ground	66
4 MPH, level ground	99
Walking downstairs, steady pace	50
Walking upstairs, slow steady pace	151

*Energy costs are calculated for persons weighing 150 pounds. For each 10 pounds more or less than 150 pounds, add or subtract 7 percent from these figures.

You may find that being active becomes more enjoyable if you cultivate a variety of activities and alternate among them. You are likely to meet different people in each. Good combinations of activities involve different muscle groups, and, interestingly enough, the cardiovascular endurance you develop in one activity is not spread equally to others. This is a good reason to cultivate a number of activities.

For example, walking and jogging develop the muscles in the lower body, the circulation to that part of the body improves, and the muscles involved adapt to the demands of exercise by storing more fuel so that they can respond more efficiently. But the upper body does not keep pace—the training effect is quite specific. This became clear to me as a jogger and tennis player. During a period in which I developed a severe case of tennis elbow, I took a vacation from the game for several weeks. I increased my jogging from my customary two or three miles a day to five or six. I even did intervals and practiced the quick side to side, and back-and-forth sprints of several steps at a time that are required in tennis. I thought I would be in excellent shape when I resumed playing that game. Not so. The first time I got on the court, served, sprinted to the net, and had to hit two overhead smashes in a row, I was out of breath.

My upper body had become deconditioned. Fortunately, because of my prior level of conditioning and level of cardiovascular endurance, it was only a matter of a few days, during which I practiced hitting overheads, before I was back in shape.

Is there a best time of day for exercise?

There certainly is. It's the time of day that is most convenient for you and when it gives you the most enjoyment.

As for clock time, some research says that early in the morning, before breakfast, when your body is in fat-burning mode, is the time you burn a few extra fat calories. Other research says a walk after meals—as simple a thing as a fifteen-minute walk back to work from lunch—can increase the thermic effect of food. That is, a comfortably paced walk after a meal increases the metabolic cost of digestion and walking by a couple of percentage points. Other research says exercise in the late afternoon, when metabolic rate tends to be a few percentage points higher than at other times of the day, will burn a few extra calories. So, as far as I am concerned, take your choice. You're a winner when you exercise at any time of the day!

There is only one exception to this recommendation. While almost everyone finds walking at a cruise pace after dinner can help digestion and be quite relaxing, strenuous activity can interfere with sleep. So I would avoid doing anything more than a gentle amble after your evening meal.

A word about equipment for walking. Unfortunately, a great many overweight people develop shin splints when they start walking. This is more likely to occur if you walk on pavement or the hard surfaces in malls, and less likely if you can walk on trails, running tracks, and dirt roads. However, you can do a great deal to prevent shin splints by starting off gradually, *and being sure you have good walking shoes.* In almost every case of shin splints that occurred among walkers in my weight groups, the cause was bad shoes! We were able to remove the cause by finding the correct kind of walking shoe to fit the persons' individual walking styles, foot and ankle alignment, and the requirements of the surface they walked on. We were fortunate enough to find a shoe store that was willing to take the time to do this with the participants in our program. I suggest that when you go to purchase walking or jogging shoes, find a sympathetic and knowledgeable salesperson and explain your needs, especially if you are experiencing any foot, ankle, leg, hip, or even lower back problem when you walk.

EXERCISE AND APPETITE

Depending upon a number of factors, exercise can either decrease or increase appetite.

In sedentary persons who are outeating their energy needs and gaining weight, exercise may help reduce nonhunger-related overeating. Exercise, by raising body temperature, decreasing the flow of saliva, and diverting blood from the internal organs to the muscles, decreases appetite in the short term. Then, when appetite returns following exercise, it seems to be better attuned to the amount of energy you are expending each day than it is in the sedentary person. In other words, people who exercise tend to eat in a way that does not lead to an increase in weight. It's as though Mother Nature, in ways that we are unaware of, keeps our bodies adapted to the physical demands we make on them. The active person needs a thinner body in order to be efficient in activity, so appetite becomes regulated to keep you thin. This mysterious adaptive mechanism goes out of whack in the sedentary person.

But certain forms of exercise, under certain conditions, can also increase appetite over its accustomed level. This can happen if the exercise drastically depletes your glycogen stores. With a steady, ongoing exercise program to which we have become accustomed, glycogen stores fluctuate within the accustomed range, as does appetite, and all is in balance. But we can exceed the usual range and really turn on when we make a drastic change in the nature of our activity.

This was brought home to me many years ago the very first time I did a complete strength-training workout under the guidance of an instructor at the YMCA. He was demonstrating the equipment in the weight room, so that I would know what to do on future visits, and I did several sets of exercises covering both the lower and upper body. I did all exercises to virtual exhaustion for all the muscle groups. (Normally you would do upper body on one day, lower body on another.)

I went to my office at the university after the workout, and about an hour or so after arriving, I became ravenous. I have rarely had such an appetite in my life. It was a completely different sensation compared with other times in which I have been hungry after going a long time between meals. It reduced me to near-criminal activity:

I went sneaking around the psychology department, looking for food in my colleagues' offices and in the secretaries' offices. I think the almost complete depletion of my muscle glycogen stores was responsible for this. In addition, there may have been an increased need for some protein for muscle repairs, since this was the first time I had ever lifted weights.

Fortunately, one of the secretaries had a package of peanut butter crackers (!), which she gave to me, and my appetite was satisfied until lunch. But by the end of the day, I had eaten enough so that my glycogen stores were replenished above baseline and I ended up a couple of pounds heavier the next day.

Will strength training interfere with weight loss and fat loss on the T-Factor 2000 Diet?

Power lifting—that is, heavy weight lifting with quick explosive movements to exhaustion for each muscle group—burns primarily carbohydrate. If you want to lose weight and body fat, and include power lifting in your regimen, you must be sure that you follow the T-Factor 2000 Diet in order to replenish carbohydrate without an overconsumption of fat, since power lifting is not a fat-burning activity. At one point, the young man who was Mr. Tennessee came into the Vanderbilt Weight Management Program because he was experiencing a problem taking off a few pounds of extra fat, which was making it difficult to trim down for competitions. An adjustment in his diet and the addition of a couple of miles of jogging to his power-lifting routine solved his problem.

If you decide to add power lifting to your regimen, you should do so under professional supervision, since there is a significant risk of injury. On the other hand, I want to encourage you to follow my moderate-endurance strength-training program (Appendix B) because it will tone you up and you will look and feel better for doing it. Endurance strength training with light weights will still increase your muscle mass, and since muscle is active tissue—that is, it burns a lot of calories even at rest—a few pounds of extra muscle will actually help you stay thin!

Should you walk with weights in your hands, or use some artificial "power" motion? I would approach both of these options cautiously. Carrying light weights (one pound) can help improve your cardiovascular condition more rapidly and build a little more muscular endurance, but I have known persons who sustained joint injuries and lower back pain by adding weights while they walked.

Race walking, however, has been a life saver for many joggers who have injured themselves running, so if you learn the motion correctly, you probably won't injure yourself. Simply swinging your arms while walking any old way that feels good to you can significantly increase the intensity of your workout and build endurance. Test out all changes in your natural walking style gingerly, and let your experience be your guide.

THE SWIMMING CONTROVERSY

I occasionally still come across the claim that you can't lose body fat if you take up swimming as the main component of your exercise program. This is simply not true.

The reason some experts claim that swimming is not a good exercise for weight control is that the temperature of the pool, being perhaps 20 or more degrees cooler than your body, encourages the body to retain the layer of surface fat that lies just under your skin. In thin people who may have little to begin with, swimming may help add a bit of surface fat. This occurs to help prevent heat loss as your body struggles to maintain its internal temperature at around 98.6 degrees Fahrenheit.

However, swimming, when it becomes as easy as walking or jogging for you, is a fat-burning exercise, and the struggle to maintain internal temperature is also fueled by fat to a large extent. In combination with the T-Factor 2000 Diet, you are assured of burning more fat in your fuel mixture than you are eating if you make swimming your favorite exercise. But you *will* tend to retain a bit more surface body fat than if you walk, jog, or ride a bicycle.

Although I have never learned to be comfortable in the water, I have spoken with persons for whom swimming is as easy and automatic as walking. They can become completely entranced as they glide back and forth in the pool. It's as restful and refreshing as meditation for them. If you have difficulty coordinating your breathing with your strokes and this prevents you from becoming relaxed and enjoying a swim, you may find that learning to use a snorkel will put you completely at ease.

HOW TO DETERMINE THE NUMBER OF CALORIES/FAT BURNED DURING EXERCISE

I have often been asked how a person can determine the number of calories or fat burned when they perform different exercises. The best way to do this is to use your pulse rate as your guide. It's done in this way:

Go for a walk at three miles per hour (one mile in twenty minutes), and, after about five minutes, measure your pulse rate. Walking at three miles per hour burns about three times the calories of sitting still. Assuming a fifty-fifty ratio of fat to carbohydrate in your fuel mixture, it burns three times the fat and three times the carbohydrate. Whenever you reach this pulse rate in any other activity in which you are reasonably comfortable (for example, cycling or swimming) you will be burning about the same number of calories as you do while walking at three miles per hour, and half these calories are coming out of your fat cells.

If you are capable of it, walk for five minutes at four miles per hour (one mile in fifteen minutes) and take your pulse rate. Walking at four miles per hour burns almost five times the calories of sitting still. If you are in good condition, we can again assume about a fifty-fifty mixture of fat to carbohydrate in your fuel mixture. Whenever you reach this pulse rate in any other activity in which you are reasonably comfortable, you will be burning about the same number of calories as you do while walking at four miles per hour, and about half of them will be supplied by fat. Of course, the fitter you get, the more fat you burn relative to carbohydrate.

THE COMPLETE FITNESS PROGRAM

I have focused my discussion of physical activity on its role in burning calories and body fat because that is where our main interest lies. But staying fit and healthy also requires that we maintain our flexibility and muscular strength.

The masters of yoga say, "You are as old as your spine." That's because, as we age, our spines, as well as our joints, lose flexibility. With loss of flexibility comes an increased likelihood of injury, and the chronic aches and pains associated with stiffness. To a great extent, however, we can maintain flexibility and agility with appropriate stretching and toning exercises, and in this way we preserve biological if not chronological youth.

While many of us neglect to include a good stretching routine in our fitness programs, even more fail to do anything to maintain muscular strength. The requirements of life today, for most of us, do not include much lifting, pushing, or shoving of heavy objects. In fact, the heaviest things most of us ever carry after our children are grown are the weekly bags of groceries. This means that we do not build and maintain a level of strength that can protect us from injury anytime we find it necessary to exert physical force—even moving a chair, much less a heavier piece of furniture.

You can never experience a fraction of the energy, agility, and vitality you are capable of unless you incorporate a modest level of stretching exercise and strength training into your regimen. In Appendix B I include a training routine that combines flexibility and modest strength-training exercises.

After you get a sense of what you need to do to maintain flexibility and strength, you can be creative and invent ways to do exercise of this nature and keep it interesting. Here's how I manage it.

After the alarm goes off in the morning, while still in bed and lying flat on my back, I do some leg-lifts, crunches (mini-sit-ups), back stretches, and a series of knee-strengthening and bicycle-pedaling motions (Enid is always out of bed before me, so I am not disturbing her). These exercises take about five or six minutes, and I listen to the weather report as I do them. The knee exercises are especially important, because I injured both knees as a tennis player and these exercises have kept me injury-free while walking and jogging for many years. I keep 3- and 5-kilo weights (6.6 and 11 pounds) in the den, and, at least once a day, when I take a break from sitting and writing at my computer, I go through a light strength-training routine for about five minutes. At least once a day, as I wait for the water to boil for a cup of coffee, I do some half–push-ups against the countertop in the kitchen, and some half–knee bends. Since my office is in the basement of my home, I go up and down a flight of stairs at least ten times a day (I must go up to get my weights in the den or to go out for a walk around the yard with my dogs). I have a hilly yard, so I even get in a bit of hill climbing.

I hope the facts I've given you about exercise, the other hints for incorporating exercise in your life, and my discussion of the psychological and emotional correlates of activity will motivate you to begin an effective and enjoyable exercise program. The payoff in terms of weight management and overall health from physical activity—activity of almost any kind—will be worth every moment of time invested, the cost of appropriate clothing and equipment, and physical effort.

In Chapter 11 I will show you even more evidence of the key role that activity plays in the lives of people who have lost significant amounts of weight and who have found the permanent solution to weight maintenance.

CHAPTER 10

T-Factor 2000 Principles for Healthy, Happy Kids

Jamie Pope, M. S., R. D.

At least one-third of American children are overweight or obese, representing more than a 50 percent increase since the 1960s. During the same time period, the percentage of severely obese children has risen almost 100 percent. The incidence mirrors that of adults (or may, in fact, be higher!). Children, like adults, are exposed to an abundance of high-fat and energy-dense foods that are freely advertised and have far too few opportunities to exercise. In this environment, kids with genetic vulnerability to obesity will gain inappropriate amounts of weight. Without some sort of intervention, many overweight kids will remain so or gain even more weight as they enter adulthood—about 70 percent of overweight adolescents become overweight or obese adults.

Why are so many kids overweight? It is difficult to gather reliable data on children's eating habits, because the same problems with underestimation of intake, especially of dietary fat, show up in studies with children as they do with those of obese adults. They are likely eating more fat than is recorded. A 1995 study reported that American children in general consumed 11 percent more calories than recommended. Recent studies have shown that obese children do eat more dietary fat than children whose weight is normal and, when given the option, tend to choose foods that are more fat- and calorie-laden. Just as in adults, fat is the primary dietary culprit for weight gain in children, and just like their adult counterparts, inactivity is a significant contributor. But while they do tend to be less active overall, overweight kids require more energy to move around and thus end up burning about the same number of calories as their thinner counterparts. The difference may be that given a high-fat diet and sedentary habits, kids with genetic predisposition to obesity will become overweight. Not only does genetics influence extent of body fat and its distribution, but food preferences play a part—children of obese parents naturally seem to prefer high-fat foods.

Television viewing and video games contribute directly to the fattening of American children. Kids spend on average upward of twenty-five hours a week in front of the tube. Figured on an annual basis, that's more hours than they spend in school! And certainly more hours than they spend in active play. Studies demonstrate that each of those hours adds to their risk of developing lifelong obesity. In fact, hours of television watched is predictive of children's increasing weight. Television puts children into a veritable trance, reducing their metabolic rate by some 16 percent more than other sedentary activities. At the same time, commercial sponsors prompt young viewers to hunger for packaged treats that are usually high in fat and low in nutrition. The advertising has its intended effect, since parents who let their kids watch the most TV also tend to honor more of their children's shopping requests than other parents. One of the most important things you can do to aid in your child's weight management is turn off the TV!

FAMILY DYNAMICS

Kid's weight issues go beyond genetic predisposition, the fat in their diet, or how much they exercise. When a child gains excess weight, it may mean that there is something amiss in the dynamics of the family and the emotional atmosphere in the home. Kids who do not receive enough of the right kind of attention from their parents or caregivers, whether they are overindulged or emotionally neglected, may be at risk. Psychologists who study weight gain in children have found that rates of obesity tend to be lowest in families where the lines of communication are open between parents and kids. In fact, family cohesiveness seems to be a more reliable criterion than diet or exercise in predicting childhood weight! Since the unity of the family is so important in keeping kids at a healthy weight, it's not surprising that young people frequently gain weight in the face of parental divorce or death in the family, or that children from abusive families often comfort themselves with food and end up overweight. The solution for children in such situations is not to put them on a diet. Even teaching to eat low-fat foods, turn off the TV, and take up a sport, while important, are all secondary to the need for security and nurturing. Family-based therapy may be helpful.

WEIGHT-MANAGEMENT PRINCIPLES FOR CHILDREN

This chapter is included as an essential part of the T-Factor 2000 program for several reasons. Primarily because children are not mini-adults, principles of weight control for adults do not necessarily apply to children. Children need sufficient intake to provide for growth and physiological needs—plus stamina to fully participate in the social, educational, and physical aspects of their young lives. Although children confront many of the same issues adults face, they have some unique and difficult challenges. You may be reading this chapter as a parent or caretaker of an overweight child or as a parent concerned about helping your child maintain a healthy weight in the midst of a culture that fosters weight gain. If you are overweight yourself or have to work hard at keeping pounds off, your child has inherited at least part of your genetic predisposition.

It is important to differentiate between kids who are inappropriately overweight and obese and those who are large but not unusually so for their heredity, predisposition, or bone structure. Some kids are genetically larger than others and it may be natural for them to have more body fat and body weight even when eating a healthful diet and exercising consistently.

Just as in adults, the majority of weight issues for children have to do with 5, 10, or 20 extra pounds (which in children can represent a greater percentage of body weight than in adults). However, more and more children are becoming 30, 40, and 50 pounds heavier than is healthy for them. If your child is severely overweight or more than twice his or her ideal body weight, I hope you have already sought medical and professional assistance. There are some resources and programs listed at the end of this chapter.

FAMILY COOPERATION

Your personal involvement and commitment to do what it takes to help your child are essential to your child's progress. You must be willing to make changes in not only the food and activity arenas of your family life but in the interpersonal, emotional, and social realms as well. Children's weight is a family issue—never should the child be singled out or asked to make changes solo.

Within a family it is almost impossible to separate your own eating habits from those of your children or your spouse. You may have found from your own attempts at changing your diet that when you tried to go about it solo, the changes were usually short-lived. Not only is it more work and effort to do things differently for different members of the family, but the temptation of higher-fat foods and even social pressure generally prevail. More often than not, however, women are the gatekeepers for their families' food choices and eating habits. If you are in this role, you can have a powerful and positive influence on your family's eating habits, as they eat primarily what you stock and prepare. Stock a low-fat kitchen (granted there will likely be some grumbling), and, aside from meals outside the home, you will all eat less fat.

Children do not tend to be adventurous about trying new foods. And their repertoire of foods tends to be fairly limited. In a recent study of USDA survey data of over three thousand youths, ages two to nineteen, across the United States, it was found that only 1 percent met all recommendations for food group servings! It's certainly safe to conclude that the vast majority of American kids have intakes for many nutrients below recommended dietary allowance levels; at the same time, they consume excessive amounts of dietary fat and sodium.

MY OWN EXPERIENCE AS A MOM

As a mother of a three-year-old, I can name on two hands the foods I am assured of my daughter accepting and probably eating! Fortunately, her most frequent requests are for cantaloupe and grapes— and ice cream. I must reveal that I have succumbed on more than one occasion to standbys like macaroni and cheese or "Happy

Meals." But overall our cupboard and refrigerator are stocked with lots of healthful and varied options, which form the base of our food choices. As I'm writing this afternoon looking back at today, we had cereal with 1% milk for breakfast, and my daughter had ziti, cheese cubes, grapes, and raw baby carrots for lunch, with snacks of kid-size fruit yogurt and part of my banana. And since I'm working under a deadline, we likely will have cheese pizza delivered! Which I'll round off with applesauce and broccoli (she loves "little trees"!). My daughter eats pretty well, I'd say—she seems to be genetically lean and has never been a food-focused child, despite my some-times pushing foods more than I probably should. I contrast my daughter to a friend's children who seemed to be pudgy by the time they were toddlers and have continued in that direction despite participation in sports. Part of their challenge is genetics com-pounded by fast-track food in a fast-track life. Their divorced mom works full time, and between the kids' school and extracurricular de-mands, she finds little time to spend on planning, shopping, or preparing meals. Her reality is likely more the norm than my own.

WHAT CAN PARENTS DO?

Our job as parents or caregivers is to provide and offer in a positive way an array of healthful and, for the most part, low-fat foods. It's not our job to make kids eat everything on their plate or force them to eat foods they turn up their noses at (even if they are "good" for them!). Offer new and varied foods and GUIDE them toward a healthful diet. Even if your child refuses once to eat something, offer it again—and again. You might recall how you hated certain vegetables as a child, only to come to enjoy them as an adult. Food is one of those arenas in which children begin to exercise some choice and independence, and I think that their increasing self-reliance should be fostered. Do make sure your child is getting a bal-anced diet with grains, fruits, vegetables (be creative about how they are offered), low-fat dairy foods, and lean protein sources. My daughter loved milk from her bottle as an infant and now drinks only small quantities from a glass or cup, but she loves yogurt, cheese, and cottage cheese. So I don't worry. And I continue to offer milk as a beverage at many of her meals—she takes a few sips, but

I don't bribe or threaten her to finish it; nor do I remind her that there are starving people somewhere in the world.

DON'T GET OVERZEALOUS ABOUT CUTTING FAT FOR KIDS

You need to be cautious in dealing with fat in a child's diet. Babies and young children need some fat. So while you might encourage your adolescent to drink skim or 1% milk, your two-year-old should drink 2% milk. For a child under two years of age, your pediatrician would likely encourage whole milk. I cringe when I hear stories of parents restricting young children in hopes of preventing excessive weight gain and raising them on low-fat frozen dinners and reduced-fat convenience foods. These children can suffer physical and emotional consequences from overly diet-conscious parents.

The way to encourage low-fat foods is not through lecturing or ultimatums. It is, quite simply, to limit the high-fat and calorie-dense, nutrient-poor foods you keep around the house. Children of parents who try to control and dictate food choices, even in the name of health or weight control, are less able to regulate their own eating as they grow older. So don't pressure—instead, stock up on snacks like fruit, whole-grain cereal and breads, frozen yogurt or ice milk, low-fat puddings, pretzels, and popcorn. Beware of fat-free or reduced-fat cookies, desserts, pastries, and the like—in some instances they make sense as substitutes for higher-fat counterparts as long as children limit themselves to a serving as recommended on the package. I've had overweight kids tell me, "But I only eat those cookies and stuff that have no fat, so they don't really count." They do, for the reasons already discussed in earlier chapters, so I recommend not keeping them around all the time. Buy lean cuts of luncheon meats and reduced-fat cheeses. Pack nutritious lunches for school or camp. Modify favorite family recipes so that they are lower in fat, or experiment with new, leaner recipes (vegetarian, for example) at suppertime. Between meals, encourage your kids to eat whatever's on hand whenever they are hungry. If no high-fat snacks are available, there's little need to restrict them or worry about between-meal pantry raids.

It is better to emphasize wholesome, low-fat choices than to dwell on what not to eat. Children need not "count," per se; after all, families eat food, not fat grams. Older kids should understand how to construct a fairly balanced diet, read food labels, and have a general idea of what is low or high in fat. It is also advisable not to dwell on weight as the "reason" for eating healthier or for getting more active. This can just add to the discomfort and shame your child may already be feeling. Instead, focus on healthful eating for energy, fitness, and health.

Even if the family embraces nutritional redirection and the principles of the T-Factor 2000 Diet, do not expect to see a big difference in what your children order at restaurants or what they eat at their friends' homes. However, when the family goes out together, shift the emphasis toward restaurants that offer more healthful and lower-fat choices. Unless your children do the majority of their eating elsewhere, there's no real need to worry about what they eat when they're away. It's what they eat at home that makes the most difference in their weight, present and future. As they grow more accustomed to leaner eating, many children will gradually lose some of their affection for high-fat items and will naturally begin to make different choices most of the time.

ESTABLISHING A POSITIVE FOCUS

Focusing on controlling an overweight child's food intake or forcing activity do little good in the long run and can be harmful, particularly if the chief cause of overeating is a poor family dynamic—which, of course, will have a profound influence on your child's interactions with friends, teachers, and so forth. Singling out the child from the family makes for minimal success.

Reduced physical activity and movement can precipitate weight gain but can also be a result of excess body fat. Overweight children find it more challenging physically and socially to participate in sports. Children can be just as self-conscious as adults about wearing exercise clothing or "performing" in front of others. A friend described a traumatic incident with her twelve-year-old daughter as they tried to find a bathing suit to fit her during an impromptu visit to the beach. Lots of tears later, the preteen refused to join her friends and read a book alone on the boardwalk, watching everyone else splash and play. And just as for many adults, food becomes the temporary solace and comfort.

The time to create a lifetime exercise habit is childhood. Active preschoolers have been found to be leaner later than their less active counterparts. Kids have a number of fitness advantages over grown-ups. They tend to be more flexible. Their bodies are smaller, more compact, and more resilient. Children seem to learn new skills and adapt to new and different body movements more easily than adults can. Finally, as kids are naturally learning and trying new experiences all the time, they are more likely to try a new form of exercise—even if they don't do it well—than most adults are.

There is also evidence that people are more likely to continue sports later in life if they start playing them as children. This is particularly true of organized team sports, which have complicated rules of play and expected conduct. It also seems true of sports such as swimming, which involve subtleties of form. People who learned to swim as children, particularly those who swam on teams, tend as adults to be much faster, more efficient, and more comfortable in the water than people who begin swimming later in life.

The most compelling reason to get your children into the habit of exercising is simply that fitness is good for everyone at every age. Regular physical activity will make them stronger, leaner, faster, and better coordinated. It will help them think clearly and sleep well. It will boost their self-esteem and reduce feelings of stress. Join in their activities—you'll reap the same benefits yourself!

Parents of overweight children who themselves are or have been overweight much of their lives are especially sensitive to the pain, prejudice, and self-recrimination that often accompany obesity in our thin-obsessed society. They want to spare their children what they themselves might have experienced. Lean parents of overweight children also do not want their children to grow up with the added burden that excess body fat can bring.

Whether you are trying to help your overweight child curtail further weight gain or sustain your child at a healthy weight, it's critical that you appreciate the stigma children attach to fatness. From a very young age kids learn that excess weight can be a source of tremendous shame. Elementary school students in several studies ranked obesity as a fate worse than being handicapped or disabled. Overweight children are often ridiculed by and alienated from their peers, and the negative attitudes of their peers will be internalized by the overweight child. When asked to name the "worst thing about being fat," sixth-grade girls answered that it would make them unattractive and unpopular, feel bad about themselves, and vulnerable to teasing. Just as kids are using drugs and alcohol, smoking, and having sex at earlier ages, so, too, are younger and younger children obsessing about their weight.

Of course, the problem is most serious with girls, because they pattern their behavior after the female role models in their lives. They see attractive and thin women on TV bemoaning the condition of their bodies. They see glamorous celebrities touting weight-loss products. They come to the conclusion: It's a sign of sophistication to hate their bodies and want to lose weight. I recall being asked to talk about nutrition to a class of fifth graders several years ago. What stands out in my mind is that in introducing me, the slim and attractive female teacher said, "Jamie is a dieting expert, and do I ever need to hear what she has to say" as she patted her narrow hips. I could just imagine these young girls thinking that if this lovely woman thought she was fat and needed to lose weight, what did that say about them as they added the natural padding and body fat that comes with pubescence? We have to be careful not to transfer our skewed ideas about weight, food, and body ideals to our children. In a study of 239 third-grade students, the children expressed weight, dieting, and physique concerns that reflect Western sociocultural values and preoccupation with body weight and dieting.

Some 60 percent of girls between grades one and six fear they are fatter than they really are. A study of public school students in a middle-class area of Boston found that more than half had dieted by age twelve and still wanted to lose more weight—even though most described their weight as "about right." An even more recent survey found that 80 percent of fourth-grade girls reported that they had dieted in order to control or lose weight!

These girls had already absorbed the societal message that would pursue them into adulthood: Women should never eat normally or be satisfied with their bodies as they are. They had also adopted a thoroughly "female" dieting mentality. Even among those girls who were not concerned about their weight, most restricted their eating in front of other people; more than half felt "guilty" about overeating; almost all were familiar with fat and calorie counts, tried to avoid calorie-dense foods, worried about eating, and thought of exercise as a way to lose weight. As for the punishing consequences of dieting—the fatigue, poor concentration, listlessness, and declining grades caused by chronic hunger, the distractions and anxiety caused by the obsession with weight, and the low self-esteem caused by constant self-criticism—these girls, like older, seasoned dieters, accepted it all as part of being a woman.

It is not within the scope or purpose of this chapter to deal with eating disorders in children and adolescents. If your child seems overly obsessed with her weight and size or begins to restrict her intake or exercise inappropriately, then take note and seek professional help. Eating disorders are serious and sometimes deadly, if intervention isn't begun early and adequately.

In conclusion, feed your children well—not only nutritionally but emotionally, spiritually, and intellectually. A healthful diet and active lifestyle that you and the rest of your family embrace in a positive and caring atmosphere promotes not only a healthy body but a sound mind and character. Your children's genetics may mean they will never be "thin," but they can be healthy and happy as they grow into their own unique bodies—whatever their dimensions.

POSITIVE PARENTING PRINCIPLES FOR HEALTHY AND HAPPY KIDS

1. Feed children well
   - Emphasize wholesome, healthful, and appealing foods that are naturally low in fat.
   - Design an eating environment conducive to healthful, low-fat choices.
   - Limit availability of appetite turn-on foods if your child has a weight problem.
   - Offer snacks at predictable times.
   - Keep serving dishes off the table. The habit of reaching for another helping may be triggered more by the convenient presence of food than by hunger.
   - Establish regular mealtimes, and include the children in dinner-table conversation. Don't use mealtimes as a battleground or a forum for discipline!
   - Include your children in food shopping and preparation as much as possible.
   - Teach them to appreciate and enjoy good food by exposing them to a wide variety of dishes, but don't insist they eat everything you put before them.
   - Don't establish a "clean plate club." Let your kids eat until they are satisfied, even if that requires only a few

bites (which for very young children is often the case).
- Don't rely on food as a reward, pacifier, or babysitter.
- Try to be conscientious rather than controlling in your switch to low-fat nutrition; don't "police" the kitchen.
- Remember your children's growing bodies may require more food than you do. Feed them without overfeeding yourself.
- Set a good example for your family by selecting healthy foods and moderate portions for yourself at home and away.
- Model a positive yet "self-regulated" attitude toward food.
- Acquaint your child with the Food Guide Pyramid and how to build a healthy diet. Put positive emphasis on eating *more* (vegetables, fruits, whole grains, beans . . .) instead of on less (processed, calorie-dense foods; fats; fried foods; high-fat meats, etc.).

2. Provide opportunities for active movement
   - Get the kids out of the house from a young age. Take walks, go to local playgrounds and parks.
   - Take advantage of shopping malls for climate-controlled walks.
   - Play together. Start with roughhousing when kids are small, then play ball, practice sports, and take family bike rides.
   - Join a local YMCA or other fitness facility that offers programs for younger members of the family. Have your children accompany you—they can walk on the indoor track or take a swimming class while you work out.
   - Keep jump ropes, hula hoops, skates, and basketballs (with a hoop) available for activity possibilities at home.
   - Involve your child in yard work and gardening.
   - Do not use TV as the family babysitter.
   - Limit television viewing and video game time, and have plenty of safe (preferably active) alternatives readily available. Some parents set daily limits on or have their children "earn" TV hours through chores and good behavior.
   - Make play dates for your children; kids tend to be much more physically active in pairs or groups than they are alone but do not often take the initiative in lining up playmates.

- Encourage and facilitate participation in team sports. The benefits go far beyond fitness and calorie burning. Kids on teams learn to work within a structure of rules and to cooperate toward a common goal—and make friends!
- Make sure any after-school or summer program offers ample opportunity for active play, organized athletic games, and physical skill development. Sports camps or clinics may be a preferable option to traditional day camps.
- Plan active family vacations. Hike, bike, camp, ski, or explore new destinations by foot.
- Present your personal view of exercise as fun, not drudgery.

3. Nurture the whole child
   - Pay ample (and then some) personalized attention to each young member of the family.
   - Listen to your children with your full attention and respect. Encourage them not to hold feelings inside and to express emotions appropriately.
   - Resist the urge to criticize. Look for constructive ways to foster behavior changes. Offer praise liberally.
   - Pay attention to significant changes in your child's eating and activity level.
   - Set reasonable limits for your children in all areas—they need room to make mistakes and the security of boundaries to feel loved and safe.
   - Provide for social, emotional, and spiritual needs.
   - Allow your children to grow up into bodies that reflect their genetic endowment.

When help is needed, check first with your pediatrician or registered dietitian. To obtain additional information for healthy weight management, you can contact the following resources:

American Academy of Pediatrics
www.aap.org

American Dietetic Association/National Center for Nutrition and
   Dietetics Consumer Hot Line
1-800-366-1655
www.eatright.org

Child Nutrition and Health Campaign Food Guide Pyramid for
   Children
www.eatright.org/child/pyramid

Committed to Kids Pediatric Weight Management Program
1-888-809-2701
www.committed-to-kids.com

Shapedown Pediatric Weight Loss Programs
1-888-724-5245
www.shapeup.org

Shapers (Kaiser Permanente)
1-888-7-SHAPERS

CHAPTER 11

Let Successful People
Tell You How They Do It

I opened the Introduction to *The T-Factor 2000 Diet* by saying that while losing weight is hard enough, keeping it off is a **very** hard thing to do.

Yet some people do it!

What's their secret? What enables or motivates these successful people to do what it takes when so many others have failed?

When you read the interviews with successful people that I reproduce in this chapter, I think you will discover that the secret to success lies deep within your own mind and character. It is already there, hidden within you. And I think you can find it if you want to.

Once they resolve to do it, successful people create a new mental and emotional environment for themselves. They make a decision about priorities—what's truly important to achieve in their lives. If losing weight and keeping it off is one of the top priorities, then they begin to think and act in a way that will help them achieve that goal.

As far as actions are concerned, there is *no* secret about the behavioral changes that are required to lose weight and keep it off. I want to deal briefly with the behavioral aspect first. Then, I hope the interviews will help you discover that you, too, have the power within you to do what it takes, just as these successful persons have done.

From a dietary standpoint, all of the research shows that people can *lose* weight effectively on any low-calorie diet that they can stick with. But, once lost, *a low-fat diet is the easiest and most effective way to keep weight off.* Maintenance diets among successful people average about 25 percent of total calories in fat. In general, successful people tend to reduce their consumption of red meat, and include more poultry and fish in their diet to replace it. They also increase their consumption of fruit and vegetables. I've tried to show you how to make the dietary changes with the T-Factor 2000 Diet.

All of the research also points to the key role played by physical activity. Over 90 percent of the people who have been successful in losing a significant amount of weight (at least 30 pounds) and keeping it off for a minimum of a year report a significant increase in their physical activity. The increase in energy expenditure among successful people amounts to an average of 2800 calories a week, which is the equivalent of four miles of walking a day. People reach that energy expenditure by devoting an average of eighty minutes a day to whatever activity or activities they've chosen to do.

But this research doesn't tell us the most important things we need to know. What we really need to know is *why* successful people continue to do what it takes to keep their weight off—*why* they follow a low-fat diet and *why* they exercise. What's the payoff? And we need to know both *why* and *how* they deal with all of the circumstances in their previous lives that led them to become overweight. In most cases, these circumstances don't just disappear.

Throughout this book I have taken the opportunity to tell you what I did to lose 70 pounds thirty-five years ago, and why I did it. I also talked about what keeps me motivated to do what I do today to remain successful. But I have become convinced through the years of trying to help overweight people that those who have been successful are motivated for many different reasons. While successful people find new rewards for doing what it takes to keep the weight off, and the rewards sustain their motivation, the payoffs are different for different people. As the saying goes, it's different strokes for different folks. One thing in particular stands out, however, and that is, there is a change in the way people talk to themselves and think about their actions that helps them to be successful. They create for themselves a positive mental environment that assures their success. I'll show you how they do this in the following interviews that I've had with a number of people who have lost a great deal of weight and have kept it off for many years.

3 0 0 0   S U C C E S S F U L   P E O P L E

While writing this book I was fortunate to have a series of conversations and an ongoing correspondence with the aforementioned Dr. James Hill,* one of the principal investigators on the National Weight Control Registry (NWCR) research project. He was kind enough to arrange for me to interview some of the successful participants in the registry. With permission, I recorded all of the conversations, so I am able to report verbatim comments.† I was already aware of Dr. Hill's published research, and he was kind enough to send me a selection of articles that had not yet appeared but were in press in leading scientific journals. So, first a brief summary of the formal research.

There are now (as of December 1998) over 3000 successful persons in the NWCR. The average weight loss is 67 pounds, and five years is the average length of time these successful people have maintained their losses.

Almost 90 percent of the participants in the registry reported that they limit the intake of certain types or classes of foods, just as I had done on my rotation plan thirty-five years ago. While many of the people in the registry had dieted a number of times before only to regain weight, in this last, successful effort, they tended to be more severe in their limitations. In Dr. Hill's words, "It's almost a little bit like good food/bad food . . . " While losing weight, successful people tend to eliminate certain high-fat and high-calorie foods from their diet, or to control them tightly. *They continue to limit these foods in order maintain their losses.* In fact, the percentage of people reporting that they limit certain classes of foods goes up over 90 percent in maintenance.

From one-third to one-half of the registrants in the NWCR report using one or more of several other behavioral strategies *both while losing weight and in maintenance.* In addition to eliminating or severely limiting certain foods, they may *limit the size of food portions, limit the percentage of daily energy from fat, and count calories and count fat grams.* As with limiting certain types and

---

*James O. Hill, Ph. D., is professor of pediatrics and medicine at the University of Colorado Health Sciences Center in Denver, Colorado.

†I have taken some small liberties either for grammatical purposes or for clarity. However, I have not attempted to alter the way successful persons expressed themselves in our telephone interviews (except for clarification) because I wanted to retain the original, unique flavor of the conversations. While I did have prepared questions, the conversations were informal, and, except for the opening and final questions, I generally followed my interview subjects' lead.

classes of foods, the percentage of successful losers using these other strategies, one or more in combination, also tends to go up in maintenance.

In other words, successful people demonstrate that it takes the same kind of vigilance to maintain a weight loss as it takes to lose weight! This makes sense, of course. You must do something that keeps you from going back to old habits. However, just about all successful persons do deviate from plans on occasion. The reason they remain successful is that they know how to compensate. They go back quickly to a kind of mini-diet to compensate for any deviation, which, together with an increase in physical activity, prevents a lapse from turning into a relapse or a complete collapse.

When I asked Dr. Hill what he thought motivates people to continue to use these behavioral strategies for so many years, he had no ready answer but remarked, "There's nothing new here (referring to the behavioral strategies). What we are telling people is right. If you do it, it works. The burning question is *how these people are able to maintain healthy behaviors in an environment that isn't supportive. They are having to make heroic efforts in order to do it.*" He went on to say, "What people have to do [in maintenance] is fight the environment a little bit. I think that people who really want to do it can do it. These people in the registry are handling maintenance all on their own. I think they have created their own mini-environment within the bigger environment. We need to tell people how to do that—how to make their own little environment no matter what their larger environment is."

What this means, of course, is that one of the most important steps you can take to ensure your success is to have a safe eating "mini-environment" in your home. Enid and I tend to keep such an environment in our home. We are not perfect; but neither are most successful people. Indeed, just as my taste for peanut butter changed and I can now enjoy it without overeating, similar changes seem to occur in other successful people. They find, at least to a certain extent, that they can allow some formerly "dangerous" foods in the house without these foods interfering with maintenance. Nevertheless, except for a few items or infrequent occasions, successful people make drastic changes in their home eating environments.

But what about eating out? I seem to carry a portable version of my mini-eating environment with me. I have a kind of "Star Trek" shield around me that protects me from foods I consider to be unhealthy.

When I look at the menu, the shield goes up, and only things like fish, salads, and vegetarian pastas can penetrate. My rule is to limit alcohol to two drinks and I rarely deviate from it because, as my festive dinner at Caesar's proves, the shield can be dissolved by three glasses of wine. Then it can take two days to repair the damage. Successful people do occasionally choose to have high-fat/high-calorie meals, but they don't stray far from the dietary regimen they have designed for themselves. When they do stray, they get quickly back on track.

Now I'd like to let some successful people inform you and motivate you with their success stories. I interviewed all of the following people in the three weeks before Christmas 1998.

My first interview was with Bonnie Holmes, 46. She lost 65 pounds and has kept them off for five years.

We talked first about her family and early weight history.

It runs in my family. My mother—she's definitely overweight—and my younger sister is way overweight. I was heavy in high school. I wasn't fat but I wasn't a tiny person and it was like my mother was always after me. I've always dieted, but off and on. *(Bonnie, as is true of the other people that I interviewed, has a familial predisposition to obesity.)*

I asked Bonnie how overweight she was when she embarked on her last, successful diet, and what motivated her.
Now I'm still overweight, by standards. I was up to 235 and I now weigh 170.* It was a healthy loss. It took me quite a while to lose it. I did it fairly slowly, but the big thing is that I've kept it off. It began when my mother insisted that I needed to go to Weight Watchers. I told her I did not want to go to Weight Watchers. I'm kind of a stubborn person. I'm a registered nurse, and I work odd hours, and it just didn't fit into my lifestyle, and I told her no and that when I wanted to lose weight I would do it but I would do it my way. She just told me that I couldn't do it, then, that I would never lose weight, then, and that it was very sad. *(I think that this challenge from her mother got Bonnie's dander up—there was a little irritation in her voice as she said it.)* This started it. My second thing,

*I want to point out that "success" is a very individual matter. It is not necessarily being as thin as the image on a women's magazine cover or even at suggested weight according to medical standards. You are successful when you reach a weight at which you are healthy and happy, and which you can realistically maintain within the context of your life situation.

though, that really started me into knowing that I needed to lose weight was that one night when I was running up and down the hall I got sort of out of breath, and that was embarrassing. You know, when you are going to take care of people . . . you don't want a nurse huffing and puffing when she comes up to take care of you. And, you know, I'm also a single person, and I'm by myself, so I have to take care of myself. *(There was concern in her voice here— and she had now given three reasons why she was at the ready point.)* So that's what did it, and at that point that's when I decided I'm going to start cutting back on the fat. I'm a very social person, and social is food. So I didn't diet. I don't like that word and I don't like people to use it. I never use it and I'm not going to say I'm on a diet because people, I think, sabotage you. It's like, "Oh, you can just have one. Just have this little piece," or something, so I decided I'm not going to let anyone know I'm doing this. *(For Bonnie, changing her eating habits is her own business. She doesn't want to be nagged about it or have to fight negative influences from other people in addition to her own weakness for certain foods.)*

How do you deal with social situations?
I just cut back my portions, or I would just say, "I've already eaten," and as far as alcohol is concerned, I don't drink. *(I think little white lies—anything to get people off your back about eating—are just fine!)* Maybe an occasional glass of wine now and then. I would do club sodas. It worked. But I think the basic thing that really, really helped me was that I got into an exercise. *(You are going to hear this over and over again.)* But you know what, that's the other thing. Everybody goes, "Oh, you went to a gym," and I said "No, I did not." I bought a used alpine walker from a girlfriend, an alpine climber, like a Stairmaster, and I can honestly tell you that the first time I got on it, it was for two minutes, and I thought I was going to die. I just kept working at it. Every night I'd come home and I'd do a few more minutes and I started building up and I'm now to the point I can do forty minutes solid! *(It's pretty obvious that when Bonnie decides something is worth doing, she has the determination to succeed. Forty minutes on a Stairmaster is a physical achievement to be proud of.)* I do different things, like I started incorporating a couple of Richard Simmons tapes, because they're fun, and I like music. I make myself exercise by just incorporating it—if I'm watching TV I have to be exercising. That's my reward. I tape my shows and then I get to watch them while I'm on my Stairmaster.

How long did it take you to lose 65 pounds? Did you hit any plateaus?
It took me about three years. It took me a long time because it didn't come off real fast and with my exercise I was building muscle while I was losing some of the fat. If I got disappointed sometimes [with weight not coming off fast enough], I changed my exercise. I started getting five-pound weights and just started doing different things. If I noticed my arms were getting flabby I went from aerobics to more reps [with the weights]. I think if you do different things, your body is working harder and then you do lose. Yes, I did a lot of up and down in the three years, because, like I said, I never went on what you'd call a diet, and I didn't want to quit eating sweets or quit eating desserts. I didn't quit going out. I do like going out, and it's hard to go out and stay on a diet.

I knew when I made the appointment with Bonnie that she was going out to lunch with a friend before the interview. I asked what had happened at lunch.
Today I actually had dessert, and I couldn't believe it, because I need to lose 5 pounds, but I thought, this is my day off and tonight I will not eat that much. I'll probably cook a pork chop or something on the grill and have a salad—something light. *(Bonnie has a plan in place to compensate for any dietary excess—it's obviously worked for several years.)* And then I'm gonna exercise because I just feel like doing that today. I've found that when I eat a big meal I want to exercise. I want to! And endorphins. You know how you read about endorphins? They are for real! There is such a good high that comes from when you reach that point. *(She was in high gear—exuberant—just talking about it.)* People think I'm crazy, but I've never done drugs. Don't need to. Don't need those diet pills or anything.

I commented that it seemed to me that the main dietary change seemed to be controlling portions, so I asked if she had ever counted calories or fat grams.
No, I didn't count. I never kept a record. I'm kind of a lazy dieter. I didn't want to go to all the work of doing the calories or the grams. I just cut back. And when I was full, I quit eating. Sometimes I do eat larger portions, but when I do, then I don't eat as often. *(Everything she says about her eating habits shows that Bonnie has devised her own plan—a way that is exactly right for her. Whatever way you*

go *about it, must be* your *way—it doesn't have to fit anyone else's prescription!)*

Have you ever injured yourself in physical activity?
I did injure a knee, but not badly. I just sprained one of my tendons and had one of the docs look at it at work and wore a brace for a while and did quit exercising—and it drove me crazy because that's when I noticed a weight gain. I hate that. But it's a neverending battle. You can't ever quit exercising. In fact, I got back from Hawaii about three weeks ago, and the girls I went with . . . we ate in five-star restaurants every night. I decided I was on vacation and I decided I was going to eat whatever I wanted to. And I did a lot of walking and a lot of hiking and stuff but I still wound up gaining this 5 pounds. So I'm consciously exercising five times a week instead of three. *(This is what successful people do!)*

How do you manage to eat a nutritious diet, cooking for one at home?
I don't have to cook three meals a day. I think if you have a family or a husband you still feel the need to have regular scheduled meals for them. I've been very lucky that way. I'm very good about buying prepackaged small meats. I get all my steaks individually wrapped; same thing with pork chops; same thing with chicken breasts—so I can take them out one at a time. I use the grill all year round. I can throw an individual hamburger, chicken breast, whatever on the grill, make myself a salad. I buy the frozen asparagus and things like that and I throw it in the microwave and that's not too tough. *(People who live alone have difficulty preparing an interesting and nutritious diet for themselves. I think Bonnie has some ideas worth copying if you live alone.)*

I asked her how many years ago it was that she started losing weight.
It's been eight years. I was thirty-eight years old. I started a year after my divorce. I blossomed right after my divorce. I ate my way right through my depression. It was just like, "OK, I got rid of him, now I can eat whatever I want. Blah, blah, blah." I put on a lot of weight while I was married . . . and then in the year after I got divorced, I gained probably about 20 pounds. *(I think emotional triggers can go either way. Some folks gain, others lose. One successful woman reported that she got motivated to lose weight because the lawyer in her divorce case said bluntly, "The reason your husband left you is that*

you're too fat.") I really blossomed and didn't even weigh myself. I
still don't weigh myself a lot, because when I was dieting I weighed
myself pretty much every week and now I'm about at every three
weeks. I just look at how my clothes are fitting. *(Again, choose your
strategy for weighing—for years, as long as I was burning between
700 and 1000 calories a day in physical activity, I didn't need to
weigh myself. After having to cut back on activity to about 500 calories a day, I now weigh myself every day and give myself a two-
pound window.)*

Has your life changed since losing weight?
I've gotten more social. But I was always social. I guess I didn't really ever have a problem. I was always able to date and things like
that. I guess I just feel better about myself. I enjoy shopping for
clothes. For big girls back in those days they did not have cool-
looking clothes.

Do you have any big challenges in maintaining your weight?
I'm pretty much OK with what I have to do. Exercise, like I say, I
fit into my schedule. I've been thinking I might take a belly dancing class. *(We joked about this, and I encouraged her to do it. My
daughter is a belly dancer and gets a big kick out of it, as well as
great exercise.)* I'm just really happy. I think I'm probably the hap-
piest I've ever been in my life. I like my job. I'm very lucky in that
respect. There're a lot of nurses out there who I do not think are as
happy, but I do like what I do. I have a very nice family and I am
a happy single person.

*Have you changed your home eating environment—are the same
foods there as before?*
No, I have changed that. I keep a lot more carrots and celery
around. I do try and buy a lot of low-fat things. I don't count the
grams, but I'm conscious when I do shop to buy low-fat, and it's so
easy to do. It's just not a challenge anymore. *(Once you've remade
your home eating environment you will have a major part of the
problem solved.)*

Do you keep certain foods out of the house?
I do not. Anything can come in. I just watch my portions. I just
bought six gallons of ice cream because I've got company coming
at Christmas—my nieces and nephews and mom and dad—and I

buy everything for them and I have found that I do not have to eat it. I say to myself, "Bonnie, if you're really hungry you can have a bite of ice cream. Just do a little bit of it." I don't deprive myself of anything. I think life's too short. I think if you want a little ice cream, it's OK, but just do a little bit of it and don't do it all the time. If sometimes I overindulge—maybe one out of five or six times when I eat ice cream—then I double exercise. *(Bonnie has one food in her home that might tempt her to overeat, but it happens rarely and she has a compensating strategy in place.)*

Do you ever hold conversations with yourself?
I do talk to myself. I don't talk out loud, but I do talk. I think a big thing is staying positive. *(Successful people accent the positive. They direct their minds to positive thoughts, and it works.)* If I am depressed—I don't get depressed very often—I tell myself how lucky I am. I may not be lucky in all ways, but I'm lucky to have a very nice home, to be comfortable, to have a good job, to have a loving family. I get depressed when I don't exercise. I went to visit my parents for two weeks and was very busy and I didn't exercise. When I got home I was down. I find that every time I haven't exercised at least once or twice a week I get down and I talk myself out of it by exercising and thinking about the positives in my life. *(For some reason, exercise makes it easier to create a positive frame of mind—perhaps it really is the endorphins!)*

And you know what else I do . . . what else is a high for me? I like to clean! I like to clean house. If I'm getting depressed, I'll wipe down a floor or something. That's an upper for me. It's another thing that I can do because I know that it will lift my spirits.

For people like yourself, do you have any words of encouragement or advice?
I have many obese friends, and they do come to me and tell me things and ask advice. It's kind of ironic. They come to me and they all go, "I'm going to do this and I'm going to do that," and I say, "That's wonderful if that's what works for you." I've got one girlfriend who has gone through Weight Watchers three times now, and she is horribly obese, and healthwise she is going to be hurt, and all I said to her, again, was, "I really don't think you should tell anybody that you're doing this—maybe your family—and I don't think you should change your diet like you usually do." All these people that change their diets . . . I have one girlfriend who went

to this Jenny Craig. She did all the exact diet like they did and she lost 150 pounds and she looked dynamic and she was exercising and then she quit Jenny Craig and she started eating—just normal foods—not a lot but she may have been cheating at home, but I never saw her eat a lot and she is now up and over. I think she gained it all back and another 50. It's so sad, because all that money and all that time and she is just huge. So she's another one that has come to me, and all I can tell them is, "Just watch your fat intake and exercise. Just start walking. Start with five minutes a day." *(Bonnie says it all in this last line.)*

———

Terri Boyle, 45, lost 145 pounds three years ago and has kept off 135 of those pounds.

Does obesity run in your family?
I would say yes, my father has always been overweight and has had a big problem with that, and I am my father's daughter, not only by body build but by looks. I was large when I was in high school. I was a size 14, 16, somewhere around there, so I was overweight at that point and then got progressively bigger as I had kids and got older.

Did you try to diet before this last successful time?
No, I never really dieted. My family—my immediate family (my sister and mother) would occasionally say, "You know, you're really heavy," and I'd say, "When I'm really ready to lose the weight, I'll lose the weight and until I'm ready to lose it I'm not going to do anything about it." *(I remember getting pretty annoyed when people nagged me about my weight—after making me clean my plate because of the starving people in Armenia, my mother would always remind me that I was too fat and had to go on a diet—from the age of twelve on. The determination to be successful in the weight-loss battlefield has to come from within.)*

What motivated you when you finally decided?
Well, there were a lot of changes that were going on in my life. There was a move to another state, and the family was going to be separated for a while, and I decided I wanted to find "me." I was kinda tired of being somebody's mom and somebody's wife. There was a Terri out there somewhere, and I sure didn't know who she was. I just wanted to find me. *(The changes Terri so briefly alludes*

to influenced every moment of her daily life. The separation from her husband enabled her to take command, as you will see.)

How old were you at that time?
I was forty-two.

What did you do to go about losing the weight?
I slowly changed my eating patterns. I sat down and decided that I knew what a healthy diet was because my then-husband had been diagnosed as diabetic several years before, and I'd been to nutritionists over and over again, learning how to take care of him. So I knew what a healthy diet was. I knew what I should be eating, and I made a conscious effort to change how I ate and what I ate. I had three teenage kids, age fifteen to twenty-two, and I basically looked at them and said, "This is what I am going to eat. I'll be more than happy to make enough for all of us, but if you don't want what I'm going to eat, there's the kitchen and you can go fix your own food." *(How about that! How many overweight wives and mothers feel they can take a stand like that? Some of the determination she must have felt at that time was still in her voice this moment.)*

You said your "then-husband."
We're in the throes of a divorce, actually, right now. I'm a much happier person right now.

Has the divorce caused any problems in managing your weight?
On occasion it has. There is a lot of stress related to that and I occasionally go into little pity parties and say, "I don't care. I'm going to eat that doughnut. I don't care." Then I kick myself and say, "You really gotta get back."

How much did you lose in the first place, and how did you go about doing it?
Total loss down to my lowest point was about 145 pounds. I did it all on my own. No pills, no diets, no doctors, no nothing. I cut out almost all my breads, I cut out all fried foods, I ate very little meat, I ate tons and tons of vegetables, and I actually ate quite a few baked potatoes. I pretty much had half a baked potato just about every day. I cut out butter and things like that when I had a baked potato. I used to have a baked potato with my butter, but I cut it out and had it with salsa or with onions or with something like that. I

didn't need the butter. I cut out all snacking things like potato chips and stuff like that, although I was a big fan (and still am) of baked tortilla chips. That was my chip. I learned the magic word "no." I also did not deprive myself. If I really, really wanted something . . . I always kept candy in the house, I kept my stash of chocolate and it was mine and I could have a piece if I really wanted it. I haven't missed the French fries and the Big Macs and things. I ate a lot of salad. I love salad. I went to things that I really enjoyed eating—and why I didn't eat them before in the amount I do now was, I think, because I didn't like myself. I was in an unhappy place in my life and food was a great comfort to me. Now I definitely like myself a whole lot better.

Were there any adverse effects of your dieting?
I did have a problem in my left leg, a kind of palsy, that was due to such rapid weight loss. I lost about 130 pounds in a year. It was an average of about 10 pounds a month, but I never starved myself. People used to ask me, "Aren't you hungry?" and I'd say, "No, I'm not hungry. I eat like a fiend." My daughter, who is now about nineteen, so she was sixteen, seventeen, eighteen . . . her friends would say, "Your mother starves herself," and she goes, "Oh, my God, my mother has food in her hands all the time!" So it wasn't that I wasn't eating. I was. I nibbled constantly. Carrots, celery, cauliflower—especially as snacks. *(As long as you cultivate a taste for "safe" foods, you really can nibble all day long.)*

Did you get support or collaboration from your family and your children and friends?
Nobody noticed, because I started out at 255 plus, and my husband and I hadn't seen each other . . . he left in March and I saw him at the end of May and I had lost about 30 pounds, and 30 pounds on my frame at that time, you couldn't tell. The next time I saw him I had lost 60 pounds, and at that point in time you could tell. I had support from my daughter. My daughter and I stayed in Texas an extra year while the rest of my family moved to Colorado. I worked with computers in the technology department of a school district and I had a year-round contract. But I stayed down there so she could graduate from high school. She was very active in her school and I couldn't move her. She supported me quite a bit, and the people at work, once they noticed, supported me. I will tell you I had a win-win-win situation. I started my weight loss in March, and

by the time school was out at the end of May I had lost 30 pounds, and that was great, but nobody really noticed. I thought, "Well, during the summer if I continue to lose weight, that's great; but if I don't lose any more weight, I've at least lost 30 pounds; and if I gain it all back, nobody is going to notice it. So I'll only know if I've failed. So I'm in a win-win-win situation." Like I said, I continued to lose weight, so when everybody came back from summer break they went, "Whoa!" So I had all that support plus my daughter. To be really honest, my husband never really recognized the fact and never praised me, never asked me about losing weight or anything, and that was a stumbling block for me.

How about physical activity while you were dieting?
I did absolutely nothing for six months. Then I started slowly doing crunches and things like that. Not a lot. About nine months after I started, I started walking and I became an avid walker. I walked about two miles every day, and normally a little bit longer on Sundays. I was religious on that. I had my time to walk, and I enjoyed it, and it didn't matter if it was 110 degrees or if it was 40. I enjoyed my walk. Then, when I moved to Colorado, the change in temperature really kinda blew me. I found other ways. I joined a step aerobic class and I attended . . . I say attended because right now I am really not doing a lot. I was in a bad car accident and I hurt my back and my shoulders so I'm going through PT [physical therapy], which is called Pain and Torture. This has also caused a problem in how I eat, especially with holidays. Not being active and seeing all this food is not easy.

How are you dealing with that? You're in a tough situation. You can't exercise, you're surrounded by foods, the holiday . . .
Well, actually, what I do now is walk stairs every day during work. I'm now a business analyst with the local phone company. I interact between the clients, when they call to say they have a problem, and the programmers, and describe the problem so they can fix it. There's a group of four of us that usually meet at a certain point in the morning to walk the stairs, and then we go back to work. It takes twenty minutes or so. I walk 14 flights of stairs every day, up and down and around my building and back to my floor. They have been doing it for several years, and I am almost at the one-year mark. My physical therapist says walking is OK, and I occasionally

get a walk in, but with it getting dark so early and with the temps and everything I find that much more difficult. Seeing that I haven't been able to do my regular exercise I have really kept up with the stair climbing.

I guess we just have to stay motivated and find something when circumstances change.
Yes, yes—when our phone company went on strike—I was transplanted to Salt Lake City, and at four o'clock every morning I was down on the treadmill because I didn't know where to walk. So, yes, you always find a means somehow if you really want to do it.

Has your life changed since losing all this weight?
I've become a much happier person. I think those around me have become much happier, although my marriage has broken up. That wasn't due to my weight loss. The one thing that I still have problems with—I walk past a window and see my reflection and I have to double-take because I still don't believe it's me. I still see a fat Terri in there, and I have a problem with that. *(Many overweight people have this problem. I did. In fact, only after I became a runner and ran my first quarter-mile in ninety seconds did the illusion of still being fat pass. Physical activity, especially of a vigorous nature, will give you a better sense of your body than a mirror will.)* But I love buying clothes. *(Said with a great deal of pleasure!)* I got down to 111, and at five-feet-five I looked emaciated. I am normally 122 to 125. *(This puts her toward the bottom of the range of suggested weights for height in government guidelines.)*

Did you ever count calories or fat grams?
I read labels, and, yes, I will put things down that have a large amount—but counting them and keeping track of them, no. I realized what was fat, what wasn't fat. I was thinking of limiting fat and limiting sugar, so in essence I guess I was limiting calories because I cut out chocolate cake and things like that. And I've been able to bake and not eat cookies. In fact, there's fudge sitting out in my kitchen right now. I think I've had half a piece since it's been out there for two weeks.

What would you say are your biggest challenges right now?
Exercise. The frustration of not being able to exercise.

Have you brought much more food into your home for the holidays, or is it just at work and when you go out?
A lot of it is at work, and there are occasions that we have been going out at work. That's not so bad. I can go out and get soup and salad. That's not hard for me to do, but what is really, really difficult for me are the potlucks. Everybody brings their stuff to work and I have a real . . . I live to eat; I don't eat to live. I love food.

Do you still limit certain foods most of the time?
I have no wants or desires for McDonald's or French fries. I limit fried foods—fried chicken totally turns me off now. I don't eat chips. I still limit my meat. I will fix hamburgers and chicken and all kinds of things for the kids, but then I don't generally eat it. I pick out all the vegetables and leave the meat for the kids.

How about fish?
I do like fish, but I don't cook fish very well. I will have it when I go out on occasion. If it's on the menu and it looks good, and if it's grilled. I will not eat fried fish.

Are you careful about portion sizes?
Generally I am, but I let myself gorge on vegetables.

Vegetables are one thing; but how about anything that has a lot of fat or sugar—the things that people normally think put on weight?
On Sundays we always have had a family ritual of chocolate chip pancakes with butter and powdered sugar, and I will tell you that I never limited myself completely. I cut back. Instead of having three pancakes, now I have one. It's either that or French toast on Sundays, and that's one thing that I said if I'm good all week long I can have.

Are there still some times when you have finished a meal and you say to yourself that you did overeat? Or does that never happen anymore?
Oh, no, it happens. I'm terrible, especially going out to [my favorite local] all-you-can-eat buffet. We even have a super salad at the buffet I like, and I'll just go in and get salads but I'll eat so much I'll almost get sick. But if I'm that full I won't eat later. Especially if it's a lunchtime meal, I won't eat dinner because I'm just too full. I don't eat when I'm not hungry normally. *(Terri's description of her eating*

environments at home, work, and at the buffet illustrates the kind of battle all of us face. As Dr. Hill says, "The environment is not supportive." Terri knows how to win most of the battles, and when she loses one, she regroups and wins the next several!)

Do you hold conversations with yourself?
Oh, yes! A lot of times I kick myself for eating the wrong things, and about three weeks ago I had had, I guess, about a week of too much nibbling, and I sat myself down on a Friday and I talked to myself. I said "Terri, I give you permission to eat anything you want all weekend, in any quantity you want, it doesn't matter what you eat. You have free permission to go and do whatever you want." And I did. And on Monday I got up and I felt fantastic and then I didn't budge. I stuck to it. I really had success of having several weeks of not having to—to—appease myself. I think every now and then you have to give yourself permission. *(I agree—if you are going to deviate, put it under your conscious control. Most of the time you won't get carried away if you do this. But before Terri gave herself permission for the weekend, she had a plan for Monday and the days after, and she was confident she would be able to carry out her plan.)* I do occasionally look at myself and say, "You do look good." I guess I take better care of myself totally, not just bodily, but I do give myself better strokes. I do tell myself I look good even though sometimes I do see a fat person. I treat myself—to an extra nice blouse or something—where I wouldn't have before. *(There's that positive frame of mind, and she feels good enough about herself to give herself a well-deserved reward.)*

I think hearing the things you are saying would be so helpful to folks just starting out.
I will tell you that I went to a focus group meeting on Monday night through the Weight Loss Registry. It was eight women and it was fascinating because I'd never been through this before. All of us had the same theme in our wants and desires and our successes in losing weight, and that was a lifestyle change. There were a couple of women who had tried diet programs or whatnot, but they failed with them. And then when they made the conscious effort, that they knew that they were going to have to find a way to eat and live with that pattern for the rest of their lives, that was the only successful way that we all found that we could lose weight. We thought that

was fascinating. *(And it's obviously one of the conditions necessary for success. You've got to think in terms of the rest of your life.)*

What kind of advice would you give to somebody about losing and maintaining from your experience?
About losing, that was one question that was asked of us—like if it was a 300-pound person saying, "What do I do?" One of my things is not to focus on the negative. There's always a thing that you like about yourself. It may be your nose. But there is always something that you like. Concentrate on that, and be happy with that, and then try to improve other things. Don't try to improve everything, because you have to take it slow. Make small steps. Don't say you're going to lose 100 pounds. That is self-defeating right there. Make small steps and don't be disappointed when things don't go the way you want them to. Realize that there are going to be disappointments, there's going to be setbacks and there's going to be times where you overeat and you don't like yourself. But you get over it. So it's OK. Every now and then, everybody's going to fall. I would say find an exercise that you like, because everybody does need to exercise. You need to move. *(This last paragraph is worth copying and putting up on your refrigerator door. In fact, if you have a long way to go, it might be worth making several copies and putting them up on your bedroom and bathroom mirrors, posting one at work, and keeping a copy in your purse.)*

Katherine Banks is thirty-three years old. She lost 55 pounds and has kept them off for three years. Her way to success is quite different from that of the other two women. Her physical activity has become so central to her life that it has become part of her identity.

We started talking about her family and weight history.
My father's about 100 pounds overweight, my sisters are all about between 50 and 75 pounds overweight. I started gaining weight in my twenties—I was fat in my twenties. I really didn't realize how big I was. It gradually just got more and got more and more until I realized I wasn't wearing pants anymore and dresses and things that were real comfy and I thought, "Ooooo." My highest point was 190 pounds. I tried all the little tricks to lose weight, to no avail. I'd try a little bit of this diet or that diet, and I'd lose a couple here and there and then gain them back and then gain more. But I was only

successful this last time. This last time, I made life changes. I was turning thirty and I didn't like how I was feeling. So I just made lifestyle changes. When I was fat, it was taking a lot of calories for me to maintain that weight—like maybe 2500—and to lose the weight. I'm a little over five-foot-two—1200 calories would be more like maintenance.

I asked if she counted calories on this last diet.
No, I just stuck with eating a small serving of lunch and sometimes prepared meals like Lean Cuisine. I didn't count, but it was under 700 calories a day because it was a set diet. Like a Lean Cuisine, an apple, and a yogurt. I kept eating the same things. *(Using a limited diet of this kind, with low-calorie foods, is probably closest to my own early rotation plan. It will lead to a quick weight loss. You need to be sure you make a wise selection of foods if you plan to do it for any length of time.)*

Did you cut out certain foods?
I cut out bread. I can have a potato but I can't eat bread. Bread is my downfall. Just plain bread. But I've stopped doing that. I began leaning more toward the meat and fruits and vegetables and low-calorie carbohydrates. But I could have rice and potatoes, they were OK. *(This sounds like a pretty good selection.)*

How long ago did you lose the weight?
I just had my three-year anniversary on the fifteenth of December. I lost 52 pounds and I've been able to keep all off and then some more. I stay down below it, but I don't freak out if I'm up a little bit, because my workouts have gotten more . . . I work out a lot and so I don't worry. My clothes fit. The numbers don't bother me any more.

What motivated you this last time, when you were successful?
My mother had three heart attacks, one after the other, at thirty-two. She threw blood clots. *(I believe blood clots that had formed elsewhere in her body traveled to her heart and lungs.)* I didn't want to have that—I have four small children and I wanted to get the weight off before I turned thirty-five.

How long did it take you?
Fourteen weeks.

That sounds like you were pretty severe in restricting yourself.
Yes, I was. *(She said this in such a matter-of-fact way—no special emphasis in her voice at all, as though this was the only natural way to do it.)*

Were there any adverse effects?
No. I limited my caffeine because I like sugar in my coffee and sugar is also an activator for my appetite. So that caused a little bit of a headache. Now and again, I would take some Advil, but I did this drug-free. I didn't follow anybody's diet, per se. I did what worked for me.

How about other people? How did they respond to your losing weight?
Since I'm a hair stylist, I deal with about 400 people every six weeks. There were some people, like my friend Amy, she said to me last week, "Kathy, at one moment we were weight woeing, and then the next time I saw you, you were a bombshell." People were very, very neat about the whole thing. Very responsive, positive. I had a couple of people that were a little bit envious. They tried to play sabotage. They'd say, "You look too thin. I brought this sandwich for you. I know you skipped lunch." It was more of . . . I don't know if some of it was envy. Like when it came to parties at the salon, I would not have the cake. For one, I don't like cake. But there were just a couple of girls who were just a little catty about the situation. Overall, I'd say 98 percent were incredible. My husband is just ecstatic. He loves it. He loves it that I feel so good. *(If you are married and plan to stay that way, I think the cooperation, support, and encouragement of your spouse are very important. But as you have already seen, if you are divorced or getting a divorce, you can find the cooperation, support, and encouragement you need from other significant persons around you.)*

Did you get active? You said you work out.
That's how the weight kept coming down. I didn't cut more food out—I started amping up my workouts. I started building on them and really making them special for me. I started the first week when I started my new lifestyle. I started at three half-hour workouts a week at a club—a twenty-four-hour workout place. I found a workout partner. I work with Donna. She was going to her gym and I was going to my gym and I said, "Why don't we just start going to this

one and go together?" So we started going to classes together, then we started doing weights together, then we started doing elliptical trainers, and it was really nice because it's on the days you say to yourself, "I really don't want to go," Donna goes, "I'm ready," and it was extremely helpful.

What is your typical workout now?
I went from an hour and a half a week to ten hours a week. Two hours, five times—a complete workout, and I started teaching there. *(If you set yourself up as a teacher, you will have a pretty high standard to live up to, and it will add greatly to your motivation.)*

I told her that I thought it was great that she had started teaching and asked if she had ever had any injuries due to exercise.
None. I didn't sustain any injuries. When I was a teenager I danced, and I was never heavy until I hit my twenties. It was like going back [to her teens]. To me injury is just not being responsible to your form and listening to your body and watching everything and not overdoing.

Has your life changed?
My husband is pleased. My children are just . . . to be able to keep up with them and carry them up the stairs and not be winded . . . everyone's just been so wonderful. The people that didn't know me back then don't even know that I had lost this weight, so I show them pictures and they're just amazed. I say, "Aren't these great? Look at these! Look at the before and look at the after." And they say, "That's not you." I say, "Yes, that's me." *(Talk about pride and joy! I wish I could play my recording of the interview for you so you could hear the enthusiasm and excitement in her voice.)*

Do you face any challenges to keeping that weight down?
No. To be honest, I don't watch it now. I just make sure that I'm feeling good. I haven't weighed myself in probably six months. Not even at the club—I just know. *(With her workout schedule plus teaching, who would need to weigh?)*

Do you keep any particular foods out of your diet?
I don't ever limit my variety. I do allow myself a couple of bites of, say, a piece of cheesecake. I do allow myself a cookie. But I don't really like that stuff.

Did you ever like it? Is this a change in food preference?
It's a change in food preferences. My taste has gone from creamier things to more zest, more herbs. *(If you go about experimenting with herbs and spices, I think the same thing will happen to you.)*

Do you keep everything in the house, or do you keep some things out of the house?
I keep everything in the house. I just watch the portions, and I'm teaching my children also.

How about eating out?
I eat out. I just watch my breads when I eat out. I watch my creamy soups. If there's a choice of baked potato soup and vegetable soup, I take the vegetable soup where before I'd take the potato soup "and please add some cheese."

Are you eating more fruits and vegetables?
I have become a salad gourmet. I am just really into different tastes and different textures and seeing how many different ways I can surprise my taste buds.

How about fat-free desserts, cookies, pastries, and things?
Nope. To me, I'd rather eat a bite of something yummy than a whole piece of something that's yukka. *(I couldn't say it any better.)*

Do you hold conversations with yourself?
Yes, I do. A conversation that I would have about food would be at night. Actually, I do control my intake at night. I try not to eat because I have bad dreams if I eat too close to bedtime. I tell myself to put it off until tomorrow. I talk to myself about my exercise—that's the first thing I think of when I wake up.

How do you keep yourself motivated?
Hmmm, hmmm, what motivates me? People ask me all the time. They are surprised at me because I have a full-time job, four children, and I am going to the gym a minimum of ten hours a week (five days a week, two-hour workouts) and then all the running around that they [the children] have to do. I suppose my health. I like to feel good. And that makes me feel good. *(This also could not be better put. It's fundamental. You must find something that feels good, and makes you feel good about yourself.)*

When you were a heavier woman, did eating made you feel good?

Eating made me feel wonderful! A full tummy. Ohhh! I just loved a full tummy. That was just the most satisfying feeling. *(She drew out the word "won-der-ful," and her voice communicated what must have been deep sensual satisfaction. I can only think that her intense activity and healthier diet yield feelings that surpass even the gratification she must have felt from a full tummy.)* And then it was really, really funny—about a year or so ago I changed something else: now I do not finish my plate. I leave food on the plate. I never clean my plate. And I don't make my children finish everything on their plates either.

Since that is something usually suggested in weight-management classes, I asked if she had read about doing that someplace or someone had suggested it to her.

My mother and father are heavy people, and I was brought up in a home where you finished everything that was given to you, and you did not leave the table until your plate was clean. So, no. I just started to do that to prove to myself that I didn't have to have that. That I didn't really need that and that that's OK. *(I think she is demonstrating both her strength of character and independence with this control over an appetite that once had control over her.)*

What kind of advice would you give people like yourself?

In your weight-loss program, make small successes for yourself. Attainable goals. Be realistic. But don't cave in to your old lifestyle, because if you're heavy for so long it's going to take a little while to change the clock. So do not set expectations so high that you're setting yourself up for a fall. In maintaining, whatever you're doing your last week of whenever you hit your goal, you need to maintain that much activity. I was at two hours a workout, five times a week. You have to maintain your last week's activity as your minimum activity level. *(The advice to keep up your activity at the level that helped you lose weight is very important. If you maintain your level of activity, it reinforces your motivation to stick with a healthful weight-maintenance diet. As a member of one of my weight groups once said when asked what motivated him to stick with his diet, "I'm not going to blow it after I've invested an hour of my time walking today!")*

Susan Carpenter is forty-one years old and works in the Treasury Department of the Tennessee state government. She was adopted as an infant and does not know her biological parents. She told me that she did not start to gain weight until her late twenties.

I asked her what brought on the weight gain.
I attribute most of it to stress. There were a lot of problems in my adoptive family—I'm pretty much the caretaker and I get involved. I was not taking as good care of myself as I should have.

That was in your late twenties? Did you start dieting then?
I tried to do quick-fix things. I tried exercising here and there. I didn't stick to anything. I tried to eat quick on the run, fast meals and all that. It just gradually added up.

What motivated you this last time?
I was feeling terrible. I couldn't get into any of the clothes that I liked and found myself getting bigger and bigger clothes. Just one day I got up and said to myself, "This is just not gonna get it. This is terrible. What am I doing to myself?" I weighed 195 pounds. I'm pretty tall [she is five-foot-nine], but that was about 45 pounds over-weight. So I made up my mind to start—it was last December, about the day before New Year's Eve. I decided I was going to do a jour-nal of everything that I ate and that I would start a walking program. That's what I did, and that's what I stuck to. *(Susan is a very at-tractive woman, and I feel certain that gaining weight was a blow to her self-esteem. She was the first person I interviewed to indicate the use of a journal.)*

Was the journal an eating record? Did you keep track of anything be-sides the food you were eating?
I was trying to keep up with what I felt when I wanted to eat for all of the wrong reasons. I was trying to keep up with what I felt at cer-tain times of the day—when my danger times were. When I found out, I prepared to do something else as opposed to eating. I would go out and take a quick walk or pick up a book and start reading—something different rather than eat something that wasn't good for me. *(Like most people who keep a record of their eating, she quickly found the times of day when she would eat in a way that contributed not only to her weight gain, but to feelings of anger, frustration, and depression. What she did instead of eating helped her deal with her feelings at the same time.)*

Did you use any special diet this time?

To tell you the truth, no. I just pretty much got together everything I had read. But I pretty much decided on my own regimen. I just tried to eat a lot more vegetables and fruit. Cutting down on meat. I've never been that much of a meat eater anyway, but I just really tried to kinda watch my fat grams.

Did you actually count fat grams?

I didn't really count them. I watched the fat, but I wasn't real strict on watching every gram or anything like that. I just kind of watched how many vegetables and fruits I was eating every day. I was trying to "up" on that. *(Like other successful people who do it on their own, Susan knows where the fat is in her foods and designs a diet that fits her own unique needs. Her emphasis is positive—she is focusing more on what she wanted to "up" rather than on the fat she was reducing in her diet.)*

Would you say that you were limiting foods—that you were cutting certain things out of your diet?

Yes—I was trying to cut out a lot of dairy foods and I was trying to cut out some of the cheeses and mayo and some of the breads and starches. I love potatoes and bread and all that good stuff and I knew that I was eating too much of it.

How about today? Are you still limiting foods?

I've found that I've become, through this year of doing this, almost automatically aware of what I eat, and if I allow myself certain things I realize later on that I have to make up for that. It has kinda become my own little system.

Do you think in terms of some foods are good and some foods are bad?

Yes. I sure do. *(Susan is the first to put it quite so bluntly. But as you'll see, thinking in terms of good/bad has no ill effects for her. She has a compensation strategy that allows her to occasionally eat "bad" foods without going off the deep end or feeling particularly guilty or bingeing.)*

And what do you do about "bad" foods? Do you keep them in the house?

I try not to. Through my year of watching myself and putting everything in a journal, I've found that at certain times of the day—and it's usually afternoon when I get home from work—that's when I find myself doing the weirdo eating. Of grabbing potato chips or crackers or anything quick. But sometimes my husband will bring things in that I don't really want, and sometimes I do have some. Then I try to always walk a little bit extra or really, really limit myself the rest of the day, or maybe the first of the next day. I will, somehow or other, keep myself from having any more of it or just really try to eat things that are not as bad the rest of the day.

Going back to this past year, when you were watching your diet, have you had any problems sticking with it—problems with people or your schedule?
No, not really. At the very first I found myself turning down lots of offers to go out or things that I would have done before just because I knew that tempting things would be there. I was really trying to start out hard core on all of it, and I found myself doing that and not seeing some of my friends as much as I had before because of the things that we ate together. I knew that I just couldn't do that then. Now I go out and stick with it. Sometimes not totally, but I find myself limiting. I'm very aware of what I'm eating, as opposed to before. I had no idea until I started writing it down. I had NO idea. *(This is something most people will find out if they take the trouble to observe themselves carefully and truthfully.)*

When you write things down, do you do it before you eat or afterwards?
That's a good question, because sometimes I'd cheat and not even want to write down what I would eat. Usually it was after. And there were times, though, when I did before. I was trying at certain times to plan my meals and go to the grocery store and get the things together, and I'd try to stick to what I knew that I wanted and needed to eat.

Did that help you?
It did. I like having strict guidelines. For me, it works. Don't always stick to them, but I'm trying to go that route.

Was this the first time that you had tried to get active?
No. I've tried to work out with other people, go to health clubs and different things that I ended up not sticking to, but I have found with the walking (I walk at home now and I walk at other places too) that

it's something that I really enjoy and that I can stick to. I do four to five miles a day, average.

What keeps you motivated to stay active?
The way that it makes me feel better. The energy that it gives me. It's meant a lot to me spiritually. When I miss a few days or when the weather is too bad or whatever, there is a big difference in how I feel and my mood, my energy level, everything. And even, really, how I eat. *(Susan is as committed to walking as I am, even without having a contract to do so with three dogs. She's out there in all kinds of weather, except for electrical storms.)*

Being active helps with better control over your eating habits?
Absolutely. It's really true for me.

Did you ever have any injuries while you were walking this past year?
Not really. I noticed, though, there were times that maybe the knee would hurt a little or the ankle or whatever and it would make me kind of ease up for a little while, but, no, I haven't had any injuries. The only thing was my feet—when I first started out I was walking so much, and I ended up spending quite a bit of money on good walking shoes. It made a big difference. *(This is an important point. As I said earlier in the book, most aches and pains people get from walking are due to shoes that are not correct for their leg, foot, and ankle alignment.)*

Has your life changed since losing weight?
I'm feeling so much better, resting better, just wanting to be more active in general.

Do you face any challenges in maintaining your activity and in sticking to your regimen?
There are times when the weather seems to affect my joints, with swelling and things like that, and that's the biggest challenge for me to go ahead and get up and go out and walk anyway, when I'm having some pain. But I find that if I go ahead and do it, it's almost like it's a natural painkiller, because it goes away.

Are there any foods that you used to eat that you do not eat anymore?
I do not eat pork. I've limited red meat to very, very little. Probably once a month. I eat a lot of chicken and fish, and I watch portions.

How about eating out? Is that a challenge?
I love to eat out, and that is a challenge. I like Japanese food a lot. Japanese, Chinese, and really this whole year I haven't been eating out much just because it's easier for me to watch what I eat and get it together myself at home. *(Successful people report eating the great majority of their meals at home, not out. They frequently brown-bag to work.)*

Has your husband been cooperative?
He's done fairly well this time. We've been through this before. This time I told him, I said, "You know, I've got to do this, and I'm going to do this, and I want you to do it with me, but if you can't, please try to be supportive because this is the way it's got to be," and he's been pretty good about it. And of course he's been really happy to see that I've lost. *(If you have not always gotten the level of support from your spouse that you would like, you need to sit down and discuss your needs. If you cannot reach an understanding, I think you will both be very unhappy. Perhaps you will find that doing "fairly well" and being "pretty good" are enough.)*

What do you think is more important, watching food or staying active?
Staying active. I've benefited from both, and I think they both work together, but as far as being active, for me I think I've benefited most from that. I really do. I think once I finally get all of the weight off— I want to lose another 15 to 20 pounds—I'll maintain it this time. I think walking will do it.

Do you hold any conversations with yourself?"
I'm telling myself, "You can do it." And, "This is a new day." I'm very positive, very positive.

What kind of advice would you give to other people to help them succeed?
You just have to come to a point where you really want to do it. I realize that now. There's nothing that can make you do that but yourself. And I would definitely advise them to write down what they ate and why. When I did that, so much came to me. I couldn't believe what I was eating, and it all came to me why I had the weight on me. *(As I have said before, I think this is an excellent*

idea, and if you do it before you eat, it may help you even more to gain a sense of control.)

Some observations on these successful weight-loss stories.

The printed word does not do justice to the excitement and happiness I heard in the voices of these women as they answered my questions. They are pleased with themselves, and they deserve to be. It takes great determination to accomplish what they have accomplished—they are the weight-loss heroes. Kathy was absolutely gleeful when she recounted showing her before and after pictures to friends who never knew her as a fat person. All of the conversations were filled with youthful laughter—they all were just bubbling over—and it was clear that they all enjoyed talking about their success. I believe talking about your success reinforces your motivation and commitment.

The first three women, from the NWCR, are doing it on their own, as is Susan Carpenter, a neighbor. Each has devised her own regimen, and I say "doing it" rather than "did it" because it is an ongoing, never-ending process. The only weight-management approach that will work for you is one that you tailor-make for yourself and that you can live with for the rest of your life. Take good ideas from wherever they originate, but *make them your own.*

Notice, however, that everyone is ending up in the same place—a permanent low-fat diet and a big increase in physical activity. And while it's a low-fat diet, we don't all eat the same foods; nor do we all engage in the same physical activities. You must find your own way.

Why do successful people do what they do?

In part, it's because the payoff is especially great when you find your own way. It fits you. And because it's your own, there is an even greater sense of accomplishment and pride. Of course, being successful, you feel better and you like yourself better. You like the way you look, and you are physically and mentally more vigorous. Just feeling good about yourself—that's the bottom line.

If there is one thing that is essential to your plan, it's finding a way to deal with the almost unavoidable deviations. You must devise a plan that gives you confidence that you can make the right choices. For example, you can make a choice to have a weekend like Terri's, but you must have a plan to compensate before it develops into a downward spiral and continued bouts of overeating. Successful people quickly go back on a mini-diet, and everyone I've talked with adds a little bit more activity until they return to where they want to be. Think of it as a positive cycle: getting quickly back on track increases your confidence in your plan, and with increased confidence in yourself, you quickly put your plan into action when you need it because you know it works. End result: success.

I hope that what we have had to say in this book will be helpful to you and that you, too, will join the ranks of the weight-loss heroes. I am very happy to hear from readers. I read all my mail and *always* answer, often with Jamie's help. Please be patient, since it may take several weeks if we are away from home. (I cannot do it by phone because of the tremendous number of calls.)

Martin Katahn, Ph.D.
4607 Belmont Park Terrace
Nashville, TN 37215

Additional Scientific Background for the T-Factor 2000 Diet

A great many studies support the contention that high-fat diets promote obesity in persons with a familial predisposition to obesity and that a high-carbohydrate diet may be crucial in the prevention and treatment of obesity (Astrup, 1993; Astrup and Raben, 1996; Astrup, Toubro, Raben, and Skov, 1997). Many studies show that as the proportion of carbohydrate in total energy intake goes up, body weight goes down (Astrup and Raben, 1995).

High-fat diets promote overconsumption because, in contrast to carbohydrate, fat has a weak effect on satiation—that is, the consumption of fat does not generate strong physiological signals to turn off a person's appetite in the course of a meal at the point when energy intake is adequate to maintain energy balance. In addition, calorie for calorie, fat has a disproportionately weak effect on satiety compared with protein and carbohydrate—that is, consuming a high-fat meal does not reduce subsequent hunger and future eating compared to a high-carbohydrate meal in which far fewer calories have been consumed (Blundell and MacDiarmid, 1997). When given a choice of a range of high-fat foods or high-carbohydrate foods and the opportunity to consume as much as they wished, obese subjects took in twice as much energy from the selection of high-fat foods as from the high-carbohydrate foods (1336 calories and 677 calories, respectively). There was no significant difference in the amount of food eaten as snacks later in the day, or in the amount of food eaten in subsequent meals during the following day (Blundell, Burley, Cotton, and Lawton, 1993). This same study suggested that when obese persons are hungry, they are likely to overeat on high-fat foods, not high-carbohydrate foods. While laboratory experiments show that consistent high-fat or low-fat food manipulations lead to weight gain or weight loss, respectively, obesity in humans in free living conditions may develop gradually as a result of only occasional high-fat meals—for example, on just one or two days each week (Blundell and MacDiarmid, 1997; MacDiarmid, Cade, and Blundell, 1996).

THE SECOND LAW OF ENERGY BALANCE

The First Law of Energy Balance states that *energy in* must equal *energy out* to maintain a stable weight. Obese individuals must therefore have ingested more energy than they expended over some period of time in order for them to have expanded their fat stores and gained weight.

The Second Law of Energy Balance evolved from research that showed that there is a complex relationship between each of the macronutrients that affect energy expenditure such that each must be in balance for a stabilized body weight. "Carbohydrate, fat and protein are regulated separately, with no conversion taking place between fats and carbohydrates" (Astrup, 1993, p. S32). Both protein and carbohydrate are tightly regulated in a way that results in whatever is eaten being oxidized in the body's fuel mixture. Fat is oxidized in the fuel mixture to fill the gap between the energy supplied by protein and carbohydrate in the diet and the body's total energy needs (Flatt, 1988; Flatt, 1995c).

Acheson et al. demonstrated that while a 2000-calorie carbohydrate load resulted in the temporary conversion of 81 calories to fat, at the end of twenty-four hours, the subjects were in negative fat balance (they burned the 81 calories and a couple hundred more withdrawn from fat stores). The authors conclude that the conversion of fat to storage "remains too limited even after such large CHO [carbohydrate] intakes to cause an increase in the body's fat content" (Acheson et al., 1984, p. E62).

Another experiment (Flatt, Ravussin, Acheson, and Jequier, 1985) showed that the amount of protein and carbohydrate in a meal will be oxidized in the body's fuel mix whatever the fat content. Subjects consumed a breakfast containing about 120 calories in protein and about 292 calories in carbohydrate on each of two days. On one day it also contained 54 calories in fat, and on the other day it contained 414 calories in fat. The fat content of the breakfast had no effect on carbohydrate and protein oxidation. On both days, approximately 120 calories in protein and 292 calories in fat were burned in the fuel mix. Regardless of the fat content of the breakfast, the body also burned about 360 calories in fat to meet energy needs. When only 54 calories in fat were contained in the breakfast, approximately 306 were withdrawn from fat stores to be oxidized in the body's fuel mix. When 414 calories in fat were contained in the breakfast, the body burned about 360 calories supplied by fat in the breakfast, which left a surplus of dietary fat of about 54 calories to be added to the body's fat stores.*

It takes continual, greatly excessive intake of carbohydrate energy to force the body to convert an appreciable amount of carbohydrate to fat for storage. Acheson et al. fed subjects 1500 calories in excess of their energy needs for a period of seven days. On the second day, about 270 calories of carbohydrate were converted to fat, while on the fourth day the figure reached 720 calories. Had the experiment continued beyond seven days, the researchers estimated that some 70 to 75 percent of the excess intake would be retained in fat storage. However, this phenomenon is not likely to be seen under normal circumstances, since the body resists the conversion of carbohydrate to fat by greatly increasing the metabolic rate in an attempt to burn off the excess carbohydrate. In the present case, the increase amounted to 35 percent, which in turn required the subjects to ingest over 5000 calories a day when their original energy needs on day one were only 2100 calories. Such massive overfeeding causes a great deal of discomfort, and few people are likely to do this except under research conditions (Acheson et al., 1988).

But carbohydrate does have an indirect effect on the body's ability to burn fat. Right after a meal, the body switches to carbohydrate in its fuel mix and suppresses fat oxidation. This occurs even if the meal contains only a small amount of carbohydrate. An excessive amount of carbohydrate consumption on a continual basis may re-

*An extremely high intake of fat—for example, 80 grams (720 calories)—may cause a slight increase in fat oxidation (perhaps about 10 percent of the intake) and an equal reduction in carbohydrate oxidation.

sult in heavily loaded glycogen stores, which, in turn, may put continual pressure on the body to favor carbohydrate oxidation over fat oxidation. To put it another way, as carbohydrate consumption increases, the gap between total energy needs and combined carbohydrate and protein intake narrows. Since whatever carbohydrate and protein is consumed will be burned in the fuel mix, if the fat intake is less than the gap, it will be withdrawn from fat stores and burned to meet the body's needs. If the fat intake exceeds the gap, it goes into storage (Flatt, 1995a; Flatt, 1995c; Flatt, 1996a; Flatt, 1996b). An enlargement of the body's fat mass "causes an increase in fatty acid release, which leads to higher fatty acid concentrations, and to a type of insulin resistance susceptible to enhancing fat oxidation relative to glucose oxidation"; and " . . . the problem of body weight regulation can, in effect, be focused on the issue: How fat does one have to be to oxidize as much fat as one eats?" (Flatt, 1995d, p. 956S).

Schutz et al. found that fat oxidation decreased by 20 grams a day in the fasting state after a weight loss of 22 pounds of fat in obese women, suggesting that 22 pounds of fat on the human body enables the oxidation of 20 grams of fat in the diet (Schutz, Tremblay, Weinsier, and Nelson, 1992). Other studies give values of as little as 11 and 13 grams of fat for 22 pounds of fat (Astrup, Buemann, Christensen, and Madsen, 1992; Astrup et al., 1994). There are wide individual differences, and some individuals can consume a high-fat diet without getting fat. What these studies show is that " . . . in susceptible individuals the expansion of fat stores is a prerequisite to increase the oxidative fat energy to an amount commensurate with a high percentage of dietary fat energy" (Astrup et al., 1994, p. 350). On the other hand, "Since the steady-state of weight maintenance is achieved with less body fat in physically active individuals, exercise is a substitute for an enlarged fat mass in bringing about rates of fat oxidation commensurate with fat intake" (Flatt, 1995b, p. S31). Since the average individual will burn at least 20 grams of fat in an hour of moderate physical activity such as walking, it is clear that exercise can play a major role in the prevention of obesity and the maintenance of a lower weight after a significant weight loss in the obese.

In a review of the role of low-fat diets in weight management, Astrup et al. list eleven studies in which low-fat diets with *ad libitum* consumption of carbohydrates resulted in spontaneous weight loss (Astrup et al., 1997). On average, a reduction of 10 percent fat energy produces an average weight loss of 12 pounds in obese persons. The review of the literature suggests that the greatest potential for a low-fat diet with *ad libitum* consumption of carbohydrates, in addition to the prevention of obesity, is in maintaining weight following weight loss achieved by any reduced energy diet. It appears to be more successful than calorie counting (Toubro and Astrup, 1997).

As the results from the National Weight Control Registry show, individuals who have lost a great deal of weight and have been successful in maintaining their losses combine the two strategies for weight management I have been discussing: a low-fat diet with exercise (Klem, Wing, McGuire, Seagle, and Hill, 1997).

SUMMARY OF RESULTS OBTAINED BY THE NATIONAL WEIGHT CONTROL REGISTRY

The National Weight Control Registry is the largest ongoing study of individuals who have been successful at long-term maintenance of weight loss ever to be undertaken. As of December 1998 there were over 3000 registrants, the average weight loss was 67 pounds, and the average length of time that the loss had been maintained was five years.

The goal of the registry is to determine what strategies successful persons use to lose weight and, perhaps of greater importance, what they do to maintain their losses. Participants in the registry report losing weight in a variety of different ways. In the first published study, which reported results for the 784 participants then enrolled, about 55 percent reported using a formal program or professional assistance to lose weight, and about 45 percent reported doing it on their own (Klem et al., 1997). In making dietary changes, almost 90 percent of the participants reported restricting intake of certain types or classes of foods, which, according to Dr. Hill, meant eliminating certain foods (for example, fried foods) during the period of weight loss or severely limiting them. Between one-third and one-half of the participants ate all foods but limited quantities; counted calories; or limited percent of energy from fat. Approximately 20 percent of the sample used liquid formula as part of their weight-loss effort. About 90 percent of the sample reported an increase in physical activity during their weight loss. Compared with previous unsuccessful attempts at losing weight, in their successful attempt, participants said they were more committed to losing weight and making behavioral changes, were more strict in their dietary approach, and engaged in physical activity to a greater extent.

In maintenance, participants report consuming 24 percent of total calories from fat. They eat out rather infrequently (less than once a week in fast food restaurants, and between two and three times a week in sit-down restaurants). The main strategy used to limit dietary intake in maintenance remains restricting intake of certain types or classes of foods (92 percent of persons). Fully 50 percent of the sample report they still count calories, fat grams, or both calories and fat grams to maintain their loss. *Thus the same strategies used to lose weight remain important in maintenance for successful losers.*

As to the quality of diet in successful losers, a recent study indicates a greater intake of calcium and vitamins A, C, and E than found for the average person in the NHANES III, probably because of a greater than average intake of fruits, vegetables, and low-fat sources of calcium. While intake of iron does not meet the RDA, it is comparable to the national sample (Shick et al., 1998).

Perhaps the most striking change in the behavior of successful persons is the increase in physical activity. Average energy expenditure in some form of exercise is 2800 calories, or 400 calories per day. Walking is the main activity, but a large number of participants report engaging in medium-intensity activities such as stationary and road cycling and use of a treadmill. Among the heavier-intensity activities are weightlifting, running or jogging, stair-stepping, and step aerobics. Another study confirms that the threshold for weight maintenance after a significant loss of weight appears to be at eighty minutes per day of activities equivalent to walking (Schoeller, Shay, and Kushner, 1997).

The questionnaires used by the researchers were not designed to get at the reasons successful persons continue to do the same things they did while losing weight to maintain their losses. However, questions about the effect of weight loss on other areas of their lives are suggestive. Over 90 percent of the participants report that their quality of life has improved, they have increased energy and greater mobility, their general mood has improved, and they are more self-confident. Perhaps these benefits underlie their willingness to continue to monitor their eating behavior and stay so active. Researchers in charge of the registry are gathering data through interviews and focus groups that may help understand more clearly the incentives and rewards that maintain successful weight-maintenance behaviors in an environment that encourages the development of obesity.

ADDITIONAL RESEARCH BACKGROUND

The artificial sweetener controversy. Is the substitution of noncaloric artificial sweeteners for sugar and other caloric sweeteners helpful in the short-term control of appetite? In a review of the literature investigating this question, Blundell and Green state, " . . . it appears to be now agreed (even among researchers who formerly held different view) that the substitution of sweet carbohydrates with high intensity sweeteners does induce caloric compensation. That is, people tend to eat more later to make up for the energy saved." But is a high intake of sugar associated with obesity? The authors go on to say, "Epidemiological studies indicate that a low body mass index is inversely associated with the intake of sugar" (Blundell and Green, 1996, p. S15). Two recent studies (Bolton-Smith, 1996; Bolton-Smith and Woodward, 1994) confirm that sugar intake is not correlated with obesity—indeed, the opposite is true. "Dietary sugars have frequently been linked with excess body weight and poor quality diets. A review of the recent research in this area reveals no basis for a causative association between sugar intake and obesity. Rather, a diet which contains a high percentage of energy from carbohydrate (starch and sugars) may assist in weight loss if the proportion of energy from fat is low" (Bolton-Smith, 1996, p. S31).

Are Americans eating less fat? The data indicating that Americans have increased their intake of fat since the 1970s are taken from Ernst et al., 1997. Another, more recent report from the USDA Center for Nutrition Policy and Promotion indicates that between 1990 and 1995, fat consumption in the United States increased by about 7 percent, with the major part of the increase (over 10 percent) occurring in the diets of men (*Insight* 5, April 1998).

Do people really know what they eat? While underreporting of food intake is common, it is especially great in overweight people. "Snack-type foods may be preferentially forgotten when obese people omit food items in dietary reporting. These results seem to match the general assumption that obese people tend to underreport fatty foods and foods rich in carbohydrates rather than underreport their total dietary intake" (Heitmann and Lissner, 1995). But underestimation of calories and fat is not limited to the obese (or lay persons). In October 1996, in a survey conducted by New York University and the Center for Science in the Public Interest, 203 dietitians were shown five typical restaurant meals at the American Dietetic Association's national convention in San Antonio, Texas. A tuna salad sandwich was estimated to contain 374 calories and 18 grams of fat, whereas the sandwich actually contained 720 calories and 43 grams of fat. A hamburger with onion rings was estimated to contain 863 calories and 44 grams of fat, whereas the meal contained 1550 calories and 101 grams of fat. A porterhouse steak dinner was estimated to contain 1239 calories and 64 grams of fat, whereas the actual dinner contained 1860 calories and 125 grams of fat. All in all, on the average, the dietitians underestimated calories by 37 percent and fat by 49 percent. The size of the meals shown had previously been determined to represent the *average*-size portions of meals served in restaurants. Obviously, portion sizes are out of control, and it seems plausible that only one or two meals such as these each week could contribute to the gradual development of obesity. The fact that trained persons can underestimate calories and fat to such an extent indicates how difficult it is for anyone to estimate how much energy they consume each day.

Additional bibliography. I have included in the bibliography that follows the reference list additional sources that were consulted while researching the scientific background for this book.

References

Acheson, K. J., Y. Schutz, T. Bessard, K. Anantharaman, J. P. Flatt, and E. Jequier. 1988. Glycogen storage capacity and de novo lipogenesis during massive carbohydrate overfeeding in man. *Am. J. Clin. Nutr.* 48, 240–247.

Acheson, K. J., Y. Schutz, T. Bessard, E. Ravussin, E. Jequier, and J. P. Flatt. 1984. Nutritional influences on lipogenesis and thermogenesis after a carbohydrate meal. *Am. J. Physiol* 246, E62–E70.

Astrup, A. 1993. Dietary composition, substrate balances and body fat in subjects with a predisposition to obesity. *Int. J. Obes. Relat. Metab. Disord.* 17, Suppl. 3, S32–S36; discussion S41–S42.

Astrup, A., B. Buemann, N. Christensen, and J. Madsen. 1992. 24-hour energy expenditure and sympathetic activity in postobese women consuming a high-carbohydrate diet. *Am. J. Physiol.* 262 (3), Pt. 1, E282–E288.

Astrup, A., B. Buemann, P. Western, S. Toubro, A. Raben, and N. Christensen. 1994. Obesity as an adaptation to a high-fat diet: evidence from a cross-sectional study. *Am. J. Clin. Nutr.* 59 (2), 350–355.

Astrup, A., and A. Raben. 1995. Carbohydrate and obesity. *Int. J. Obes. Relat. Metab. Disord.* 19, Suppl. 5, S27–S37.

Astrup, A., and A. Raben. 1996. Glucostatic control of intake and obesity. *Proc. Nutr. Soc.* 55 (1B), 485–495.

Astrup, A., S. Toubro, A. Raben, and A. Skov. 1997. The role of low-fat diets and fat substitutes in body weight management: what have we learned from clinical studies? *J. Am. Diet. Assoc.* 97, Suppl. 7, S82–S87.

Blundell, J., V. Burley, J. Cotton, and C. Lawton. 1993. Dietary fat and the control of energy intake: evaluating the effects of fat on meal size and postmeal satiety. *Am. J. Clin. Nutr.* 57, Suppl. 5, S772–S777; discussion S777–S778.

Blundell, J., and S. Green. 1996. Effect of sucrose and sweeteners on appetite and energy intake. *Int. J. Obes. Relat. Metab. Disord.* 20, Suppl. 2, S12–S17.

Blundell, J., and J. MacDiarmid. 1997. Fat as a risk factor for over-consumption: satiation, satiety, and patterns of eating. *J. Am. Diet. Assoc.* 97, Suppl. 7, S63–S69.

Bolton-Smith, C. 1996. Intake of sugars in relation to fatness and micronutrient adequacy. *Int. J. Obes. Relat. Metab. Disord.* 20, Suppl. 2, S31–S33.

Bolton-Smith, C., and M. Woodward. 1994. Dietary composition and fat to sugar ratios in relation to obesity. *Int. J. Obes. Relat. Metab. Disord.* 18 (12), 820–828.

Ernst, N. D., E. Obarzanek, M. B. Clark, R. R. Briefel, C. D. Brown, and K. Donato. 1997. Cardiovascular health risks related to overweight. *J. Am. Diet. Assoc.* 97, Suppl. 7, S47–S51.

Flatt, J. P. 1988. Importance of nutrient balance in body weight regulation. *Diabetes Metab. Rev.* 4, 571–581.

———. 1995a. Body composition, respiratory quotient, and weight maintenance. *Am. J. Clin. Nutr.* 62, 1107S–1117S.

———. 1995b. Integration of the overall response to exercise. *Int. J. Obes. Relat. Metab. Disord.* 19, Suppl. 4, S31–S40.

———. 1995c. McCollum Award Lecture, 1995: Diet, lifestyle, and weight maintenance. *Am. J. Clin. Nutr.* 62, 820–836.

———. 1995d. Use and storage of carbohydrate and fat. *Am. J. Clin. Nutr.* 61, 952S–959S.

———. 1996a. Carbohydrate balance and body-weight regulation. *Proc. Nutr. Soc.* 55, 449–465.

———. 1996b. Glycogen levels and obesity. *Int. J. Obes. Relat. Metab. Disord.* 20, Suppl. 2, S1–S11.

Flatt, J. P., E. Ravussin, K. J. Acheson, and E. Jequier. 1985. Effects of dietary fat on postprandial substrate oxidation and on carbohydrate and fat balances. *J. Clin. Invest.* 76, 1019–1024.

Heitmann, B. L., and L. Lissner. 1995. Dietary underreporting by obese individuals—is it specific or non-specific? *BMJ* 311, 986–989.

Klem, M. L., R. R. Wing, M. T. McGuire, H. M. Seagle, and J. O. Hill. 1997. A descriptive study of individuals successful at long-term maintenance of substantial weight loss. *Am. J. Clin. Nutr.* 66 (2), 239–246.

MacDiarmid, J., J. Cade, and J. Blundell. 1996. High and low fat consumers, their macronutrient intake and body mass index: further analysis of the National Diet and Nutrition Survey of British Adults. *Eur. J. Clin. Nutr.* 50 (8), 505–512.

Schoeller, D. A., K. Shay, and R. F. Kushner. 1997. How much physical activity is needed to minimize weight gain in previously obese women? *Am. J. Clin. Nutr.* 66 (3), 551–556.

Schutz, Y., A. Tremblay, R. L. Weinsier, and K. M. Nelson. 1992. Role of fat oxidation in the long-term stabilization of body weight in obese women. *Am. J. Clin. Nutr.* 55, 670–674.

Shick, S. M., R. R. Wing, M. L. Klem, M. T. McGuire, J. O. Hill, and H. Seagle. 1998. Persons successful at long-term weight loss and maintenance continue to consume a low-energy, low-fat diet. *J. Am. Diet. Assoc.* 98 (4), 408–413.

Toubro, S., and A. Astrup. 1997. Randomised comparison of diets for maintaining obese subjects' weight after major weight loss: ad lib, low fat, high carbohydrate diet v. fixed energy intake. *BMJ* 314, 29–34.

Bibliography

Acheson, K. J., J. P. Flatt, and E. Jequier. Glycogen synthesis versus lipogenesis after a 500 gram carbohydrate meal in man. *Metabolism* 31 (1982), 1234–1240.

Almeras, N., N. Lavallee, J. P. Despres, C. Bouchard, and A. Tremblay. Exercise and energy intake: effect of substrate oxidation. *Physiol. Behav.* 57 (1995), 995–1000.

Ballor, D. L., J. R. Harvey-Berino, P. A. Ades, J. Cryan, and J. Calles-Escandon. Decrease in fat oxidation following a meal in weight-reduced individuals: a possible mechanism for weight recidivism. *Metabolism* 45 (2; 1996), 174–178.

Black, A. E., G. R. Goldberg, S. A. Jebb, M. B. Livingstone, T. J. Cole, and A. M. Prentice. Critical evaluation of energy intake data using fundamental principles of energy physiology: 2. Evaluating the results of published surveys. *Eur. J. Clin. Nutr.* 45 (1991), 583–599.

Black, A. E., A. M. Prentice, G. R. Goldberg, S. A. Jebb, S. A. Bingham, M. B. Livingstone, and W. A. Coward. Measurements of total energy expenditure provide insights into the validity of dietary measurements of energy intake. *J. Am. Diet. Assoc.* 93 (1993), 572–579.

Bouchard, C., and A. Tremblay. Genetic effects in human energy expenditure components. *Int. J. Obes.* 14 (1990), Suppl. 1, S49–S55; discussion S55–S58.

Bouchard, C., A. Tremblay, J. P. Despres, A. Nadeau, P. J. Lupien, S. Moorjani, G. Theriault, and S. Y. Kim. Overfeeding in identical twins: 5-year postoverfeeding results. *Metabolism* 45 (1996), 1042–1050.

Bouchard, C., and A. Tremblay. Genetic influences on the response of body fat and fat distribution to positive and negative energy balances in human identical twins. *J. Nutr.* 127 (1997), 943S–947S.

Brownell, K. D., and T. A. Wadden. Etiology and treatment of obesity: understanding a serious, prevalent, and refractory disorder. *J. Consult. Clin. Psychol.* 60 (4; 1992), 505–517.

Buemann, B., and A. Tremblay. Effects of exercise training on abdominal obesity and related metabolic complications. *Sports Med.* 21 (1996), 191–212.

Burstein, R., A. M. Prentice, G. R. Goldberg, P. R. Murgatroyd, M. Harding, and W. A. Coward. Metabolic fuel utilisation in obese women before and after weight loss. *Int. J. Obes. Relat. Metab. Disord.* 20 (3; 1996), 253–259.

Colman, E., L. I. Katzel, E. Rogus, P. Coon, D. Muller, and A. P. Goldberg. Weight loss reduces abdominal fat and improves insulin action in middle-aged and older men with impaired glucose tolerance. *Metabolism* 44 (11; 1995), 1502–1508.

Colvin, R. H., and S. B. Olson. A descriptive analysis of men and women who have lost significant weight and are highly successful at maintaining the loss. *Addict. Behav.* 8 (3; 1983), 287–295.

Cowburn, G., M. Hillsdon, and C. R. Hankey. Obesity management by life-style strategies. *Br. Med. Bull.* 53 (2; 1997), 389–408.

Dengel, J. L., L. I. Katzel, and A. P. Goldberg. Effect of an American Heart Association diet, with or without weight loss, on lipids in obese middle-aged and older men. *Am. J. Clin. Nutr.* 62 (4; 1995), 715–721.

Dengel, D. R., R. E. Pratley, J. M. Hagberg, E. M. Rogus, and A. P. Goldberg. Distinct effects of aerobic exercise training and weight loss on glucose homeostasis in obese sedentary men. *J. Appl. Physiol.* 81 (1; 1996), 318–325.

Deriaz, O., G. Fournier, A. Tremblay, J. P. Despres, and C. Bouchard. Lean-body-mass composition and resting energy expenditure before and after long-term overfeeding. *Am. J. Clin. Nutr.* 56 (1992), 840–847.

Doucet, E., and A. Tremblay. Food intake, energy balance and body weight control. *Eur. J. Clin Nutr.* 51 (1997), 846–855.

Doucet, E., N. Almeras, M. D. White, J. P. Despres, C. Bouchard, and

A. Tremblay. Dietary fat composition and human adiposity. *Eur. J. Clin. Nutr.* 52 (1998), 2–6.

Drewnowski, A., C. L. Kurth, and J. E. Rahaim. Taste preferences in human obesity: environmental and familial factors. *Am. J. Clin. Nutr.* 54 (1991), 635–641.

Drewnowski, A., and J. Holden-Wiltse. Taste responses and food preferences in obese women: effects of weight cycling. *Int. J. Obes. Relat. Metab. Disord.* 16 (1992), 639–48.

Drewnowski, A., C. Kurth, J. Holden-Wiltse, and J. Saari. Food preferences in human obesity: carbohydrates versus fats. *Appetite* 18 (1992), 207–221.

Drewnowski, A. Why do we like fat? *J. Am. Diet. Assoc.* 97 (1997), S58–S62.

———. Taste preferences and food intake. *Annu. Rev. Nutr.* 17 (1997), 237–253.

Eckel, R. H., T. J. Yost, and D. R. Jensen. Sustained weight reduction in moderately obese women results in decreased activity of skeletal muscle lipoprotein lipase. *Eur. J. Clin. Invest.* 25 (6; 1995), 396–402.

Ewbank, P. P., L. L. Darga, and C. P. Lucas. Physical activity as a predictor of weight maintenance in previously obese subjects. *Obes. Res.* 3 (3; 1995), 257–263.

Ferguson, K. J., P. J. Brink, M. Wood, and P. M. Koop. Characteristics of successful dieters as measured by guided interview responses and Restraint Scale scores. *J. Am. Diet. Assoc.* 92 (9; 1992), 1119–1121.

Ferraro, R., S. Lillicja, A. M. Fontvieille, R. Rising, C. Bogardus, and E. Ravussin. Lower sedentary metabolic rate in women compared with men. *J. Clin. Invest.* 90 (1992), 780–784.

Ferraro, R. T., R. H. Eckel, D. E. Larson, A. M. Fontvieille, R. Rising, D. R. Jensen, and E. Ravussin, Relationship between skeletal muscle lipoprotein lipase activity and 24-hour macronutrient oxidation. *J. Clin. Invest.* 92 (1993), 441–445.

Flatt, J. P. Conversion of carbohydrate to fat in adipose tissue: an energy-yielding and, therefore, self-limiting process. *J. Lipid. Res.* 11 (1970), 131–143.

———. Body weight, fat storage, and alcohol metabolism. *Nutr. Rev.* 50 (1992), 267–270.

———. Dietary fat, carbohydrate balance, and weight maintenance. *Ann. N. Y. Acad. Sci.* 683 (1993), 122–140.

————. Influence of body composition on food intake. *Adv. Exp. Med. Biol.* 352 (1994), 27–44.

Flynn, M. A., D. D. Sugrue, M. B. Codd, and M. J. Gibney. Women's dietary fat and sugar intakes: implications for food based guidelines. *Eur. J. Clin. Nutr.* 50 (1996), 713–719.

Forbes, G. B. Diet and exercise in obese subjects: self-report versus controlled measurements. *Nutr. Rev.* 51 (1993), 296–300.

Foster, G. D., T. A. Wadden, J. L. Mullen, A. J. Stunkard, J. Wang, I. D. Feurer, R. N. Pierson, M. U. Yang, E. Presta, T. B. Van Itallie. Resting energy expenditure, body composition, and excess weight in the obese. *Metabolism* 37 (5; 1988), 467–472.

Foster, G. D., T. A. Wadden, Z. V. Kendrick, K. A. Letizia, D. P. Lander, and A. M. Conill. The energy cost of walking before and after significant weight loss. *Med. Sci. Sports. Exerc.* 27 (6; 1995), 888–894.

Foster, G. D., T. A. Wadden, R. A. Vogt, and G. Brewer. What is a reasonable weight loss? Patients' expectations and evaluations of obesity treatment outcomes. *J. Consult. Clin. Psychol.* 65 (1; 1997), 79–85.

Garrow, J. S., and C. D. Summerbell. Meta-analysis: effect of exercise, with or without dieting, on the body composition of overweight subjects. *Eur. J. Clin. Nutr.* 49 (1; 1995), 1–10.

Gatenby, S. J., J. I. Aaron, G. M. Morton, and D. J. Mela. Nutritional implications of reduced-fat food use by free-living consumers. *Appetite* 25 (1995), 241–252.

Gebhard, R. L., W. F. Prigge, H. J. Ansel, L. Schlasner, S. R. Ketover, D. Sande, K. Holtmeier, and F. J. Peterson. The role of gallbladder emptying in gallstone formation during diet-induced rapid weight loss. *Hepatology* 24 (3; 1996), 544–548.

Geliebter, A., S. Schachter, C. Lohmann-Walter, H. Feldman, and S. A. Hashim. Reduced stomach capacity in obese subjects after dieting. *Am. J. Clin. Nutr.* 63 (2; 1996), 170–173.

Gibney, M. Sugar and obesity. *J. Ir. Dent. Assoc.* 39 (1993), 98.

Gibney, M., M. Sigman-Grant, J. L. Stanton, Jr., and D. R. Keast. Consumption of sugars. *Am. J. Clin. Nutr.* 62 (1995), 178S–193 S; discussion 194S.

Gibney, M. J. Epidemiology of obesity in relation to nutrient intake. *Int. J. Obes. Relat. Metab. Disord.* 19 (1995), Suppl. 5, S1–3.

Gibney, M. J., and T. M. Wolever. Periodicity of eating and human health: present perspective and future directions. *Br. J. Nutr.* 77, Suppl. 1 (1997), S3–5.

Gibson, S. A. Are high-fat, high-sugar foods and diets conducive to obesity? *Int. J. Food. Sci. Nutr.* 47 (1996), 405–415.

Golay, A., C. Eigenheer, Y. Morel, P. KuJawski, T. Lehmann, and N. de Tonnac. Weight-loss with low or high carbohydrate diet? *Int. J. Obes. Relat. Metab. Disord.* 20 (12; 1996), 1067–1072.

Goldberg, G. R., A. E. Black, S. A. Jebb, T. J. Cole, P. R. Murgatroyd, W. A. Coward, and A. M. Prentice. Critical evaluation of energy intake data using fundamental principles of energy physiology: 1. Derivation of cut-off limits to identify under-recording. *Eur. J. Clin. Nutr.* 45 (1991), 569–581.

Grilo, C. M., S. Shiffman, and R. R. Wing. Coping with dietary relapse crises and their aftermath. *Addict. Behav.* 18 (1; 1993), 89–102.

Grodstein, F., R. Levine, L. Troy, T. Spencer, G. A. Colditz, and M. J. Stampfer. Three-year follow-up of participants in a commercial weight loss program. Can you keep it off? *Arch. Intern. Med.* 156 (12; 1996), 1302–1306.

Harvey, J., R. R. Wing, and M. Mullen. Effects on food cravings of a very low calorie diet or a balanced, low calorie diet. *Appetite* 21 (2; 1993), 105–115.

Heitmann, B. L., and L. Lissner. Dietary underreporting by obese individuals—is it specific or non-specific? *BMJ.* 311 (1995), 986–989.

Heitmann, B. L., L. Lissner, T. I. Sorensen, and C. Bengtsson. Dietary fat intake and weight gain in women genetically predisposed for obesity. *Am. J. Clin. Nutr.* 61 (1995), 1213–1217.

Heshka, S., A. Spitz, C. Nufiez, A. M. Fittante, S. B. Heymsfield, and F. X. Pi-Sunyer. Obesity and risk of gallstone development on a 1200 kcal/d (5025 Kj/d) regular food diet. *Int. J. Obes. Relat. Metab. Disord.* 20 (5; 1996), 450–454.

Hill, J. O. Dealing with obesity as a chronic disease. *Obes. Res.* 6, Suppl 1 (1998), S34–S38.

Hill, J. O., and J. C. Peters. Environmental contributions to the obesity epidemic. *Science* 280 (5368; 1998), 1371–1374.

Hill, J. O., H. M. Seagle, S. L. Johnson, S. Smith, G. W. Reed, Z. V. Tran, D. Cooper, M. Stone, and J. C. Peters. Effects of 14d of covert substitution of olestra for conventional fat on spontaneous food intake. *Am. J. Clin. Nutr.* 67 (6; 1998), 1178–1185.

Horton, T. J., and J. O. Hill. Exercise and obesity. *Proc. Nutr. Soc.* 57 (1; 1998), 85–91.

Ikeda, T., T. Gomi, N. Hirawa, J. Sakurai, and N. Yoshikawa. Improvement of insulin sensitivity contributes to blood pressure reduction after weight loss in hypertensive subjects with obesity. *Hypertension* 27 (5; 1996), 1180–1186.

Jakicic, J. M., R. R. Wing, B. A. Butler, and R. J. Robertson. Prescribing exercise in multiple short bouts versus one continuous bout: effects on adherence, cardiorespiratory fitness, and weight loss in overweight women. *Int. J. Obes. Relat. Metab. Disord.* 19 (12; 1995), 893–901.

Jebb, S. A., G. R. Goldberg, W. A. Coward, P. R. Murgatroyd, and A. M. Prentice. Effects of weight cycling caused by intermittent dieting on metabolic rate and body composition in obese women. *Int. J. Obes.* 15 (1991), 367–374.

Jebb, S. A., R. J. Osbome, A. K. Dixon, N. M. Bleehen, and M. Elia. Measurements of resting energy expenditure and body composition before and after treatment of small cell lung cancer. *Annu. Oncol.* 5 (1994), 915–919.

Jebb, S. A., and A. M. Prentice. *Is* obesity an eating disorder? *Proc. Nutr. Soc.* 54 (1996), 721–728.

Jebb, S. A. Aetiology of obesity. *Br. Med. Bull.* 53 (1997), 264–285.

Jeffery, R. W., R. R. Wing, and S. A. French. Weight cycling and cardiovascular risk factors in obese men and women. *Am. J. Clin. Nutr.* 55 (3; 1992), 641–644.

Jeffery, R. W., W. L. Hellerstedt, S. A. French, and J. E. Baxter. A randomized trial of counseling for fat restriction versus calorie restriction in the treatment of obesity. *Int. J. Obes. Relat. Metab. Disord.* 19 (2; 1995), 132–137.

Jenkins, A. B., T. P. Markovic, A. Fleury, and L. V. Campbell. Carbohydrate intake and short-term regulation of leptin in humans. *Diabetologia* 40 (3; 1997), 348–351.

Kant, A. K., and A. Schatzkin. Consumption of energy-dense, nutrient-poor foods by the U.S. population: effect on nutrient profiles. *J. Am. Coll. Nutr.* 13 (3; 1994), 285–291.

Kant, A. K., R. Ballard-Barbash, and A. Schatzkin. Evening eating and its relation to self-reported body weight and nutrient intake in women, CSFII 1985–86. *J. Am. Coll. Nutr.* 14 (4; 1995), 358–363.

Kant, A. K., B. I. Graubard, A. Schatzkin, and R. Ballard-Barbash. Proportion of energy intake from fat and subsequent weight change in the NHANES I Epidemiologic Follow-up Study. *Am. J. Clin. Nutr.* 61 (1; 1995), 11–17.

Kant, A. K., A. Schatzkin, and R. Ballard-Barbash. Evening eating and subsequent long-term weight change in a national cohort. *Int. J. Obes. Relat. Metab. Disord.* 21 (5; 1997), 407–412.

Keim, N. L., D. J. Canty, T. F. Barbieri, and M. M. Wu. Effect of exercise and dietary restraint on energy intake of reduced-obese women. *Appetite* 26 (1; 1996), 55–70.

Keller, C., D. Oveland, and S. Hudson. Strategies for weight control success in adults. *Nurse Pract.* 22 (3; 1997), 33, 37–38, 40 passim.

Kern, P. A. A prudent and practical approach to the treatment of obesity. *J. Ark. Med. Soc.* 94 (5; 1997), 191–197.

Kimm, S. Y. The role of dietary fiber in the development and treatment of childhood obesity. *Pediatrics* 96 (5; 1995), Pt. 2, 1010–1014.

King, N., A. Tremblay, and J. Blundell. Effects of exercise on appetite control: implications for energy balance. *Med. Sci. Sports Exerc.* 29 (8; 1997), 1076–1089.

Kushi, L. H., E. B. Lenart, and W. C. Willett. Health implications of Mediterranean diets in light of contemporary knowledge *Am. J. Clin. Nutr.* 61 (1995), Suppl., Pts. 1 and 2, S1407–S1427.

Kushi, L. H., R. M. Fee, A. R. Folsom, P. J. Mink, K. E. Anderson, and T. A. Sellers. Physical activity and mortality in postmenopausal women. *Jama* 277 (16; 1997), 1287–1292.

Lappalainen, R., A. Saba, L. Holm, H. Mykkanen, and M. J. Gibney. Difficulties in trying to eat healthier: descriptive analysis of perceived barriers for healthy eating. *Eur. J. Clin. Nutr.* 51, Suppl. 2 (1997), S36–S40.

Larson, D. E., R. Rising, R. T. Ferraro, and E. Ravussin. Spontaneous overfeeding with a "cafeteria diet" in men: effects on 24-hour energy expenditure and substrate oxidation. *Int. J. Obes. Relat. Metab. Disord.* 19 (1995), 331–337.

Lawton, C. L., V. Burley, J. Wales, and J. E. Blundell. Dietary fat and appetite control in obese subjects: weak effects on satiation and satiety. *Int. J. Obes. Relat. Metab. Disord.* 17 (7; 1993), 409–416.

Lawton, C. L., and I. E. Blundell. The role of reduced fat diets and fat substitutes in the regulation of energy and fat intake and body weight. *Curr. Opin. Lipidol.* 9 (1998), 41–45.

Lean, M. Why is losing weight so hard? *Practitioner* 241 (1574; 1997), 253–256.

Lichtman, S. W., K. Pisarska, E. R. Berman, M. Pestone, H. Dowling, E. Offenbacher, H. Weisel, S. Heshka, D. E. Matthews, and S. B. Heymsfield. Discrepancy between self-reported and actual caloric intake and exercise in obese subjects. *N. Engl. J. Med.* 327 (27; 1992), 1893–1898.

Lissner, L., L. Sjostrom, C. Bengtsson, C. Bouchard, and B. Larsson. The natural history of obesity in an obese population and associations with metabolic aberrations. *Int. J. Obes. Relat. Metab. Disord.* 18 (1994), 441–447.

Lissner, L., and B. L. Heitmann. Dietary fat and obesity: evidence from epidemiology. *Eur. J. Clin. Nutr.* 49 (2; 1995), 79–90.

Lissner, L., and B. L. Heitmann. The dietary fat: carbohydrate ratio in relation to body weight. *Curr. Opin. Lipidol.* 6 (1995), 8–13.

Lissner, L., B. L. Heitmann, and C. Bengtsson. Low-fat diets may prevent weight gain in sedentary women: prospective observations from the population study of women in Gothenburg, Sweden. *Obes. Res.* 5 (1997), 43–48.

Low, C. C., E. B. Grossman, and B. Gumbiner. Potentiation of effects of weight loss by monounsaturated fatty acids in obese NIDDM patients. *Diabetes* 45 (5; 1996), 569–575.

McCargar, L. J., J. Sale, and S. M. Crawford. Chronic dieting does not result in a sustained reduction in resting metabolic rate in overweight women. *J. Am. Diet. Assoc.* 96 (11; 1996), 1175–1177.

Melville, S., M. A. McNurlan, B. A. McGaw, K. C. McHardy, L. M. Fearns, and P. J. Garlick. Carbohydrate oxidation: do we eat ourselves or our food? *Scott. Med. J.* 33 (1988), 203–204.

Nicklas, B. J., E. M. Rogus, and A. P. Goldberg. Exercise blunts declines in lipolysis and fat oxidation after dietary-induced weight loss in obese older women. *Anl. J. Physiol.* 273 (1; 1997), Pt. 1, E149–E155.

Owens, J. F., K. A. Matthews, R. R. Wing, and L. H. Kuller. Can physical activity mitigate the effects of aging in middle-aged women? *Circulation* 85 (4; 1992), 1265–1270.

Pagliassotti, M. J., E. C. Gayles, and J. O. Hill. Fat and energy balance. *Annu. N. Y. Acad. Sci.* 827 (1997), 431–448.

Pascale, R. W., R. R. Wing, B. A. Butler, M. Mullen, and P. Bononi. Effects of a behavioral weight loss program stressing calorie restriction versus calorie plus fat restriction in obese individuals with NIDDM or a family history of diabetes. *Diabetes Care* 18 (9; 1995), 1241–1248.

Poppitt, S. D. Energy density of diets and obesity. *Int. J. Obes. Relat. Metab. Disord.* 19 (1995), Suppl. 5, S20–S26.

Poppitt, S. D., and A. M. Prentice. Energy density and its role in the control of food intake: evidence from metabolic and community studies. *Appetite* 26 (2; 1996), 153–174.

Prentice, A. M., G. R. Goldberg, S. A. Jebb, A. E. Black, P. R. Murgatroyd, and E. O. Diaz. Physiological responses to slimming. *Proc. Nutr. Soc.* 50 (1991), 441–458.

Prentice, A. M., and S. A. Jebb. Obesity in Britain: gluttony or sloth? *BMJ* 311 (1995), 437–439.

Price, R. A., A. J. Stunkard, R. Ness, T. Wadden, S. Heshka, B. Kanders, and A. Cormillot. Childhood onset (age less than 10) obesity has high familial risk. *Int. J. Obes.* 14 (2; 1990), 185–195.

Proserpi, C., A. Sparti, Y. Schutz, V. Di Vetta, H. Milon, and E. Jequier. Ad libitum intake of a high-carbohydrate or high-fat diet in young men: effects on nutrient balances. *Am. J. Clin. Nutr.* 66 (1997), 539–545.

Raben, A., N. Christensen, and A. Astrup. Postprandial responses in substrate oxidation and appetite in post-obese subjects. *Int. J. Obes. Relat. Metab. Disord.* 17 (1993), Suppl. 3, S37–S40; discussion S41–S2.

Raben, A., H. Andersen, N. Christensen, J. Madsen, J. Holst, and A. Astrup. Evidence for an abnormal postprandial response to a high-fat meal in women predisposed to obesity. *Am. J. Physiol.* 267 (4; 1994), Pt. 1, E549–E559.

Raben, A., and A. Astrup. Manipulating carbohydrate content and sources in obesity prone subjects: effect on energy expenditure and macronutrient balance. *Int. J. Obes. Relat. Metab. Disord.* 20 (1996), Suppl. 2, S24–S30.

Racette, S. B., D. A. Schoeller, R. F. Kushner, K. M. Neil, and K. Herling-Iaffaldano. Effects of aerobic exercise and dietary carbohydrate on energy expenditure and body composition during weight reduction in obese women. *Am. J. Clin. Nutr.* 61 (3; 1995), 486–494.

Racette, S. B., D. A. Schoeller, R. F. Kushner, and K. M. Neil. Exercise enhances dietary compliance during moderate energy restriction in obese women. *Am. J. Clin. Nutr.* 62 (2; 1995), 345–349.

Ravussin, E., and C. Bogardus. A brief overview of human energy metabolism and its relationship to essential obesity. *Am. J. Clin. Nutr.* 55 (1992), S242–S245.

Ravussin, E., and B. A. Swinburn. Pathophysiology of obesity. *Lancet* 340 (1992), 404–408.

Ravussin, E., A. M. Fontvieille, B. A. Swinburn, and C. Bogardus. Risk factors for the development of obesity. *Annu. N. Y. Acad. Sci.* 683 (1993), 141–150.

Ravussin, E., M. E. Valencia, J. Esparza, P. H. Bennett, and L. O. Schulz. Effects of a traditional lifestyle on obesity in Pima Indians. *Diabetes Care* 17 (1994), 1067–1074.

Ravussin, E. Low resting metabolic rate as a risk factor for weight gain: role of the sympathetic nervous system. *Int. J. Obes. Relat. Metab. Disord.* 19 (1995), Suppl. 7, S8–S9.

————. Metabolic differences and the development of obesity. *Metabolism* 44 (1995), 12–14.

Ravussin, E., and P. A. Tataranni. The role of altered sympathetic nervous system activity in the pathogenesis of obesity. *Proc. Nutr. Soc.* 55 (1996), 793–802.

————. Dietary fat and human obesity. *J. Am. Diet. Assoc.* 97 (1997), Suppl. S42–S46.

Rising, R., S. Alger, V. Boyce, H. Seagle, R. Ferraro, A. M. Fontvieille, and E. Ravussin. Food intake measured by an automated food-selection system: relationship to energy expenditure. *Am. J. Clin. Nutr.* 55 (1992), 343–349.

Rising, R., I. T. Harper, A. M. Fontvielle, R. T. Ferraro, M. Spraul, and E. Ravussin. Determinants of total daily energy expenditure: variability in physical activity. *Am. J. Clin. Nutr.* 59 (1994), 800–804.

Rising, R., P. A. Tataranni, S. Snitker, and E. Ravussin. Decreased ratio of fat to carbohydrate oxidation with increasing age in Pima Indians. *J. Am. Coll. Nutr.* 15 (1996), 309–312.

Robison, J. I., S. L. Hoerr, K. A. Petersmarck, and J. V. Anderson. Redefining success in obesity intervention: the new paradigm. *J. Am. Diet. Assoc.* 95 (4; 1995), 422–423.

Rolls, B. J. Carbohydrates, fats, and satiety. *Am. J. Clin. Nutr.* 61 (1995), Suppl. 4, 960S–967S.

Saris, W. H. Exercise with or without dietary restriction and obesity treatment. *Int. J. Obes. Relat. Metab. Disord.* 19 (1995), Suppl. 4, S113–S116.

Schlundt, D. G., J. O. Hill, J. Pope-Cordle, D. Arnold, K. L. Virts, and M. Katahn. Randomized evaluation of a low fat ad *libitum* carbohydrate diet for weight reduction. *Int. J. Obes.* 17 (1993), 623–629.

Schutz, Y., J. P. Flatt, and E. Jequier. Failure of dietary fat intake to promote fat oxidation: a factor favoring the development of obesity. *Am. J. Clin. Nutr.* 50 (1989), 307–314.

Schutz, Y., A. Tremblay, R. L. Weinsier, and K. M. Nelson. Role of fat oxidation in the long-term stabilization of body weight in obese women. *Am. J. Clin. Nutr.* 55 (1992), 670–674.

Schutz, Y. Abnormalities of fuel utilization as predisposing to the development of obesity in humans. *Obes. Res.* 3 (1995), Suppl. 2, S173–S178.

Shah, M., and A. Garg. High-fat and high-carbohydrate diets and energy balance. *Diabetes Care* 19 (10; 1996), 1142–1152.

Skender, M. L., G. K. Goodrick, D. J. Del Junco, R. S. Reeves, L. Darnell, A. M. Gotto, and J. P. Foreyt. Comparison of 2-year weight loss trends in behavioral treatments of obesity: diet, exercise, and combination interventions. *J. Am. Diet. Assoc.* 96 (4; 1996), 342–346.

Skov, A., S. Toubro, B. Buemann, and A. Astrup. Normal levels of energy expenditure in patients with reported "low metabolism." *Clin. Physiol.* 17 (3; 1997), 279–285.

Snitker, S., D. E. Larson, P. A. Tataranni, and E. Ravussin. Ad libitum food intake in humans after manipulation of glycogen stores. *Am. J. Clin. Nutr.* 65 (1997), 941–946.

Spirt, B. A., L. W. Graves, R. Weinstock, S. J. Bartlett, and T. A. Wadden. Gallstone formation in obese women treated by a low-calorie diet. *Int. J. Obes. Relat. Metab. Disord.* 19 (8; 1995), 593–595.

Steen, S. N., T. A. Wadden, G. D. Foster, and R. E. Andersen. Are obese adolescent boys ignoring an important health risk? *Int. J. Eat. Disord.* 20 (3; 1996), 281–286.

Stubbs, R. J., P. R. Murgatroyd, G. R. Goldberg, and A. M. Prentice. Carbohydrate balance and the regulation of day-to-day food intake in humans. *Am. J. Clin. Nutr.* 57 (1993), 897–903.

Stubbs, R. J., P. Ritz, W. A. Coward, and A. M. Prentice. Covert manipulation of the ratio of dietary fat to carbohydrate and energy density: effect on food intake and energy balance in free-living men eating ad libitum. *Am. J. Clin. Nutr.* 62 (1995), 330–337.

Stubbs, R. J., C. G. Harbron, and A. M. Prentice. Covert manipulation of the dietary fat to carbohydrate ratio of isoenergetically dense diets: effect on food intake in feeding men ad libitum. *Int. J. Obes. Relat. Metab. Disord.* 20 (1996), 651–660.

Stubbs, R. J., A. M. Prentice, and W. P. James. Carbohydrates and energy balance. *Annu. N. Y. Acad. Sci.* 819 (1997), 44–69.

Stunkard, A., R. Berkowitz, T. A. Wadden, C. Tanrikut, E. Reiss, and L. Young. Binge eating disorder and the night-eating syndrome. *Int. J. Obes. Relat. Metab. Disord.* 20 (1; 1996), 1–6.

Surwit, R. S., M. N. Feinglos, C. C. McCaskill, S. L. Clay, M. A. Babyak, B. S. Brownlow, C. S. Plaisted, and P. H. Lin. Metabolic and behavioral effects of a high-sucrose diet during weight loss. *Am. J. Clin. Nutr.* 65 (4; 1997), 908–915.

Swinburn, B., and E. Ravussin. Energy balance or fat balance? *Am. J. Clin. Nutr.* 57 (1993), S766–S770; discussion S770–S771.

————. Energy and macronutrient metabolism. *Baillieres Clin. Endocrinol. Metab.* 8 (1994), 527–548.

Tataranni, P. A., and E. Ravussin. Effect of fat intake on energy balance. *Annu. N. Y. Acad. Sci.* 819 (1997), 37–43.

Tremblay, A., I. P. Despres, J. Maheux, M. C. Pouliot, A. Nadeau, S. Moojani, P. J. Lupien, and C. Bouchard. Normalization of the metabolic profile in obese women by exercise and a low fat diet. *Med. Sci. Sports Exerc.* 23 (1991), 1326–1331.

Tremblay, A. Human obesity: a defect in lipid oxidation or in thermogenesis? *Int. J. Obes. Relat. Metab. Disord.* 16 (1992), 953–957.

Tremblay, A., J. P. Despres, G. Theriault, G. Fournier, and C. Bouchard. Overfeeding and energy expenditure in humans. *Am. J. Clin. Nutr.* 56 (1992), 857–862.

Tremblay, A., N. Almeras, J. Boer, E. K. Kranenbarg, and I. P. Despres. Diet composition and postexercise energy balance. *Am. J. Clin. Nutr.* 59 (1994), 975–979.

Tremblay, A., and N. Almeras. Exercise, macronutrient preferences and food intake. *Int. J. Obes. Relat. Metab. Disord.* 19 (1995), Suppl. 4, S97–S101.

Tremblay, A. Differences in fat balance underlying obesity. *Int. J. Obes. Relat. Metab. Disord.* 19 (1995), Suppl. 7, S10–S14; discussion S15–S16.

Tremblay, A., E. Wouters, M. Wenker, S. St-Pierre, C. Bouchard, and J. P. Despres. Alcohol and a high-fat diet: a combination favoring overfeeding. *Am. J. Clin. Nutr.* 62 (1995), 639–644.

Tremblay, A., and B. Buemann. Exercise-training, macronutrient balance and body weight control. *Int. J. Obes. Relat. Metab. Disord.* 19 (1995), 79–86.

Tremblay, A., A. Nadeau, I. P. Despres, and C. Bouchard. Hyperinsulinemia and regulation of energy balance. *Am. J. Clin. Nutr.* 61 (1995), 827–830.

Tremblay, A., B. Buemann, G. Theriault, and C. Bouchard. Body fatness in active individuals reporting low lipid and alcohol intake. *Eur. J. Clin. Nutr.* 49 (1995), 824–831.

Tremblay, A., and S. St-Pierre. The hyperphagic effect of a high-fat diet and alcohol intake persists after control for energy density. *Am. J. Clin. Nutr.* 63 (1996), 479–482.

Turner, L. W., M. Q. Wang, and R. C. Westerfield. Preventing relapse in weight control: a discussion of cognitive and behavioral strategies. *Psychol. Rep.* 77 (2; 1995), 651–656.

Valtuena, S., J. Salas-Salvado, and P. G. Lorda. The respiratory quotient as a prognostic factor in weight-loss rebound. *Int. J. Obes. Relat. Metab. Disord.* 21 (9; 1997), 811–817.

Valtuena, S., R. Solà, and I. Salas-Salvadó. A study of the prognostic respiratory markers of sustained weight loss in obese subjects after 28 days on VLCD. *Int. J. Obes. Relat. Metab. Disord.* 2 (4; 1997), 267–273.

Viswanathan, M., C. Snehalatha, V. Viswanathan, P. Vidyavathi, J. Indu, and A. Ramachandran. Reduction in body weight helps to delay the onset of diabetes even in non-obese with strong family history of the disease. *Diabetes Res. Clin. Pract.* 35 (1997), 107–112.

Wadden, T. A., G. D. Foster, K. A. Letizia, and J. L. Mullen. Long-term effects of dieting on resting metabolic rate in obese outpatients. *Jama* 264 (6; 1990), 707–711.

Wadden, T. A. Treatment of obesity by moderate and severe caloric restriction. Results of clinical research trials. *Annu. Intern. Med.* 119 (7; 1993), Pt. 2, 688–693.

Wadden, T. A., G. D. Foster, A. J. Stunkard, and A. M. Conill. Effects of weight cycling on the resting energy expenditure and body composition of obese women. *Int. J. Eat. Disord.* 19 (1; 1996), 5–12.

Wadden, T. A., R. A. Vogt, R. E. Andersen, S. J. Bartlett, G. D. Foster, R. H. Kuehnel, J. Wilk, R. Weinstock, P. Buckenmeyer, R. I. Berkowitz, S. N. Steen. Exercise in the treatment of obesity: effects of four interventions on body composition, resting energy expenditure, appetite, and mood. *J. Consult. Clin. Psychol.* 65 (2; 1997), 269–277.

Walsh, M. F., and T. J. Flynn. A 54-month evaluation of a popular very low caloric diet program. *J. Fam. Pract.* 41 (3; 1995), 231–236.

Weinsier, R. L., T. A. Wadden, C. Ritenbaugh, G. G. Harrison, F. S. Johnson, and J. H. Wilmore. Recommended therapeutic guidelines for professional weight control programs. *Am. J. Clin. Nutr.* 40 (4; 1984), 865–872.

Weinsier, R. L., L. J. Wilson, and J. Lee. Medically safe rate of weight loss for the treatment of obesity: a guideline based on risk of gallstone formation. *Am. J. Med.* 98 (2; 1995), 115–117.

Westerterp, K. R. Food quotient, respiratory quotient, and energy balance. *Am. J. Clin. Nutr.* 57 (1993), S759–S764; discussion S764–S765.

White, M. D., G. Bouchard, B. Buemann, N. Almeras, J. P. Despres, C. Bouchard, and A. Tremblay. Energy and macronutrient balances for humans in a whole body metabolic chamber without control of preceding diet and activity level. *Int. J. Obes. Relat. Metab. Disord.* 21 (1997), 135–140.

Willett, W. C., G. R. Howe, and L. H. Kushi. Adjustment for total energy intake in epidemiologic studies. *Am. J. Clin. Nutr.* 65 (1997), Suppl. 4, S1229–S1231.

Wing, R. R., C. Carrol, and R. W. Jeffrey. Repeated observation of obese and normal subjects eating in the natural environment. *Addict. Behav.* 3 (3–4; 1978), 191–196.

Wing, R. R., and R. W. Jeffery. Differential restaurant patronage of obese and nonobese people. *Addict. Behav.* 3 (2; 1978), 135–138.

Wing, R. R. Behavioral treatment of obesity. Its application to type II diabetes. *Diabetes Care,* 16 (1; 1993), 193–199.

Wing, R. R., E. H. Blair, M. Marcus, L. H. Epstein, and J. Harvey. Year-long weight loss treatment for obese patients with type II diabetes: does including an intermittent very-low-calorie diet improve outcome? *Am. J Med.* 97 (4; 1994), 354–362.

Wing, R. R., E. H. Blair, P. Bononi, M. D. Marcus, R. Watanabe, and R. N. Bergman. Caloric restriction per se is a significant factor in improvements in glycemic control and insulin sensitivity during weight loss in obese NIDDM patients. *Diabetes Care,* 17 (1; 1994), 30–36.

Wing, R. R., J. A. Vazquez, and C. M. Ryan. Cognitive effects of ketogenic weight-reducing diets. *Int. J. Obes. Relat. Metab. Disord.* 19 (11; 1995), 811–816.

Wing, R. R., R. W. Jeffery, and W. L. Hellerstedt. A prospective study of effects of weight cycling on cardiovascular risk factors. *Arch. Intern. Med.* 155 (13; 1995), 1416–1422.

Wing, R. R. Use of very-low-calorie diets in the treatment of obese persons with non-insulin-dependent diabetes mellitus. *J. Am. Diet. Assoc.* 95 (5; 1995), 569–572; quiz 573–574.

Zachwieja, J. J. Exercise as treatment for obesity. *Endocrinol. Metab. Clin. North Am.* 25 (4; 1996), 965–968.

Zelasko, C. J. Exercise for weight loss: what are the facts? *J. Am. Diet. Assoc.* 95 (12; 1995), 1414–1417.

Zurlo, F., K. Larson, C. Bogardus, and E. Ravussin. Skeletal muscle metabolism is a major determinant of resting energy expenditure. *J. Clin. Invest.* 86 (1990), 1423–1427.

Zurlo, F., S. Lillioja, A. Esposito-Del Puente, B. L. Nyomba, I. Raz, M. F. Saad, B. A. Swinburn, W. C. Knowler, C. Bogardus, and E. Ravussin. Low ratio of fat to carbohydrate oxidation as predictor of weight gain: study of 24-h RQ. *Am. J. Physiol.* 259 (1990), E650–E657.

Rounding Out Your T-Factor Fitness Program

Cardiovascular fitness is only part of the fitness picture. A total physical activity program also includes flexibility, and muscular strength and endurance.

First, let's talk about flexibility.

Stretching loosens you up before a walk or a jog, and cools you down after vigorous exercise. A good stretching routine works the most important areas of the body for active people: calves, hamstrings (the muscles at the rear of your legs), stomach, and lower back. The T-Flex Routine, described below, will also address the areas where most of us hold a lot of our tension: the upper shoulders and neck and, again, the lower back.

Remember to stretch comfortably; don't push yourself to the point of pain. In time, with practice, your flexibility will increase naturally.

T-FLEX ROUTINE

This entire series of stretches takes only minutes to perform. Add to it some hatha-yoga postures if you wish for even greater flexibility, health, and relaxation.

T-Flex for the Neck and Shoulders

These first four movements are best performed while standing in the shower with hot water pouring down on your neck.

1. *Shoulder lift.* With head straight and neck relaxed, slowly lift your shoulders toward your ears. When shoulders are as high as they can comfortably go, roll them back, pushing your shoulder blades gently together. Hold for about ten seconds, then reverse your movements, rolling your shoulders forward to the starting position, then lowering them. Repeat.

2. *Neck roll.* From the same starting position as above, slowly let your neck roll forward and your head drop down, trying to touch your chin to your chest without straining. Hold for several seconds, then roll your head up until you're looking at the ceiling. Hold for several seconds, then return to starting position. Repeat.

3. *Head roll.* From starting position, facing forward, let your head slowly drop sideways to the left. Try to touch your left ear to your left shoulder; you can lift your left shoulder slightly to give yourself an added stretch. Don't strain. Return to starting position and repeat on the other side.

4. *Neck twist.* Facing forward, turn your head slowly to the left as if to look over your shoulder. Hold for several seconds. Return to starting position, then look to your right. Repeat.

T-Flex Floor Routine

1. *Sitting stretch.* Sit on the floor with your legs crossed. Bend forward from the hips, keeping your back relaxed but straight. Reach forward as far as you can to touch the floor with your hands. Stretch your shoulder joints as well as your hips. Hold for ten to twenty seconds, then relax.

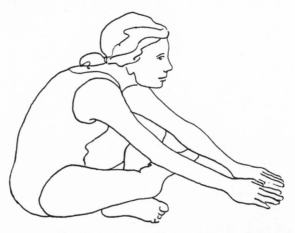

2. *Sitting toe-touch*. This one is good for the hip joints, calves, and hamstrings. While still sitting, straighten your legs out in front of you. Bend forward from the hips, aim your toes back toward your head, and reach for your toes. Many people can only reach to their ankles or calves when they first do this exercise. If this is true for you, don't force yourself to go beyond the point of comfort. Hold the stretch for ten to twenty seconds.

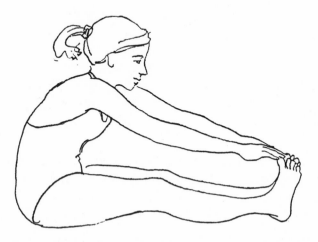

3. *Resting twist*. This will increase your lower back flexibility and relieve stiffness. Lie flat on the floor, arms straight out to the sides, legs together. Bend your right knee and place your right foot under your left knee. Keep your shoulders flat to the floor and rotate your lower body to the left, from the hips. Try to touch the inside of your right knee to the floor on your left side. Turn your head to the right and look out over your extended right arm. You can gently push your right knee toward the floor with your left hand, but don't force the stretch. Hold about ten seconds. Do the other side (left foot under right knee, etc.).

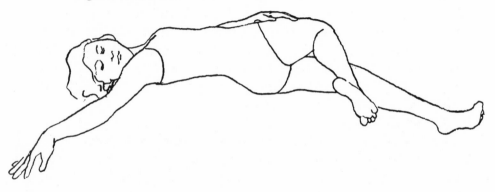

4. *Back stretch*. This also helps relieve tension in the lower back. Lie flat on the floor, legs together. Bend your right leg and bring your right knee to your chest. Hold the knee with both hands and press it gently toward your chest. Hold for ten seconds, then reverse legs. Your head and shoulders can come up off the floor if you like, or you can use a pillow under your head for this and the next three exercises.

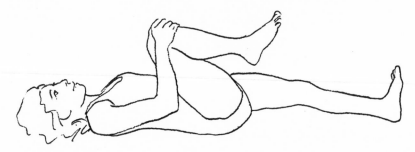

5. *Back curl*. Another excellent lower back exercise. Still lying on the floor, bring both knees to your chest, gently pressing them closer with your hands. Hold for about ten to twenty seconds. Then go right on to the next exercise.

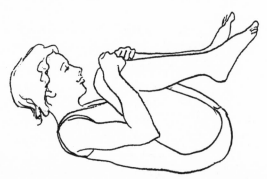

6. *Ceiling stretch*. From the position you are already in for the back curl, continue holding your right knee while grasping the big toe of your left foot with your left hand. Straighten the left leg up toward the ceiling as far as you can, continuing to hold the big toe. Hold for at least ten seconds, then do the other leg. This works the calves, hamstrings, and lower back as a unit. Return to the back curl position.

7. *Bicycle and flutter kicks*. From the back curl position, place your hands palms-down under your buttocks. With your knees about halfway to your chest, do a bicycling motion for ten seconds (or ten rotations). Then lower your legs straight out in front of you

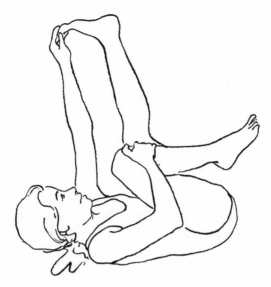

to within 6 inches of the floor and do flutter kicks for ten seconds (or ten repetitions). Repeat the bicycle motion, alternating with the flutter kicks, until you feel some strain in your stomach area. This exercise can take the place of sit-ups and is an excellent tummy toner and back exercise. *However, if you already suffer from chronic lower back pain, do not do this exercise without getting your therapist's advice. Your problem may require a different stomach muscle strengthener.*

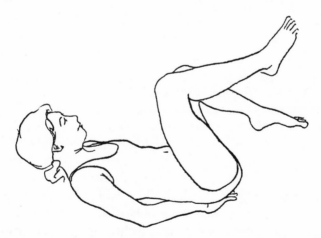

8. *Pelvic curl.* Still lying down, rest your arms flat on the floor with elbows bent and hands near your head, palms up. Bend your knees so that your feet are flat on the floor about twelve inches from your buttocks. Curl your pelvis so your lower back presses against the

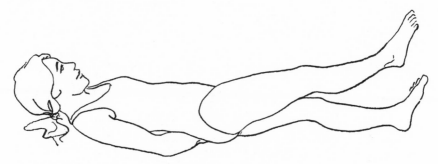

floor and your buttocks lift slightly. Hold for about ten seconds, release, and repeat. This will relieve tension in the lower back.

9. *T-Factor "shoulder stand."* Simply place your legs up on a chair and relax for thirty seconds. This is good for your circulation, helps reduce swelling around the ankles, and will relieve "drawing pains" in the legs. If you experience pain in your extremities during the night, do the T-Factor "shoulder stand" before you go to bed. If you are already fairly flexible and don't have much weight to lose, you can do the more rigorous shoulder stand: Lie flat on the floor with your arms resting along your sides. Curl your legs up as if for the back curl, but keep rolling your torso up, placing your hands on your back to help keep your balance. Straighten your legs up toward the ceiling and hold for thirty seconds. *However, if you suffer from hypertension, do not do any exercise that requires you to lift your legs up over your head, as in a shoulder stand, without consulting your physician.*

T-STRENGTH ROUTINE

In recent years, strength-training centers have been popping up everywhere: in spas, YMCAs, and private clubs. You can choose between Nautilus, Hammer Strength, Icarian, Cybex, free weights, and more for your strength-training equipment.

Which is best? Well, this is almost like asking which is the best car or television set. A lot depends on personal preference. The important thing is that you exercise each of the large muscle groups.

For women just beginning a strength-training program with free weights, it's generally best to use three-pound weights. Beginning men can go up to five or six pounds. After a few months, you may wish to increase the weights that you work with by three to six

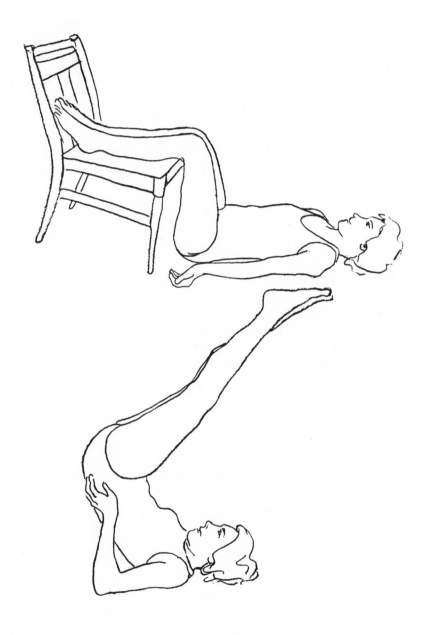

pounds, but it is generally best for most people to do more repetitions with light weights than to risk injury by using heavy weights. In addition, using light weights leads to good tone, an "alive" feeling, and nice lines without excessive bulking.

It's always a good idea to warm up with some stretching exercises before beginning any work with weights. See the previous section in this chapter on the T-Flex Routine.

T-Strength training starts by focusing on the neglected upper body, then adds a few movements for the stomach and legs. If you use free weights, such as the dumbbells that are easy to find in a department store, work up to 10 repetitions with a weight you can handle. Normally a booklet will come with the weights that will show you a number of different exercises.

Upper Body Series

1. *Two for the shoulders.* Hold arms at your sides with palms facing the rear. Keeping arms straight, raise weights forward to shoulder height and return to down position, slowly and with control. Breathe normally at all times. Work up to ten repetitions, then rest for at least one deep breath. Then, turn the weights so that your palms face your body, and raise your arms outward to the sides, up to shoulder level. Work up to ten repetitions.

2. *Biceps curl.* Stand straight with arms at sides, palms facing forward. Curl forearms up to shoulder ten times at a moderate pace.

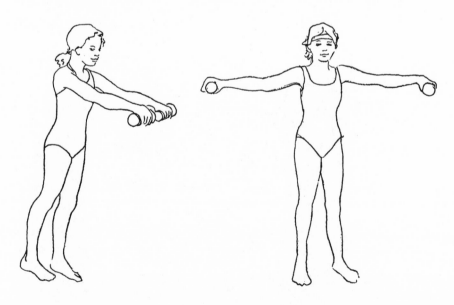

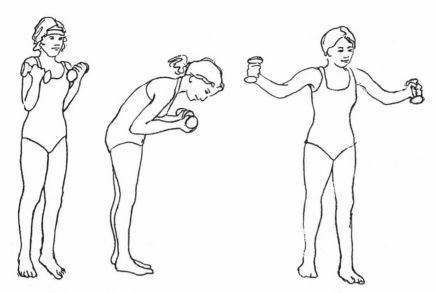

3. *Triceps.* Keep elbows next to your body, bend forward at about a sixty-degree angle from the hips, and curl forearms, bringing weights up to your shoulders. Then, keeping elbows next to your body, straighten your arms out in back behind you. Repeat until you feel some strain and stop.

This will build the muscle on the back of your arms, and help reduce the likelihood of loose skin on your upper arms if you have been losing weight.

4. *Forward, up, and out.* Standing upright, start with arms at your sides, palms facing body. Curling at the elbows, bring weights for-

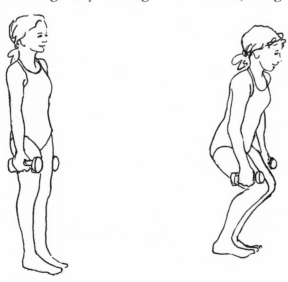

ward and up almost to the shoulders. Continuing in one uninterrupted motion, spread arms out to your sides, shoulder level, palms facing forward. Keep your arms slightly bent to avoid excessive strain. Return along the same path as you began and repeat up to ten times.

Leg Series

5. *Heel lifts.* With weights at your side, go up and down slowly on your toes several times, resting about a second at the top each time.

6. *Half squats.* (If you are more than a few pounds overweight, don't use any extra weight for this exercise.) With arms at sides, feet at shoulder width, toes facing slightly out, squat down one-third to one-half of the way to the floor. Do not go beyond the point where your thighs are parallel to the floor, and keep your knees over your feet when squatting.

Stomach Series

7. *Bent-knee sit-up.* Lie on your back with knees bent and feet close to your buttocks. Curl your head and shoulders about halfway up to

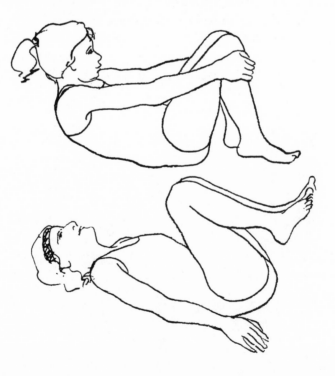

your knees to begin with. (As you get stronger, try to get closer to your knees.) Roll back down. Arms can be held out in front of you to start, and then, as you get stronger, they can be folded across your chest. Ultimately, hands are held behind your head.

8. *Reverse sit-up.* Lying flat on the floor with arms at your sides, bring your heels back to your buttocks, and then lift knees to your chest, raising hips off the floor. Return to starting position and repeat several times. Breathe normally.

Finally, one of the very best strengthening exercises of all is the push-up, but it should not be undertaken until your stomach muscles are reasonably strong and until you can do a push-up resting on your knees rather than your toes. You can practice some easier versions of the push-up by pushing off against a wall until you get stronger.

Be sure to check with your physician before beginning any new fitness program. Then, get start-up instruction from a qualified teacher at your local YMCA, club, or spa.

APPENDIX C

A Note on Noninsulin-Dependent Diabetes Mellitus

Noninsulin-dependent diabetes mellitus (NIDDM) usually develops in persons over forty years old and is the most common type of diabetes (90 to 95 percent of all cases of diabetes). Sedentary obese persons with predominantly abdominal rather than gluteal fat have an increased risk (that is, the apple body shape is more dangerous than the pear shape). The condition is marked by high blood glucose (sugar) and insulin resistance. About 8 million people have been diagnosed with NIDDM, but at least another 8 million have the disorder but have not yet been diagnosed. Many more may be in the first stages of the disease, having impaired glucose tolerance (inability to regulate blood sugar) and mild hyperglycemia (a slightly elevated amount of circulating blood glucose). However, in these early stages, symptoms associated with the disorder, such as excessive thirst and hunger, increased urination, blurred vision, fatigue, and glycosuria (sugar in the urine), may not be present.

Dietary treatment of NIDDM is aimed at controlling blood glucose levels and maximizing the effectiveness of drug therapy when that is required. The intake of carbohydrate has to be timed and distributed throughout the day in amounts that do not result in either hyper- or hypoglycemia (dangerously high or low blood glucose). This requires that carbohydrate intake also be coordinated with the impact of drugs that affect insulin secretion and insulin resistance.

Dietary treatment in NIDDM must be individualized, since all persons with NIDDM do not respond similarly. For some, a low-fat diet is appropriate (30 percent or less of total calories from fat, 55 percent of calories from carbohydrate). Recently, however, persons whose diets contain as much as 45 percent of calories from fat (25 percent monounsaturated, 10 percent polyunsaturated, and 10 percent saturated) and only 40 percent from carbohydrate have demonstrated better blood glucose and insulin levels after meals; many also show lower day-long circulating triglycerides.

Obesity often plays a key role in the development of NIDDM, and if you are overweight and suffer from NIDDM, a loss of just 10 to 20 pounds may help reverse insulin resistance, improve glucose and lipid levels, and reduce blood pressure (high blood pressure often accompanies NIDDM). Daily physical activity will add to the improvement. Experts estimate that between 80 and 90 percent of overweight people with NIDDM can control the factors that lead to the disorder through weight loss and a moderately intense program of physical activity.

If you are an overweight person suffering from NIDDM, you need to consult with your physician and a dietician certified in the treatment of diabetes to design a combined treatment program, using diet, physical activity, and, if drugs are required to achieve metabolic control, the appropriate drug dosage. Certain drugs used to treat NIDDM encourage weight gain and interfere with weight loss (e.g., insulin and the sulfonylureas). But losing weight may be essential if you are to eliminate your need for drugs. To break out of this Catch-22 situation requires strict adherence to a weight-loss diet and physical activity program.

The degree of caloric restriction and amount of physical activity required to lose weight will vary from person to person. Recommended carbohydrate foods in both kinds of diets (low-fat and high monounsaturated fat) include high-bulk vegetables and fruits and minimally processed grains. Since foods are usually eaten in combination in a mixed diet, the glycemic index of various carbohydrates (the speed with which the sugars are broken down and enter the bloodstream, which affects the height of the insulin response) may be less important than the amount of fiber at mealtimes. Snack foods not eaten in combination with other foods may require closer monitoring according to their glycemic index. Monounsaturated fats are found in large quantities in nuts, olive oil, and canola oil, and it may prove advantageous to replace some of the meat in the diet with nuts.

Instructions for Keeping a Daily Fat Gram Record and Fat Gram Counter

It's a good idea to keep a pocket notebook and record your fat gram intake until you are familiar with the fat content of the foods you normally eat. After a few weeks you will have made the required changes in your diet and committed the new knowledge to memory, and recording will become unnecessary.

Simply write down the food item on the left-hand side of the page and the fat content in grams on the right. Total after each meal and stick within your fat-gram allowance:

20 to 40 grams per day for women
30 to 60 grams per day for men

Keep a separate total of the fat grams that may be suppressed in your fuel mixture by the consumption of fat-free or reduced-fat desserts, cookies, pastries, snack foods, and candy. Figure 1 gram of fat suppressed by fat-free foods in these categories for every 10 calories above 50 in each serving. Figure the fat grams in reduced-fat foods as though they had not been reduced (that is, if fat in the food has been reduced by 33 percent compared with the original recipe, figure that an amount equal to half the remaining number of

*Nutrient values in this appendix were obtained from materials provided by the U.S. Department of Agriculture, as well as the food industry, journal articles, and computer data banks in which information is assumed to be public domain.

fat grams is being suppressed—for example, if the product contains 4 grams of fat, add 2 to the suppressed totals; if fat in the food has been reduced by 50 percent, figure an amount equal to the remaining number as being suppressed; if the product contains 4 grams of fat, add 4 to the suppressed total.) These are approximate figures and are meant only to help you keep yourself from overeating on these foods and having them interfere with your weight-management efforts.

Alcohol is burned in place of fat. Figure a suppression of 7 grams of fat per serving of an alcoholic beverage.

Do not go below 20 grams of fat in your diet if you are a woman, or 30 if you are a man. Fat supplies some essential nutrients and carries fat-soluble vitamins essential for many metabolic functions to their target areas.

Counting fat grams that are possibly suppressed in your fuel mixture is simply to help you understand why you may be having trouble managing your weight if fat-free and reduced-fat foods are included in your diet.

Since the energy in fat is so concentrated (there is a gram of fat in each 1/4 teaspoon of fat or oil, which equals 9 calories), accurate measurements of all items that contain fat are important, as well as of imitation energy-dense fat-free foods.

For your additional information, the counter also lists the fiber content of various foods. However, unless you are curious, you do not need to keep a record of fiber intake. The suggested range of 20 to 35 grams of fiber per day for women and up to 50 grams for men is easily reached on the T-Factor 2000 Diet. Slowly increase fiber until you are consuming quantities that are at the high end of the suggested range.

HOW TO USE THE COUNTER

Food items are in alphabetical order within a number of different food categories. The categories are as follows, with the page number on which you will find them:

Foods are listed in the size of portions commonly consumed. Information is given for total fat in grams, total calories, and grams of fiber. For an expanded list of foods and to obtain nutrition counts for saturated fat, cholesterol, and sodium, see *The T-Factor 2000 Fat Gram Counter.* We have included a wide sampling of generic foods and beverages. If you cannot find a product in this counter or use a specific brand, consult the nutrition labeling that appears on the food product. You'll find an extensive list of combination foods that includes representative items from different food manufacturers, or an average from several, without naming them (for example, lasagna or macaroni and cheese). Combination foods may be listed as "hmde" (homemade) or "frzn" (frozen). Values for these dishes, soups, salads, and sandwiches represent combinations of ingredients from traditional recipes. Most "lighter" versions will have nutrition counts with the recipe in cookbooks or magazines. If you create your own lower-fat recipes, simply add up nutrition counts for the ingredients and then divide by the number of servings the recipe yields.

Values for total fat are presented to the nearest tenth of a gram. Government regulations permit food processors to round to the nearest whole gram on package labels. Thus, for example, a cereal product containing 0.3 gram of fat will be rounded to 0 fat on the nutrition labeling, while another product containing 0.6 gram will be rounded up to 1. For personal monitoring it is a good idea to round to the nearest gram to simplify addition and help commit values for foods commonly eaten to memory.

We include a sampling of popular menu items from top fast food restaurants. If you eat out frequently, you'll find nutrition count listings for close to fifty national restaurant chains in *The Low-Fat Fast Food Guide,* published by W. W. Norton and available at your local bookstore. You can also obtain nutrition information from restaurants you frequent on their web sites or by requesting a nutrition brochure from the restaurant manager. An extensive listing of low- and reduced-fat brand-name products can be found in *The Low-Fat Supermarket Shopper's Guide,* also from W. W. Norton.

FAT GRAM COUNTER

Item	Serving	Total Fat (g)	Calories	Fiber (g)
BEVERAGES				
beer				
regular*	12 fl. oz.	0	148	0
light*	12 fl. oz.	0	100	0
nonalcoholic	12 fl. oz.	0	90	0
carbonated drink				
regular	12 fl. oz.	0	152	0
sugar free	12 fl. oz.	0	1	0
club soda/seltzer	12 fl. oz.	0	0	0
coffee, brewed or instant	8 fl. oz.	0	4	0
eggnog, nonalcoholic				
w/whole milk	8 fl. oz.	19.0	342	0
w/2% milk	8 fl. oz.	8.1	188	0
fruit punch	8 fl. oz.	0	107	0
gin, 90 proof*	1 fl. oz.	0	70	0
grape juice drink, canned	6 fl. oz.	0	89	0
Kool-Aid, from mix, any flavor	8 fl. oz.	0	95	0
lemonade, mix or frzn	8 fl. oz.	0	102	0
lemonade, sugar-free	8 fl. oz.	0	4	0
rum, 80 proof*	1 fl. oz.	0	70	0
tea, brewed or instant	8 fl. oz.	0	0	0
tonic water	8 fl. oz.	0	90	0
vodka, 80 proof*	1 fl. oz.	0	70	0
whiskey, 86 proof*	1 fl. oz.	0	70	0
wine*				
dessert and apertif	4 fl. oz.	0	184	0
red or rosé	4 fl. oz.	0	85	0

*Although alcohol contains no fat, scientific evidence suggests that it may facilitate fat storage and hamper your weight-loss efforts. Excessive alcohol intake is detrimental to your health. We concur with other health organizations in recommending discretion in the use of alcoholic beverages.

Item	Serving	Total Fat (g)	Calories	Fiber (g)
white, dry or medium	4 fl. oz.	0	80	0
wine cooler	8 fl. oz.	0	83	0
BREADS AND FLOURS				
bagel, cinnamon raisin	1 medium	1.2	195	2
bagel, plain	1 medium	1.1	180	2
barley flour	1 cup	3.0	600	31
biscuit				
baking powder	1 medium	6.6	156	1
buttermilk	1 medium	5.8	127	1
bread				
French/Vienna	1 slice	1.0	90	1
fruit w/nuts	1 slice	10.1	210	1
fruit w/o nuts	1 slice	5.9	150	1
Italian	1 slice	0.5	80	1
mixed grain	1 slice	0.9	70	2
multigrain, "lite"	1 slice	0.5	45	3
pita, plain	1 large	0.7	165	2
pita, whole wheat	1 large	1.2	180	7
raisin	1 slice	1.1	70	1
rye, American	1 slice	0.9	66	2
rye, pumpernickel	1 slice	0.8	82	2
sourdough	1 slice	0.8	70	1
wheat, commercial	1 slice	1.1	75	2
wheat, "lite"	1 slice	0.5	45	3
white, commercial	1 slice	1.0	75	0
white, hmde	1 slice	1.7	72	0
white, "lite"	1 slice	0.5	42	2
whole wheat, commercial	1 slice	1.2	80	3
breadcrumbs	1 cup	5.4	395	4
breadsticks				
plain	1 small	0.3	39	0
sesame	1 small	2.2	51	0
bulgur, dry	1 cup	2.0	477	25
coffee cake	1 piece	7.0	233	1

Item	Serving	Total Fat (g)	Calories	Fiber (g)
cornbread				
from mix	⅛ mix	4.0	160	1
hmde	1 piece	7.3	198	2
cornflake crumbs	1 oz.	0	100	1
crackers				
Captain's Wafers	4 crackers	2.0	60	0
cheese	5 pieces	4.9	81	0
Cheese Nips	13 crackers	3.2	70	0
cheese w/peanut butter	2 oz. pkg.	13.5	283	1
Goldfish, any flavor	12 crackers	2.0	34	0
graham	2 squares	1.3	60	0
graham, crumbs	½ cup	6.1	250	2
Hi Ho	4 crackers	4.0	70	0
matzohs	1 board	0.4	112	0
melba toast	1 piece	0.2	20	0
Norwegian flatbread	2 thin	0.2	40	0
oyster	33 crackers	3.8	143	0
rice cakes	1 piece	0.2	35	0
rice wafer	3 wafers	0	31	0
Ritz	3 crackers	3.0	53	0
Ryekrisp, plain	2 crackers	0.2	40	2
saltines	2 crackers	0.7	26	0
sesame wafers	3 crackers	3.0	70	0
soda	5 crackers	1.9	63	0
toasted w/peanut butter	1.5 oz. pkg.	10.5	212	0
Triscuit	2 crackers	1.6	40	1
Wasa crispbread	1 piece	1.0	45	1
Wheat Thins	4 crackers	1.5	35	0
wheat w/cheese	1.5 oz. pkg.	10.9	212	0
Wheatsworth	5 crackers	3.0	70	1
zwieback	2 crackers	1.2	60	0
crepe	1 medium	12.5	230	0
croissant	1 medium	11.5	167	1
croutons, commercial	¼ cup	1.8	50	1
Danish pastry	1 medium	19.3	256	1

Item	Serving	Total Fat (g)	Calories	Fiber (g)
doughnut				
cake	1 2.2 oz.	16.2	250	1
yeast	1 2.2 oz.	13.3	235	1
dumpling, plain	1 medium	1.1	42	0
English muffin				
plain	1	1.1	135	1
w/raisins	1	1.2	150	1
whole wheat	1	2.0	170	2
flour				
rye, medium	1 cup	2.2	400	13
soy	1 cup	18.0	380	2
white, all purpose	1 cup	1.2	455	4
white, bread	1 cup	3.0	401	4
white, self-rising	1 cup	1.2	436	4
whole wheat	1 cup	2.3	400	14
French toast				
frzn variety	1 slice	6.0	139	0
hmde	1 slice	10.7	172	1
funnel cake	6 in. diam.	15.3	285	1
hushpuppy	1 medium	5.5	153	1
matzoh ball	1	7.6	121	0
muffins				
all types, commercial	1 large (3 oz.)	10.3	242	1
banana nut	1 medium	5.0	135	2
blueberry, from mix	1 medium	5.1	131	1
bran, hmde	1 medium	5.8	130	3
corn	1 medium	4.8	175	2
white, plain	1 medium	5.4	135	1
pancakes				
buckwheat, from mix	3 medium	12.3	270	3
buttermilk, from mix	3 medium	10.0	270	2
hmde	3 medium	9.6	312	2
"lite," from mix	3 medium	2.0	190	5
whole-wheat, from mix	3 medium	3.0	180	6
phyllo dough	2 oz.	3.4	170	1

Item	Serving	Total Fat (g)	Calories	Fiber (g)
pie crust, plain	⅛ pie	8.0	125	0
popover	1	5.0	170	0
rice bran	1 oz.	0.4	80	2
rolls				
brown & serve	1	2.2	100	0
cloverleaf	1	3.2	89	0
crescent	1	5.6	102	1
croissant	1 small	6.0	120	0
French	1	0.4	137	1
hamburger	1	3.0	180	1
hard	1	1.2	115	1
hot dog	1	2.1	116	1
kaiser/hoagie	1 medium	2.0	190	1
pan type	1 small	1.0	80	0
parkerhouse	1	2.1	59	0
raisin	1 large	1.9	179	1
rye, dark	1	1.6	55	2
rye, light, hard	1	1.0	79	2
sandwich	1	3.1	162	1
sesame seed	1	2.1	59	1
sourdough	1	1.0	100	1
submarine	1 medium	3.0	290	2
wheat	1	1.7	72	1
white, commercial	1	2.0	80	0
white, hmde	1	3.1	119	1
whole wheat	1	1.1	85	3
yeast, sweet	1	7.9	198	1
scone	1	5.5	120	1
soft pretzel	1 medium	1.7	190	1
stuffing				
bread, from mix	½ cup	12.2	198	0
cornbread, from mix	½ cup	4.8	175	0
Stove Top	½ cup	9.0	176	0
sweet roll, iced	1 medium	7.9	198	1

Item	Serving	Total Fat (g)	Calories	Fiber (g)
toaster pastry, any flavor	1	5.0	200	0
tortilla				
corn (unfried)	1 medium	1.1	67	1
flour	1 medium	2.5	85	1
turnover, fruit filled	1	15.0	280	1
waffle				
frozen	1 medium	3.2	95	1
hmde	1 large	12.6	245	1
CANDY				
butterscotch				
candy	6 pieces	1.3	140	0
chips	1 oz.	8.3	150	0
candied fruit				
apricot	1 oz.	0.1	94	1
cherry	1 oz.	0.1	96	1
citrus peel	1 oz.	0.1	90	1
figs	1 oz.	0.1	84	2
candy bar				
Almond Joy	1 oz.	7.8	136	2
Baby Ruth	1 oz.	6.6	141	1
Bit-o-Honey	1 oz.	2.2	121	0
Butterfinger	1 oz.	5.5	131	1
Chunky	1 oz.	8.3	140	1
Heath	1 oz.	8.9	142	1
Kit Kat	1.13 oz.	9.2	162	0
Mars	1.7 oz.	11.0	240	1
milk chocolate	1 oz.	9.2	147	1
milk choc. w/almonds	1 oz.	10.1	151	2
Milky Way	1 oz.	4.3	120	0
Mounds	1 oz.	6.1	125	2
Mr. Goodbar	1 oz.	9.1	145	2
Nestle's Crunch	1.06 oz.	8.0	160	1
Snickers	1 oz.	6.5	135	1

Item	Serving	Total Fat (g)	Calories	Fiber (g)
Three Musketeers	1 oz.	3.7	120	0
Twix, caramel	1 oz.	6.7	140	0
candy-coated almonds	1 oz.	5.3	130	1
caramels				
plain or choc. w/nuts	1 oz.	4.6	120	0
plain or choc. w/o nuts	1 oz.	3.0	110	0
carob-coated raisins	½ cup	13.5	387	5
choc. chips				
milk choc.	¼ cup	11.0	218	1
semi-sweet	¼ cup	12.2	220	1
choc.-covered cherries	1 oz.	4.9	123	1
choc.-covered cream center	1 oz.	4.9	123	1
choc.-covered mint patty	1 small	1.0	40	0
choc.-covered peanuts	1 oz.	11.7	159	2
choc.-covered raisins	1 oz.	4.9	120	1
choc. kisses	6 pieces	9.0	154	1
choc. stars	7 pieces	8.1	160	1
Cracker Jack	1 cup	3.3	170	2
English toffee	1 oz.	2.8	113	0
fondant	1 piece	0.2	116	0
fudge				
choc.	1 oz.	3.4	112	0
choc. w/nuts	1 oz.	4.9	119	0
Good & Plenty	1 oz.	0.1	106	0
gumdrops	28 pieces	0.2	97	0
Gummy Bears	1 oz.	0.1	110	0
hard candy	6 pieces	0.3	108	0
jelly beans	1 oz.	0	104	0
licorice	1 oz.	0.1	35	0
M&M's				
choc. only	1 oz.	5.6	132	1
peanut	1 oz.	7.8	145	1
malted-milk balls	1 oz.	7.1	137	1
marshmallow	1 large	0	25	0

Item	Serving	Total Fat (g)	Calories	Fiber (g)
marshmallow creme	1 oz.	0.1	88	0
mints	14 pieces	0.6	104	0
peanut brittle	1 oz.	7.7	149	1
Peanut Butter Cups, Reese's	1 oz.	9.2	156	1
Peppermint Pattie	1 oz.	4.8	124	1
praline	1 oz.	6.9	130	0
sour balls	1 oz.	0	110	0
taffy	1 oz.	1.5	99	0
Tootsie Roll pop	1 oz.	0.6	110	0
Tootsie Roll	1 oz.	2.3	112	1
yogurt-covered peanuts	½ cup	26.0	387	4
yogurt-covered raisins	½ cup	14.0	313	2
CEREALS				
All Bran	⅓ cup	0.5	70	10
Alpha-Bits	1 cup	0.6	111	1
Apple Jacks	1 cup	0.1	110	1
Bran, 100%	½ cup	1.9	84	9
bran, unprocessed, dry	¼ cup	0.6	29	6
Bran Buds	⅓ cup	0.7	72	10
Bran Chex	1 cup	1.2	136	9
Bran Flakes, 40%	1 cup	0.7	127	6
Cap'n Crunch	¾ cup	3.4	121	0
Cheerios	1 cup	1.6	90	2
Cocoa Krispies	1 cup	0.5	140	0
Corn Chex	1 cup	0.1	111	1
cornflakes	1 cup	0.1	108	1
corn grits w/o added fat	½ cup	0.5	71	1
Cream of Wheat w/o added fat	½ cup	0.3	67	0
Crispix	1 cup	0	110	1
Fiber One	1 cup	2.2	128	21
Frosted Mini-Wheats	4 biscuits	0.3	100	1
Fruit Loops	1 cup	0.5	111	1
fruit squares, Kellogg's	¾ cup	0	135	3

Item	Serving	Total Fat (g)	Calories	Fiber (g)
Golden Grahams	¾ cup	1.1	109	1
granola				
commercial brands	⅓ cup	4.9	126	3
hmde	⅓ cup	10.0	184	2
low-fat, Kellogg's	⅓ cup	2.0	120	2
Grapenut Flakes	1 cup	0.4	116	2
Grapenuts	¼ cup	0.1	105	2
Kix	1½ cup	0.7	110	0
Life, plain or cinn.	1 cup	2.5	152	4
oat bran, cooked cereal				
w/o added fat	½ cup	0.5	50	2
oat bran, dry	¼ cup	1.6	82	3
oats				
instant	1 packet	1.7	108	1
w/o added fat	½ cup	1.2	72	1
Product 19	1 cup	0.2	108	1
puffed rice	1 cup	0	56	0
puffed wheat	1 cup	0.1	44	1
Raisin Bran	1 cup	0.8	156	5
Rice Chex	1 cup	0.1	110	1
Rice Krispies	1 cup	0.2	110	0
shredded wheat	1 cup	0.3	85	2
Special K	1 cup	0.1	111	0
Sugar Frosted Flakes	1 cup	0.5	147	1
Sugar Smacks	1 cup	0.7	140	1
Team	1 cup	0.5	111	1
Total	1 cup	0.7	100	2
Total raisin bran	1 cup	1.0	140	5
Wheat Chex	1 cup	1.2	169	6
wheat germ, toasted	¼ cup	3.0	108	4
Wheaties	1 cup	0.5	99	2
whole-wheat, natural,				
w/o added fat	½ cup	0.5	75	2

Item	Serving	Total Fat (g)	Calories	Fiber (g)
CHEESES				
American				
processed	1 oz.	8.9	106	0
reduced calorie	1 oz.	2.0	50	0
blue	1 oz.	8.2	100	0
brick	1 oz.	8.4	105	0
Brie	1 oz.	7.9	95	0
caraway	1 oz.	8.3	107	0
cheddar				
grated	¼ cup	9.4	114	0
sliced	1 oz.	9.4	114	0
cheese fondue	¼ cup	11.7	170	0
cheese food, cold pack	2 T	7.8	94	0
cheese sauce	¼ cup	9.8	132	0
cheese spread (Kraft)	1 oz.	6.0	82	0
Cheez Whiz	1 oz.	6.0	80	0
Colby	1 oz.	9.1	112	0
cottage cheese				
1% fat	½ cup	1.2	82	0
2% fat	½ cup	2.2	101	0
creamed	½ cup	5.1	117	0
cream cheese				
Kraft Free	1 oz. (2T)	0	25	0
"lite" (Neufchâtel)	1 oz. (2T)	6.6	74	0
regular	1 oz. (2T)	9.9	99	0
Edam	1 oz.	7.9	101	0
feta	1 oz.	6.0	75	0
Gouda	1 oz.	7.8	101	0
hot pepper cheese	1 oz.	6.9	92	0
Jarlsberg	1 oz.	6.9	100	0
Kraft American Singles	1 oz.	7.5	90	0
Kraft Free Singles	1 oz.	0	45	0
Kraft Light Singles	1 oz.	4.0	70	0
Light n' Lively singles	1 oz.	4.0	70	0

Item	Serving	Total Fat (g)	Calories	Fiber (g)
Limburger	1 oz.	7.7	93	0
Monterey Jack	1 oz.	8.6	106	0
mozzarella				
part skim	1 oz.	4.5	72	0
part skim, low moisture	1 oz.	4.9	79	0
whole milk	1 oz.	6.1	80	0
whole milk, low moisture	1 oz.	7.0	90	0
Muenster	1 oz.	8.5	104	0
Parmesan				
grated	1 T	1.5	23	0
hard	1 oz.	7.3	111	0
pimento cheese spread	1 oz.	8.9	106	0
port wine, cold pack	1 oz.	8.0	100	0
provolone	1 oz.	7.6	100	0
ricotta				
"lite" reduced fat	½ cup	4.0	109	0
part skim	½ cup	9.8	171	0
whole milk	½ cup	16.1	216	0
Romano	1 oz.	7.6	110	0
Roquefort	1 oz.	8.7	105	0
Sargento Light				
mozzarella	1 oz.	3.0	60	0
Swiss	1 oz.	4.0	80	0
smoked cheese product	1 oz.	7.0	100	0
Swiss				
processed	1 oz.	7.1	95	0
sliced	1 oz.	7.8	107	0
Velveeta	1 oz.	7.0	100	0
Velveeta Light	1 oz.	4.0	70	0
Weight Watchers, slices	1 oz.	2.0	50	0
COMBINATION FOODS				
baked beans w/pork	½ cup	1.8	134	4
beans				

Item	Serving	Total Fat (g)	Calories	Fiber (g)
refried, canned	½ cup	1.4	135	7
refried w/fat	½ cup	13.2	271	7
refried w/sausage, canned	½ cup	13.0	194	8
beans & franks, canned	1 cup	16.0	366	7
beef & vegetable stew	1 cup	10.5	218	2
beef goulash w/noodles	1 cup	13.9	335	2
beef noodle casserole	1 cup	19.2	329	2
beef pot pie, frzn	8 oz.	23.0	430	2
beef stew, canned	1 cup	8.0	184	2
beef vegetable stew, hmde	1 cup	10.5	220	2
burrito				
bean w/cheese	1 large	11.0	330	4
bean w/o cheese	1 large	6.8	225	4
beef	1 large	19.0	413	2
cabbage roll w/beef & rice	1 medium	6.0	168	2
cannelloni, meat & cheese	1 piece	29.7	420	1
casserole, meat, veg., rice, sauce	1 cup	12.2	276	3
cheese soufflé	1 cup	14.1	195	0
chicken à la king, hmde	1 cup	34.3	468	1
chicken & dumplings	1 cup	10.5	298	1
chicken & rice casserole	1 cup	18.0	365	1
chicken & veg. stir-fry	1 cup	6.9	142	3
chicken divan, frzn	8½ oz.	22.2	353	1
chicken fricassee, hmde	1 cup	18.1	318	1
chicken-fried steak	3½ oz.	23.4	355	0
chicken noodle casserole	1 cup	10.7	269	2
chicken parmigiana, hmde	7 oz.	17.0	346	2
chicken pot pie, frzn	8 oz.	23.0	430	1
chicken salad, regular	½ cup	21.2	271	0
chicken tetrazzini	1 cup	19.6	348	1
chicken w/cashews, Chinese	1 cup	28.6	409	2
chili				
w/beans	1 cup	14.8	302	6
w/o beans	1 cup	19.3	302	3

Item	Serving	Total Fat (g)	Calories	Fiber (g)
chitterlings, cooked	3½ oz.	29.4	303	0
chop suey w/o rice or noodles				
beef	1 cup	15.8	275	2
fish or poultry	1 cup	8.2	195	2
chow mein				
beef, canned	1 cup	2.3	72	2
chicken, canned	1 cup	2.3	68	2
chicken, hmde	1 cup	8.8	224	2
corned-beef hash	1 cup	24.4	374	2
crab cake	1 small	4.5	95	0
creamed chipped beef	1 cup	23.0	350	0
curry w/o meat	1 cup	6.6	138	2
deviled crab	½ cup	15.4	231	1
deviled egg	1 large	5.3	63	0
egg foo yung w/sauce	1 piece	7.0	129	1
eggplant Parmesan, traditional	1 cup	24.0	356	3
egg roll, restaurant style	1 (3½ oz.)	10.5	153	1
egg salad	½ cup	17.4	212	0
enchilada				
bean, beef, & cheese	1 piece	14.1	243	3
beef, frzn	7½ oz.	16.0	250	2
cheese, frzn	8 oz.	26.3	444	3
chicken, frzn	7½ oz.	16.1	340	4
fajitas				
chicken	1	13.5	381	4
beef	1	18.2	302	3
falafel	1 small	5.0	74	1
fettuccine Alfredo	1 cup	29.7	462	3
fish and chips, frzn dinner	5.5 oz.	14.8	325	3
fish creole	1 cup	5.4	172	2
fritter, corn	1 medium	8.5	132	1
frzn dinner				
beef tips and noodles	11 oz.	5.1	370	4
chopped sirloin	11.5 oz.	30.1	560	5

Item	Serving	Total Fat (g)	Calories	Fiber (g)
fried chicken	11 oz.	29.6	590	6
meat loaf	11 oz.	23.1	530	4
Salisbury steak	11 oz.	27.4	500	4
turkey and dressing	11 oz.	22.6	510	3
green pepper stuffed				
w/rice & beef	1 average	13.5	262	2
Hamburger Helper,				
all varieties (average)	1 cup	18.9	375	1
hamburger rice casserole	1 cup	21.0	376	3
ham salad w/mayo	½ cup	20.2	277	0
ham spread, Spreadables	½ cup	12.0	180	0
lasagna				
cheese, frzn	10½ oz.	14.0	390	5
hmde w/beef & cheese	1 piece	19.8	400	2
zucchini lasagna, lo-cal, frzn	11 oz.	8.6	301	5
lobster				
Cantonese	1 cup	19.6	334	0
Newburg	½ cup	24.8	305	0
salad	½ cup	7.0	119	0
lo mein, Chinese	1 cup	7.2	185	1
macaroni & cheese				
from package	1 cup	17.3	386	0
frzn	6 oz.	12.0	260	0
manicotti, cheese & tomato	1 piece	11.8	238	2
meatball (reg. ground beef)	1 medium	5.1	72	0
meat loaf, w/reg. ground beef	3½ oz.	20.4	332	0
moo goo gai pan	1 cup	17.2	304	1
moussaka	1 cup	8.9	210	3
onion rings	10 average	17.0	234	1
oysters Rockefeller, traditional	6–8 oysters	14.0	230	1
pepper steak	1 cup	11.0	330	1
pizza				
cheese	1 slice	10.1	270	1
combination w/meat	1 slice	17.5	272	1

Item	Serving	Total Fat (g)	Calories	Fiber (g)
deep dish, cheese	1 slice	13.5	426	4
pepperoni, frzn	¼ pizza	18.0	364	2
pork, sweet & sour, w/rice	1 cup	7.5	270	1
quiche				
Lorraine (bacon)	⅛ pie	43.5	540	1
plain or vegetable	1 slice	17.6	312	1
ratatouille	½ cup	3.0	60	2
ravioli, canned	1 cup	7.3	240	3
ravioli w/meat & tomato sauce	1 piece	3.0	49	0
Salisbury steak w/gravy	8 oz.	27.3	364	1
salmon patty, traditional	3½ oz.	12.4	239	1
sandwiches (on white bread unless otherwise noted)				
BBQ beef on bun	1	16.8	392	5
BBQ pork on bun	1	12.2	359	5
BLT w/mayo	1	15.6	282	2
bologna & cheese	1	22.5	363	2
chicken w/mayo & lettuce	1	14.4	303	2
club w/mayo	1	20.8	590	3
corned beef on rye	1	10.8	296	2
egg salad	1	12.5	279	2
french dip, au jus	1	12.2	360	2
grilled cheese	1	24.0	426	2
ham, cheese & mayo	1	16.0	350	2
ham salad	1	16.9	321	2
peanut butter & jelly	1	15.1	374	3
Reuben	1	33.3	531	6
roast beef & mayo	1	22.6	328	2
sloppy joe on bun	1	16.8	392	5
sub w/salami & cheese	1	41.3	766	3
tuna salad	1	17.5	362	2
turkey & mayo	1	18.4	402	2
turkey breast & mustard	1	5.2	285	2
turkey ham on rye	1	10.5	239	3

Item	Serving	Total Fat (g)	Calories	Fiber (g)
shepherd's pie	1 cup	24.0	407	3
shrimp creole w/o rice	1 cup	6.1	146	2
shrimp salad	½ cup	9.5	136	1
spaghetti				
w/meat sauce	1 cup	16.7	317	2
w/red clam sauce	1 cup	7.3	250	2
w/tomato sauce	1 cup	1.5	179	2
w/white clam sauce	1 cup	19.5	416	1
spanakopita	1 piece	24.1	259	2
spinach soufflé	1 cup	14.8	212	2
stroganoff				
beef w/noodles	1 cup	19.6	390	2
beef w/o noodles	1 cup	26.8	460	1
sushi w/fish & vegetables	5 oz.	1.0	210	1
taco, beef	1 medium	17.0	272	2
tamale w/sauce	1 piece	6.0	114	1
tortellini, meat or cheese	1 cup	15.4	363	1
tostada w/refried beans	1 medium	16.3	294	6
tuna noodle casserole	1 cup	13.3	315	2
tuna salad				
oil pack, w/mayo	½ cup	16.3	226	0
water pack, w/mayo	½ cup	10.5	170	0
veal parmigiana, hmde	1 cup	25.5	485	2
veal scallopini	1 cup	20.4	429	2
Welsh rarebit	1 cup	31.6	415	0
wonton w/pork, fried	1 piece	4.3	82	0
Yorkshire pudding	1 piece	2.4	56	0
DESSERTS AND TOPPINGS				
apple betty, fruit crisps	½ cup	13.3	347	3
baklava	1 piece	29.2	426	2
brownie				
butterscotch	1	6.6	150	0
choc., "light," from mix	¹⁄₂₄ pkg.	2.0	100	0

Item	Serving	Total Fat (g)	Calories	Fiber (g)
choc., plain	1	1.5	64	0
choc., w/frosting	1	9.0	210	1
choc., w/nuts	1	7.3	170	1
cake				
angel food	1/12 cake	0.1	161	0
banana w/frosting	1/12 cake	16.0	410	1
black forest	1/12 cake	14.3	279	1
butter w/frosting	1/12 cake	13.0	380	1
carrot w/frosting	1/12 cake	19.0	420	3
choc. w/frosting	1/12 cake	17.0	388	2
coconut w/frosting	1/12 cake	18.1	395	2
devil's food, "light," from mix	1/12 cake	3.5	190	0
German choc. w/frosting	1/12 cake	18.5	407	2
gingerbread	2½" slice	2.9	267	0
lemon chiffon	1/12 cake	4.0	190	0
lemon w/frosting	1/12 cake	16.0	410	1
pineapple upside-down	2½" slice	9.1	236	2
pound	1/12 cake	9.0	200	1
shortbread w/fruit	1 piece	8.9	344	1
spice w/frosting	1/12 cake	11.3	375	1
sponge	1 piece	3.1	190	0
white w/frosting	1/12 cake	14.6	369	1
white, "light," from mix	1/12 cake	3.0	180	0
yellow, "light," from mix	1/12 cake	3.5	190	0
yellow w/frosting	1/12 cake	16.4	391	1
cheesecake, traditional	1/8 pie	22.0	372	0
cobbler				
w/biscuit topping	½ cup	6.0	209	3
w/pie-crust topping	½ cup	9.3	236	3
cookie				
animal	15 cookies	4.7	152	0
anise-seed	1	4.0	63	0
anisette toast	1 slice	1.0	109	0
arrowroot	1	0.9	24	0

Item	Serving	Total Fat (g)	Calories	Fiber (g)
choc.	1	3.3	56	0
choc. chip, hmde	1	3.7	68	0
choc. chip, Pepperidge Farm	1	2.5	100	0
choc. sandwich (Oreo type)	1	2.1	49	0
fig bar	1	1.0	56	1
gingersnap	1	1.6	34	0
graham cracker, choc. covered	1	3.1	62	0
macaroon, coconut	1	3.4	60	0
molasses	1	3.0	80	0
oatmeal	1	3.2	80	0
oatmeal raisin	1	3.0	83	0
peanut butter	1	3.2	72	1
Rice Krispie bar	1	0.9	36	0
shortbread	1	2.3	42	0
sugar	1	3.4	89	0
sugar wafers	2 small	2.1	53	0
vanilla-creme sandwich	1	3.1	69	0
vanilla wafers	3	1.8	51	0
cream puff w/custard	1	14.6	245	0
cupcake				
choc. w/icing	1	5.5	159	1
yellow w/icing	1	6.0	160	1
custard, baked	½ cup	6.9	148	0
date bar	1 bar	2.0	90	1
dumpling, fruit	1 piece	15.1	324	2
eclair				
w/choc. icing & custard	1 small	15.4	316	0
w/choc. icing & whipped cream	1 small	25.7	296	0
frosting/icing				
choc.	3 T	5.3	148	0
cream cheese	3 T	6.8	170	0
"light" varieties, ready-to-spread	1/12 tub	2.0	130	0
ready-to-spread	1/12 tub	6.9	169	0
seven-minute	3 T	0	135	0

Item	Serving	Total Fat (g)	Calories	Fiber (g)
vanilla or lemon	3 T	4.0	140	0
fruitcake	1 piece	6.2	154	1
fruit ice, Italian	½ cup	0	123	0
Fudgesicle	1 bar	0.4	196	1
gelatin				
low-cal.	½ cup	0	8	0
regular, sweetened	½ cup	0	70	0
granola bar	1 bar	6.8	141	1
Hostess				
brownie	1	12.0	350	1
cupcake	1	5.0	170	1
cupcake lights	1	1.5	120	0
Ding Dong	1	9.0	160	0
fruit snack pie	1	14.4	266	2
Ho Ho	1	6.0	120	1
honey bun	1	23.0	410	2
Snoball	1	4.0	150	1
Twinkie	1	4.0	140	0
Twinkie lights	1	1.5	120	0
ice cream				
choc. (10% fat)	½ cup	7.3	145	1
choc. (16% fat)	½ cup	17.0	270	0
dietetic, sugar-free	½ cup	3.5	90	0
strawberry (10% fat)	½ cup	6.0	128	0
vanilla (10% fat)	½ cup	7.2	134	0
vanilla (16% fat)	½ cup	11.9	175	0
ice cream bar				
choc. coated	1 bar	11.5	198	0
toffee krunch	1 bar	10.2	149	1
ice cream cake roll	1 slice	6.9	159	0
ice cream cone				
(cone only)	1 medium	0.3	45	0
ice cream drumstick	1	10.0	188	1
ice cream sandwich	1	8.3	204	0

Item	Serving	Total Fat (g)	Calories	Fiber (g)
ice milk				
choc.	½ cup	2.0	100	0
soft serve, all flavors	½ cup	2.3	112	0
strawberry	½ cup	2.5	100	0
vanilla	½ cup	2.8	92	0
ladyfinger	1	2.0	60	0
lemon bars	1 bar	3.2	70	0
mousse, choc.	½ cup	15.5	189	1
napoleon	1 piece	5.3	85	0
pie				
apple	⅛ pie	16.9	347	3
banana cream or custard	⅛ pie	14.0	353	1
blueberry	⅛ pie	17.3	387	3
Boston cream pie	⅛ pie	10.0	302	1
cherry	⅛ pie	18.1	418	2
choc. cream	⅛ pie	13.0	311	3
choc. meringue, traditional	⅛ pie	18.0	378	1
coconut cream or custard	⅛ pie	19.0	365	1
key lime	⅛ pie	19.0	388	1
lemon chiffon	⅛ pie	13.5	335	1
lemon meringue, traditional	⅛ pie	13.1	350	1
mincemeat	⅛ pie	18.4	434	3
peach	⅛ pie	17.7	421	3
pecan	⅛ pie	23.0	510	2
pumpkin	⅛ pie	16.8	367	5
raisin	⅛ pie	12.9	325	1
rhubarb	⅛ pie	17.1	405	3
strawberry	⅛ pie	9.1	228	1
sweet potato	⅛ pie	18.2	342	2
pie tart, fruit filled	1	18.7	362	2
Popsicle	1 bar	0	96	0
pudding				
any flavor except choc.	½ cup	4.3	165	0
bread w/raisins	½ cup	7.4	212	1

Item	Serving	Total Fat (g)	Calories	Fiber (g)
choc. w/whole milk	½ cup	5.7	220	1
from mix w/skim milk	½ cup	0	124	0
noodle	½ cup	5.3	141	0
rice, w/whole milk	½ cup	4.4	170	1
sugar free varieties	½ cup	2.2	90	0
tapioca, w/2% milk	½ cup	2.4	150	0
pudding pop, frzn	1 bar	2.0	80	0
sherbet	½ cup	1.0	130	0
sopaipilla	1 piece	6.0	88	0
soufflé, choc	½ cup	3.9	63	0
strudel, fruit	½ cup	1.2	47	1
toppings				
butterscotch/caramel	3 T	0.1	156	0
cherry	3 T	0.1	147	0
choc. fudge	2 T	4.0	110	1
choc. syrup, Hershey	2 T	0.4	73	1
custard sauce, hmde	3 T	2.9	64	0
lemon sauce, hmde	3 T	2.1	100	0
marshmallow creme	3 T	0	158	0
pecans in syrup	3 T	2.8	168	0
pineapple	3 T	0.2	146	0
raisin sauce, hmde	3 T	3.0	126	0
strawberry	3 T	0.1	139	0
whipped topping				
aerosol	¼ cup	3.6	45	0
from mix	¼ cup	2.0	32	0
frzn, tub	¼ cup	4.8	59	0
"lite"	1 T	0.3	5	0
whipping cream				
heavy, fluid	1 T	5.6	52	0
light, fluid	1 T	4.6	44	0
turnover, fruit filled	1	19.3	226	1
yogurt, frozen				
low fat	½ cup	1.9	120	0
nonfat	½ cup	0.2	100	0

Item	Serving	Total Fat (g)	Calories	Fiber (g)
EGGS				
boiled-poached	1	5.6	79	0
fried w/ ½ t fat	1 large	7.8	104	0
omelet				
2 oz. cheese, 3 egg	1	37.0	510	0
plain, 3 egg	1	21.3	271	0
scrambled w/milk	1 large	8.0	101	0
substitute	¼ cup	0	30	0
white	1 large	0	17	0
yolk	1 large	5.6	63	0
FAST FOOD (for a more extensive listing see *The T-Factor 2000 Fat Gram Counter* or *The Low-Fat Fast Food Guide* or request a current nutrition brochure at restaurants you frequent)				
ARBY'S				
Arby Q	1	18.0	431	3
Beef 'n Cheddar	1	28.0	487	2
light menu roast beef deluxe	1	10.0	296	6
potato cakes	1 order	12.0	204	0
regular roast beef sandwich	1	19.0	388	3
Burger King				
BK Broiler chicken sandwich	1	26.0	530	2
cheeseburger	1	19.0	360	1
french fries, medium	1 order	21.0	400	4
hamburger	1	15.0	320	1
Whopper	1	40.0	660	3
Whopper w/cheese	1	48.0	760	3
Dominos Pizza				
Deep Dish Pizza, cheese only				
14" pizza	2 slices	19.7	455	3

Item	Serving	Total Fat (g)	Calories	Fiber (g)
Hand Tossed Pizza, cheese only				
14" pizza	2 slices	9.9	317	3
Thin Crust Pizza, cheese only				
14" pizza	2 slices	11.0	253	2
KFC				
Colonel's Crispy Strips	3	15.8	261	3
Extra Tasty Crispy chicken breast	1	28.0	470	1
Hot & Spicy chicken breast	1	35.0	530	2
Hot Wings	6 pieces	33.0	471	2
Original Recipe chicken breast	1	24.0	400	1
Original Recipe chicken				
sandwich	1	22.3	497	3
Tender Roast chicken breast				
w/skin	1	10.8	251	0
Tender Roast chicken w/o skin	1	4.3	169	0
McDonalds				
bacon, egg & cheese biscuit	1	28.0	470	1
baked apple pie	1	13.0	260	<1
Big Mac	1	31.0	560	3
cheeseburger	1	13.0	320	2
Chicken McNuggets	6 piece	17.0	290	0
Egg McMuffin	1	12.0	290	1
Fish Filet Deluxe	1	28.0	560	4
french fries, small	1 order	10.0	210	2
Grilled Chicken Deluxe	1	20.0	440	3
Grilled Chicken Deluxe				
w/o mayo	1	5.0	300	3
hamburger	1	9.0	260	2
Quarter Pounder	1	21.0	420	2
Quarter Pounder w/cheese	1	30.0	530	2
Pizza Hut				
cheese pizza				
hand tossed style	2 slices	20.0	560	4
pan	2 slices	28.0	600	4

Item	Serving	Total Fat (g)	Calories	Fiber (g)
pizzeria stuffed crust	2 slices	22.0	760	8
Sicilian	2 slices	26.0	580	4
Thin 'N Crispy	2 slices	18.0	420	4
Subway				
6 inch cold sandwiches (Italian white bread w/o cheese or condiments)				
cold cut trio	1	13.0	362	3
ham	1	5.0	287	3
roast beef	1	5.0	288	3
Subway Club	1	5.0	297	3
tuna	1	32.0	527	3
tuna (light mayo)	1	15.0	376	3
turkey breast	1	4.0	273	3
Veggie Delite	1	3.0	222	3
6 inch hot sandwiches (Italian white bread w/o cheese or condiments)				
meatball	1	16.0	404	3
pizza sub	1	22.0	448	3
roasted chicken breast	1	6.0	332	3
steak & cheese	1	10.0	383	3
Subway Melt	1	12.0	366	3
Taco Bell				
burritos				
bean	1	12.0	380	13
Big Beef, Supreme	1	23.0	520	11
Big Chicken, Supreme	1	20.0	500	3
grilled chicken	1	14.0	400	3
specialties				
Big Beef MexiMelt	1	15.0	290	4
Mexican pizza	1	35.0	570	8
taco salad w/shell & salsa	1	52.0	850	16
tostada	1	15.0	300	12

Item	Serving	Total Fat (g)	Calories	Fiber (g)
tacos				
grilled chicken soft taco	1	7.0	200	2
grilled steak soft taco	1	10.0	230	3
soft taco	1	10.0	220	3
taco	1	10.0	180	3
Wendy's				
breaded chicken sandwich	1	18.0	440	2
chili, small	1	7.0	210	5
french fries, small	1 order	13.0	270	3
Frosty, medium	1	11.0	440	0
grilled chicken sandwich	1	8.0	310	2
hamburger, single				
w/everything	1	20.0	420	3
jr. or kid's meal cheeseburger	1	13.0	320	2
jr. or kid's meal hamburger	1	10.0	270	2
FATS				
bacon fat	1 T	14.0	126	0
beef, separable fat	1 oz.	23.3	216	0
butter				
solid	1 t	3.8	34	0
whipped	1 t	2.6	23	0
cream				
light	1 T	2.9	29	0
medium (25% fat)	1 T	3.8	37	0
whipping, light	1 T	4.6	44	0
cream substitute				
liquid/frzn	½ fl. oz.	1.5	20	0
powdered	1 T	0.7	11	0
half & half	1 T	1.7	20	0
margarine				
liquid or soft tub	1 t	3.8	34	0
reduced calorie, tub	1 t	2.0	18	0
solid (corn), stick	1 t	3.8	34	0

Item	Serving	Total Fat (g)	Calories	Fiber (g)
mayonnaise				
fat-free	1 T	0	11	0
reduced calorie	1 T	5.0	50	0
regular (soybean)	1 T	11.0	100	0
no-stick spray				
(Pam, etc.)	2-sec spray	0.9	8	0
oil				
canola	1 T	13.6	120	0
corn	1 T	13.6	120	0
olive	1 T	13.5	119	0
safflower	1 T	13.6	120	0
soybean	1 T	13.6	120	0
pork				
backfat, raw	1 oz.	25.4	192	0
separable fat, cooked	1 oz.	23.4	216	0
pork fat (lard)	1 T	12.8	116	0
salt pork, raw	1 oz.	23.8	219	0
sandwich spread (Miracle Whip type)	1 T	4.9	57	0
shortening, vegetable	1 T	12.8	113	0
sour cream				
cultured	1 T	3.0	31	0
fat-free	1 T	0	9	0
half & half, cultured	1 T	1.8	20	0
imitation	1 T	2.8	30	0
"lite"	1 T	1.8	20	0
FISH (all baked/broiled w/o added fat unless otherwise noted)				
abalone, canned	3½ oz.	5.6	80	0
anchovy, canned in oil	3 fillets	1.2	25	0
anchovy paste	1 t	0.8	14	0
bass				
freshwater	3½ oz.	4.7	145	0

Item	Serving	Total Fat (g)	Calories	Fiber (g)
saltwater, black	3½ oz.	1.2	93	0
saltwater, striped	3½ oz.	2.5	105	0
bluefish	3½ oz.	5.4	157	0
buffalofish	3½ oz.	4.2	150	0
butterfish				
gulf	3½ oz.	2.9	95	0
northern	3½ oz.	10.2	184	0
carp	3½ oz.	6.1	138	0
catfish	3½ oz.	3.1	103	0
catfish, breaded & fried	3½ oz.	13.2	226	NA
caviar, sturgeon, granular	1 round t	1.5	26	0
clams				
canned, solids & liquid	½ cup	0.7	85	0
canned, solids only	3 oz.	1.6	118	0
meat only	5 large	1.0	80	0
cod				
canned	3½ oz.	0.8	104	0
cooked	3½ oz.	0.8	104	0
dried, salted	3½ oz.	2.3	287	0
crab				
canned	½ cup	0.9	67	0
deviled	3½ oz.	10.1	217	0
crab, Alaska king	3½ oz.	1.5	96	0
crab cake	3½ oz.	10.8	178	0
crappie, white	3½ oz.	0.8	79	0
crayfish, freshwater	3½ oz.	1.4	89	0
crooker				
Atlantic	3½ oz.	3.2	133	0
white	3½ oz.	0.8	84	0
cusk, steamed	3½ oz.	0.9	111	0
dolphinfish	3½ oz.	0.8	93	0
eel, American				
cooked	3½ oz.	18.3	260	0
smoked	3½ oz.	23.6	281	0

Item	Serving	Total Fat (g)	Calories	Fiber (g)
eulachon (smelt)	3½ oz.	6.2	118	0
fillets, frzn				
batter dipped	2 pieces	20.0	340	1
breaded	2 pieces	18.0	290	1
fish cakes, frzn, fried	3½ oz.	14.0	242	2
flatfish	3½ oz.	0.8	79	0
flounder/sole	3½ oz.	0.5	68	0
gefilte fish	3½ oz.	2.2	82	1
grouper	3½ oz.	1.3	87	0
haddock				
cooked	3½ oz.	0.6	79	0
fried	3½ oz.	14.2	284	0
smoked/canned	3½ oz.	0.4	103	0
halibut	3½ oz.	1.2	100	0
herring				
canned or smoked	3½ oz.	13.6	208	0
cooked	3½ oz.	11.3	176	0
pickled	3½ oz.	15.1	223	0
Jack mackerel	3½ oz.	5.6	143	0
kingfish	3½ oz.	3.0	105	0
lobster, northern				
broiled w/fat	12 oz.	15.1	445	0
cooked	3½ oz.	0.6	97	0
mackerel				
Atlantic	3½ oz.	13.7	204	0
Pacific	3½ oz.	7.3	159	0
muskekunge				
("muskie," "skie")	3½ oz.	2.5	109	0
mussels, meat only	3½ oz.	2.2	95	0
ocean perch				
cooked	3½ oz.	1.6	95	0
fried	3½ oz.	11.6	228	0
octopus	3½ oz.	2.1	163	0

Item	Serving	Total Fat (g)	Calories	Fiber (g)
oysters				
canned	3½ oz.	2.2	76	0
fried	3½ oz.	13.9	239	0
raw	5–8 medium	1.8	66	0
perch, freshwater, yellow	3½ oz.	0.9	91	0
pickerel	3½ oz.	0.5	84	0
pike				
blue	3½ oz.	0.9	90	0
northern	3½ oz.	1.1	88	0
walleye	3½ oz.	1.2	93	0
pollock, Atlantic	3½ oz.	1.0	91	0
pompano	3½ oz.	9.5	166	0
rainbow trout				
baked, broiled	3½ oz.	5.8	150	0
breaded, fried	3½ oz.	14.6	265	1
red snapper	3½ oz.	1.9	93	0
rockfish, oven steamed	3½ oz.	2.5	107	0
roughy, orange	3½ oz.	7.0	124	0
salmon				
Atlantic	3½ oz.	6.3	141	0
broiled/baked	3½ oz.	7.4	182	0
chinook, canned	3½ oz.	14.0	210	0
pink, canned	3½ oz.	5.1	118	0
smoked	3½ oz.	9.3	176	0
sardines				
Atlantic, in soy oil	2 sardines	2.8	50	0
Pacific	3½ oz.	8.6	160	0
scallops				
cooked	3½ oz.	1.2	81	0
frzn, fried	3½ oz.	10.5	194	0
steamed	3½ oz.	1.4	112	0
sea bass, white	3½ oz.	1.5	96	0
shrimp				
canned, dry pack	3½ oz.	1.6	116	0

Item	Serving	Total Fat (g)	Calories	Fiber (g)
canned, wet pack	½ cup	0.8	87	0
fried	3½ oz.	10.8	225	0
raw or broiled	3½ oz.	1.8	105	0
smelt	3½ oz.	2.4	100	0
sole, fillet	3½ oz.	0.5	68	0
squid				
fried	3 oz.	6.4	149	0
raw	3 oz.	1.2	78	0
surimi	3½ oz.	0.9	98	0
sushi or sashimi	3½ oz.	4.9	144	0
swordfish	3½ oz.	4.0	118	0
trout				
brook	3½ oz.	2.1	101	0
rainbow	3½ oz.	11.4	195	0
tuna				
albacore, raw	3½ oz.	7.5	177	0
bluefin, raw	3½ oz.	4.1	145	0
canned, light in oil	3½ oz.	8.1	197	0
canned, light in water	3½ oz.	0.8	115	0
canned, white in oil	3½ oz.	8.0	185	0
canned, white in water	3½ oz.	2.4	135	0
yellowfin, raw	3½ oz.	3.0	133	0
white perch	3½ oz.	3.9	114	0
whiting	3½ oz.	1.7	114	0
yellowtail	3½ oz.	5.4	138	0
FRUIT				
apple				
dried	½ cup	0.1	155	5
whole w/peel	1 medium	0.4	81	4
applesauce, unsweetened	½ cup	0.1	53	2
apricots				
dried	5 halves	0.2	83	6
fresh	3 medium	0.4	51	2

Item	Serving	Total Fat (g)	Calories	Fiber (g)
avocado				
California	1 (6 oz.)	30.0	306	4
Florida	1 (11 oz.)	27.0	339	4
banana	1 medium	0.6	105	2
banana chips	½ cup	15.5	240	4
blackberries				
fresh	1 cup	0.6	74	7
frzn, unsweetened	1 cup	0.7	97	7
blueberries				
fresh	1 cup	0.6	82	5
frzn, unsweetened	1 cup	0.7	80	4
boysenberries, frzn				
unsweetened	1 cup	0.4	66	6
breadfruit, fresh	¼ small	0.2	99	3
cantaloupe	1 cup	0.4	57	3
cherries				
maraschino	¼ cup	0.2	66	1
sour, canned in heavy syrup	½ cup	0.1	116	1
sweet	½ cup	0.7	49	2
cranberries, fresh	1 cup	0.2	46	4
cranberry-orange relish	½ cup	0.9	246	3
cranberry sauce	½ cup	0.2	209	1
dates, whole, dried	½ cup	0.4	228	8
figs				
canned	3 figs	0.1	75	9
dried, uncooked	10 figs	1.1	254	10
fresh	1 medium	0.2	37	2
fruit cocktail, canned w/juice	1 cup	0.3	112	5
grapefruit	½ medium	0.1	39	1
grapes, Thompson				
seedless	½ cup	0.1	94	1
guava, fresh	1 medium	0.5	45	7
honeydew melon, fresh	¼ small	0.1	46	1
kiwi, fresh	1 medium	0.3	46	2

Item	Serving	Total Fat (g)	Calories	Fiber (g)
kumquat, fresh	1 medium	0	12	1
lemon, fresh	1 medium	0.2	17	1
lime, fresh	1 medium	0.1	20	1
mandarin oranges, canned				
w/juice	½ cup	0	46	4
mango, fresh	1 medium	0.6	135	4
melon balls, frzn	1 cup	0.4	55	2
mixed fruit				
dried	½ cup	0.5	243	6
frzn, sweetened	1 cup	0.5	245	2
mulberries, fresh	1 cup	0.6	61	3
nectarine, fresh	1 medium	0.6	67	2
orange	1 medium	0.1	65	4
papaya, fresh	1 medium	0.4	117	3
passionfruit, purple, fresh	1 medium	0.1	18	3
peach				
canned in heavy syrup	1 cup	0.3	190	4
canned in light syrup	1 cup	0.1	136	4
fresh	1 medium	0.1	37	1
frzn, sweetened	1 cup	0.3	235	4
pear				
canned in heavy syrup	1 cup	0.3	188	6
canned in light syrup	1 cup	0.1	144	6
fresh	1 medium	0.7	98	5
persimmon, fresh	1 medium	0.1	32	3
pineapple pieces				
canned, unsweetened	1 cup	0.2	150	2
fresh	1 cup	0.7	77	3
plantain, cooked, sliced	1 cup	0.3	179	1
plum				
canned in heavy syrup	½ cup	0.1	119	4
fresh	1 medium	0.4	36	3
pomegranate, fresh	1 medium	0.5	104	2
prickly pear, fresh	1 medium	0.5	42	3

Item	Serving	Total Fat (g)	Calories	Fiber (g)
prunes, dried, cooked	½ cup	0.2	113	10
raisins				
dark seedless	¼ cup	0.2	112	3
golden seedless	¼ cup	0.2	113	3
raspberries				
fresh	1 cup	0.7	61	6
frzn, sweetened	1 cup	0.4	256	12
rhubarb, stewed, unsweetened	1 cup	0.2	26	6
star fruit/carambola	1 medium	0.4	42	2
strawberries				
fresh	1 cup	0.6	45	3
frzn, sweetened	1 cup	0.3	245	3
frzn, unsweetened	1 cup	0.2	52	3
sugar apples, fresh	1 medium	0.5	146	4
tangelo, fresh	1 medium	0.1	39	3
tangerine, fresh	1 medium	0.2	37	3
watermelon, fresh	1 cup	0.5	50	1
FRUIT JUICES AND NECTARS				
apple juice	1 cup	0.3	116	0
apricot nectar	1 cup	0.2	141	2
carrot juice	1 cup	0.4	97	2
cranberry juice cocktail				
low cal	1 cup	0	45	0
regular	1 cup	0.2	144	0
cranberry-apple juice	1 cup	0.2	170	0
grape juice	1 cup	0.2	128	1
grapefruit juice	1 cup	0.2	93	0
lemon juice	2 T	0	6	0
lime juice	2 T	0	6	0
orange-grapefruit juice	1 cup	0.2	107	1
orange juice	1 cup	0.4	105	1
peach juice or nectar	1 cup	0.1	134	1
pear juice or nectar	1 cup	0	149	1

Item	Serving	Total Fat (g)	Calories	Fiber (g)
pineapple juice	1 cup	0.2	139	1
pineapple-orange juice	1 cup	0.1	125	1
prune juice	1 cup	0.1	181	3
tomato juice	1 cup	0.2	43	2
V8 juice	1 cup	0.1	49	2
GRAVIES, SAUCES, AND DIPS				
au jus, mix	½ cup	0.7	16	0
barbecue sauce	1 T	0.3	12	0
béarnaise sauce, mix	¼ pkg.	25.6	263	0
beef gravy, canned	½ cup	2.8	62	0
brown gravy				
from mix	½ cup	0.9	38	0
hmde	¼ cup	14.0	164	0
catsup, tomato	1 T	0.1	16	0
chicken gravy				
canned	½ cup	6.8	95	0
from mix	½ cup	0.9	42	0
giblet, hmde	¼ cup	2.6	49	0
chili sauce	1 T	0	18	0
dip made with sour cream	2 T	6.0	67	0
guacamole dip	1 oz.	4.0	50	0
hollandaise sauce	¼ cup	18.0	170	0
home-style gravy, from mix	¼ cup	0.5	25	0
jalapeño dip	1 oz.	1.1	33	0
mushroom gravy				
canned	½ cup	3.2	60	1
from mix	½ cup	0.4	35	1
mushroom sauce, from mix	¼ pkg.	0.7	25	0
mustard				
brown	1 T	1.8	26	1
yellow	1 T	0.7	12	0
onion dip	2 T	6.0	67	0
onion gravy, from mix	½ cup	0.4	39	0

Item	Serving	Total Fat (g)	Calories	Fiber (g)
pesto sauce	½ cup	29.0	310	1
picante sauce	½ cup	0.8	53	2
pork gravy, from mix	½ cup	1.0	38	0
sour-cream sauce	¼ cup	7.6	128	0
soy sauce	1 T	0	10	0
soy sauce, reduced sodium	1 T	0	10	0
spaghetti sauce				
"healthy"/"lite" varieties	½ cup	1.0	60	3
hmde, w/ground beef	½ cup	8.3	145	2
Marinara	½ cup	4.7	95	3
meat flavor, jar	½ cup	6.0	100	2
meatless, jar	½ cup	2.0	70	2
mushroom, jar	½ cup	2.0	70	2
spinach dip (sour cream & mayo)	2 T	7.1	74	1
steak sauce				
A-1	1 T	0	10	0
others	1 T	0	18	0
stroganoff sauce, mix	¼ pkg.	2.9	73	0
sweet & sour sauce	¼ cup	0.1	60	0
tabasco sauce	1 t	0	1	0
taco sauce	1 T	0	5	0
tartar sauce	1 T	8.2	74	0
teriyaki sauce	1 T	0	15	0
turkey gravy				
canned	½ cup	2.4	58	0
from mix	½ cup	0.9	43	0
white sauce	¼ cup	6.8	90	0
Worcestershire sauce	1 T	0	10	0

MEATS (all cooked w/o added fat
  unless otherwise noted)
beef, extra lean, < 5% fat by
  weight (cooked)
    Healthy Choice lean ground

Item	Serving	Total Fat (g)	Calories	Fiber (g)
beef	3½ oz.	3.5	114	0
round, eye of, lean	3½ oz.	4.2	155	0
beef, lean, 5–10% fat by weight (cooked)				
arm/blade, lean pot roast	3½ oz.	9.4	207	0
flank steak, fat trimmed	3½ oz.	8.0	193	0
hindshank, lean	3½ oz.	9.4	207	0
porterhouse steak, lean	3½ oz.	10.4	225	0
rib steak, lean	3½ oz.	9.4	207	0
round				
bottom, lean	3½ oz.	9.4	207	0
roasted	3½ oz.	7.4	189	0
rump, lean, pot-roasted	3½ oz.	7.0	179	0
top, lean	3½ oz.	6.4	211	0
short plate, sep. lean only	3½ oz.	10.4	225	0
sirloin steak, lean	3½ oz.	8.9	201	0
sirloin tip, lean roasted	3½ oz.	9.4	207	0
tenderloin, lean, broiled	3½ oz.	11.1	219	0
top sirloin, lean, broiled	3½ oz.	7.9	201	0
beef, regular, 11–17.4% fat by weight (cooked)				
chuck, separable lean	3½ oz.	15.2	268	0
club steak, lean	3½ oz.	12.9	240	0
cubed steak	3½ oz.	15.4	264	0
hamburger				
extra lean	3 oz.	13.9	253	0
lean	3 oz.	15.7	268	0
rib roast, lean	3½ oz.	15.2	264	0
sirloin tips, roasted	3½ oz.	15.2	264	0
stew meat, round, raw	4 oz.	15.3	294	0
T-bone, lean only	3½ oz.	10.3	212	0
tenderloin, marbled	3½ oz.	15.2	264	0
beef, high fat,—17.4–27.4% fat by weight (cooked)				

Item	Serving	Total Fat (g)	Calories	Fiber (g)
arm/blade, pot-roasted	3½ oz.	26.5	354	0
chuck, ground	3½ oz.	23.9	327	0
hamburger, regular	3 oz.	19.6	286	0
meatballs	1 oz.	5.5	78	0
porterhouse steak lean &				
marbled	3½ oz.	19.6	286	0
rib steak	3½ oz.	14.7	286	0
rump, pot-roasted	3½ oz.	19.6	286	0
short ribs, lean	3½ oz.	19.6	286	0
sirloin, broiled	3½ oz.	18.7	278	0
sirloin, ground	3½ oz.	26.5	354	0
T-bone, broiled	3½ oz.	26.5	354	0
beef, highest fat, ≥ 27.5% fat by weight (cooked)				
brisket, lean & marbled	3½ oz.	30.0	367	0
chuck, stew meat	3½ oz.	30.0	367	0
corned, medium fat	3½ oz.	30.2	372	0
ribeye steak, marbled	3½ oz.	38.8	440	0
rib roast	3½ oz.	30.0	367	0
short ribs	3½ oz.	31.7	382	0
steak, chicken fried	3½ oz.	30.0	389	0
lamb				
blade chop				
lean	1 chop	6.4	128	0
lean & marbled	3½ oz.	26.1	380	0
leg				
lean	3½ oz.	8.1	180	0
lean & marbled	3½ oz.	14.5	242	0
loin chop				
lean	3½ oz.	8.1	180	0
lean & marbled	3½ oz.	22.5	302	0
rib chop				
lean	3½ oz.	8.1	180	0
lean & marbled	3½ oz.	21.2	292	0

Item	Serving	Total Fat (g)	Calories	Fiber (g)
shoulder				
lean	3½ oz.	9.9	248	0
lean & marbled	3½ oz.	27.0	430	0
miscellaneous meats				
bacon substitute (breakfast strip)	2 strips	4.8	50	0
beefalo	3½ oz.	6.3	188	0
frog legs				
cooked	4 large	0.3	73	0
flour-coated & fried	6 large	28.6	418	0
rabbit, stewed	3½ oz.	10.1	216	0
venison, roasted	3½ oz.	2.5	157	0
organ meats				
brains, all kinds, raw	3 oz.	7.4	106	0
heart				
beef, lean, braised	3½ oz.	5.6	175	0
kidney, beef, braised	3½ oz.	3.4	144	0
liver				
beef, braised	3½ oz.	4.9	161	0
beef, pan fried	3½ oz.	8.0	217	0
calf, braised	3½ oz.	6.9	165	0
calf, pan fried	3½ oz.	11.4	245	0
tongue				
beef, etc., pickled	1 oz.	5.8	76	0
beef, etc, potted	1 oz.	6.6	83	0
beef, med. fat, simmered	3 oz.	17.6	241	0
pork				
bacon				
cured, broiled	1 strip	3.1	35	0
cured, raw	1 oz.	16.3	158	0
blade				
lean	3½ oz.	9.6	219	0
lean & marbled	3½ oz.	18.0	290	0
Boston butt				
lean	3½ oz.	14.2	304	0

Item	Serving	Total Fat (g)	Calories	Fiber (g)
lean & marbled	3½ oz.	28.0	348	0
Canadian bacon, broiled	1 oz.	1.8	43	0
ham				
cured, butt, lean	3½ oz.	4.5	159	0
cured, butt, lean & marbled	3½ oz.	13.0	246	0
cured, canned	3 oz.	5.0	120	0
cured, shank, lean	3½ oz.	6.3	164	0
cured, shank, lean & marbled	2 slices	13.8	255	0
fresh, lean	3½ oz.	6.4	222	0
fresh, lean, marbled & fat	3½ oz.	18.3	306	0
ham loaf, glazed	3½ oz.	14.7	247	0
smoked	3½ oz.	7.0	140	0
smoked, 95% lean	3½ oz.	5.5	144	0
loin chop				
lean	1 chop	7.7	170	0
lean & fat	1 chop	22.5	314	0
picnic				
cured, lean	3½ oz.	9.9	211	0
fresh, lean	3½ oz.	7.4	150	0
shoulder, lean	2 slices	5.4	162	0
shoulder, marbled	2 slices	14.3	234	0
pig's feet, pickled	1 oz.	4.1	56	0
rib chop, trimmed	3½ oz.	9.9	209	0
rib roast, trimmed	3½ oz.	10.0	204	0
sausage				
brown and serve	1 oz.	9.4	105	0
patty	1	8.4	100	0
regular link	½ oz.	4.7	52	0
sirloin, lean, roasted	3½ oz.	10.2	207	0
spareribs roasted	6 medium	35.0	396	0
tenderloin, lean, roast	3½ oz.	4.8	155	0
top loin chop, trimmed	3½ oz.	7.7	193	0
top loin roast, trimmed	3½ oz.	7.5	187	0
processed meats				

Item	Serving	Total Fat (g)	Calories	Fiber (g)
bacon substitute				
(breakfast strips)	2 strips	4.8	50	0
beef, chipped	2 slices	1.1	47	0
beef breakfast strips	2 strips	7.0	100	0
beef jerky	1 oz.	3.6	90	0
bologna, beef/beef & pork	2 oz.	16.2	177	0
bratwurst				
pork	2 oz. link	22.0	256	0
pork & beef	2 oz. link	19.5	226	0
braunshweiger				
(pork liver sausage)	2 oz.	11.6	130	0
chicken roll	2 oz.	2.6	60	0
corn dog	1	20.0	330	0
corned beef, jellied	1 oz.	2.9	31	0
ham, chopped	1 oz.	2.3	55	0
hot dog/frank				
beef	1	13.2	145	0
chicken	1	8.8	116	0
97% fat free varieties	1	1.6	55	0
turkey	1	8.1	102	0
kielbasa (Polish sausage)	1 oz.	8.3	80	0
knockwurst/knackwurst	2 oz. link	18.9	209	0
liver pâté, goose	1 oz.	12.4	131	0
pepperoni	1 oz.	13.0	140	0
salami				
cooked	1 oz.	10.0	116	0
dry/hard	1 oz.	10.0	120	0
sausage				
Italian	2 oz. link	17.2	216	0
90% fat free varieties	2 oz.	4.6	86	0
Polish	2 oz. link	16.2	184	0
smoked	2 oz. link	20.0	229	0
Vienna	1 sausage	4.0	45	0
turkey breast, smoked	2 oz.	1.0	62	0

Item	Serving	Total Fat (g)	Calories	Fiber (g)
turkey ham	2 oz.	2.9	73	0
turkey loaf	2 oz.	1.0	62	0
turkey pastrami	2 oz.	3.5	80	0
turkey roll, light meat	2 oz.	4.1	83	0
turkey salami	2 oz.	7.8	110	0
veal				
arm steak				
lean	3½ oz.	4.8	180	0
lean & fat	3½ oz.	19.0	298	0
blade				
lean	3½ oz.	8.4	228	0
lean & fat	3½ oz.	16.6	276	0
breast, stewed	3½ oz.	18.6	256	0
chuck, med. fat, braised	3½ oz.	12.8	235	0
cutlet				
breaded	3½ oz.	15.0	319	0
round, lean	3½ oz.	12.8	194	0
round, lean & fat	3½ oz.	15.0	277	0
flank, med. fat, stewed	3½ oz.	32.0	390	0
foreshank, med. fat, stewed	3½ oz.	10.4	216	0
loin, med. fat, broiled	3½ oz.	13.4	234	0
loin chop				
lean	1 chop	4.8	149	0
lean & fat	3½ oz.	13.3	250	0
plate, med. fat, stewed	3½ oz.	21.2	303	0
rib chop				
lean	1 chop	4.6	125	0
lean & fat	1 chop	18.4	264	0
rump, marbled, roasted	3½ oz.	11.0	225	0
sirloin				
lean, roasted	3½ oz.	3.4	175	0
marbled, roasted	3½ oz.	6.5	181	0
sirloin steak				
lean	3½ oz.	6.0	204	0
lean & fat	3½ oz.	20.4	305	0

Item	Serving	Total Fat (g)	Calories	Fiber (g)
MILK AND YOGURT				
buttermilk				
1% fat	1 cup	2.2	99	0
dry	1 T	0.4	25	0
choc. milk				
2% fat	1 cup	5.0	179	0
whole	1 cup	8.5	250	0
condensed milk, sweetened	½ cup	13.3	441	0
evaporated milk				
skim	½ cup	0.4	100	0
whole	½ cup	9.5	169	0
hot cocoa				
low cal, mix w/water	1 cup	0.8	50	0
mix w/water	1 cup	3.0	110	0
w/skim milk	1 cup	2.0	158	0
w/whole milk	1 cup	9.1	218	0
low fat milk				
½% fat	1 cup	1.0	90	0
1% fat	1 cup	2.6	102	0
1.5% fat/acidophilus	1 cup	4.0	110	0
2% fat	1 cup	4.7	121	0
malt powder	1 T	1.6	86	0
malted milk	1 cup	9.9	236	0
milkshake				
choc. thick	1 cup	6.1	267	1
soft serve	1 cup	7.0	218	1
vanilla, thick	1 cup	6.9	255	0
skim milk				
liquid	1 cup	0.4	86	0
nonfat dry powder	¼ cup	0.2	109	0
whole milk				
3.5% fat	1 cup	8.2	150	0
dry powder	¼ cup	8.6	159	0
yogurt				
coffee/vanilla, low fat	1 cup	2.8	194	0

Item	Serving	Total Fat (g)	Calories	Fiber (g)
frzn, low fat	½ cup	3.0	115	0
frzn, nonfat	½ cup	0.2	81	0
fruit flavored, low fat	1 cup	2.6	225	0
plain				
low fat	1 cup	3.5	144	0
skim (nonfat)	1 cup	0.4	127	0
whole milk	1 cup	7.4	139	0
MISCELLANEOUS				
baking powder	1 t	0	3	0
baking soda	1 t	0	0	0
bouillon cube, beef or chicken	1	0.2	9	0
chewing gum	1 stick	0	10	0
choc., baking	1 oz.	15.7	148	1
cocoa, dry	⅓ cup	3.6	115	2
gelatin, dry	1 pkg.	0	23	0
honey	1 T	0	64	0
horseradish, prepared	1 t	0	2	0
icing, decorator	1 t	2.0	70	0
jam or jelly	1 T	0	50	0
marmalade, citrus	1 T	0	51	0
meat tenderizer	1 t	0	2	0
molasses	1 T	0	50	0
olives				
black	2 large	4.0	37	1
Greek	3 medium	7.1	67	1
green	2 medium	1.6	15	0
pickle relish				
chow chow	1 oz.	0.4	8	0
sweet	1 T	0.1	21	0
pickles				
bread & butter	4 slices	0.1	18	0
dill or sour	1 large	0.1	12	1
Kosher	1 oz.	0.1	7	0
sweet	1 oz.	0.4	146	0

Item	Serving	Total Fat (g)	Calories	Fiber (g)
salt	1 t	0	0	0
spices/seasonings	1 t	0.2	5	0
sugar, all varieties	1 T	0	46	0
sugar substitutes	1 packet	0	4	0
syrup, all varieties	1 T	0	60	0
vinegar	1 T	0	2	0
yeast	1 T	0	23	0
NUTS AND SEEDS				
almond paste	1 T	4.5	80	1
almonds	12–15	9.3	104	1
Brazil nuts	4 medium	11.5	114	1
cashews, roasted	6–8	7.8	94	2
chestnuts, fresh	3 small	0.8	66	4
coconut, dried, shredded	⅓ cup	9.2	135	1
hazelnuts (filberts)	10–12	10.6	106	1
macadamia nuts, roasted	6 medium	12.3	117	1
mixed nuts				
w/peanuts	8–12	10.0	109	2
w/o peanuts	2 T	10.1	110	2
peanut butter, creamy or chunky	1 T	8.0	94	1
peanuts				
chopped	2 T	8.9	104	2
honey roasted	2 T	8.9	112	2
in shell	1 cup	17.7	209	3
pecans	2 T	9.1	90	1
pine nuts (pignolia)	2 T	9.1	85	2
pistachios	2 T	7.7	92	1
poppy seeds	1 T	3.8	44	1
pumpkin seeds	2 T	7.9	93	1
sesame nut mix	2 T	5.1	65	1
sesame seeds	2 T	8.8	94	1
sunflower seeds	2 T	8.9	102	1
trail mix w/seeds, nuts, carob	2 T	5.1	87	1
walnuts	2 T	7.7	80	1

Item	Serving	Total Fat (g)	Calories	Fiber (g)
PASTA AND RICE (all measurements after cooking unless otherwise noted; 2 oz. uncooked pasta = ~ 1 cup cooked)				
macaroni				
semolina	1 cup	0.7	210	1
whole wheat	1 cup	2.0	210	5
noodles				
Alfredo	1 cup	29.7	462	3
cellophone, fried	1 cup	4.2	141	0
chow mein, canned	½ cup	8.0	150	0
egg	1 cup	2.4	212	1
manicotti	1 cup	1.0	210	1
ramen, all varieties	1 cup	8.0	190	1
rice	1 cup	0.3	140	1
romanoff	1 cup	23.0	372	3
rice				
brown	½ cup	0.6	116	2
fried	½ cup	7.2	181	1
long grain & wild	½ cup	2.1	120	2
pilaf	½ cup	7.0	170	1
Spanish style	½ cup	2.1	106	1
white	½ cup	1.2	111	0
spaghetti, enriched	1 cup	1.0	210	1
POULTRY				
chicken				
breast				
w/skin, fried	½ breast	10.7	236	0
w/o skin, fried	½ breast	6.1	179	0
w/skin, roasted	½ breast	7.6	193	0
w/o skin, roasted	½ breast	3.1	142	0
fryers				

Item	Serving	Total Fat (g)	Calories	Fiber (g)
w/skin, batter dipped, fried	3½ oz.	17.4	289	0
w/o skin, fried	3½ oz.	11.1	237	0
w/skin, roasted	3½ oz.	13.6	239	0
w/o skin, roasted	3½ oz.	7.4	190	0
giblets, fried	3½ oz.	13.5	277	0
gizzard, simmered	3½ oz.	3.7	153	0
heart, simmered	3½ oz.	7.9	185	0
leg				
w/skin, fried	1 leg	8.7	120	0
w/skin, roasted	1 leg	5.8	112	0
w/o skin, roasted	1 leg	2.5	76	0
liver simmered	3½ oz.	5.5	157	0
roll, light meat	3½ oz.	7.4	159	0
stewers				
w/skin	3½ oz.	18.9	285	0
w/o skin	3½ oz.	11.9	237	0
thigh				
w/skin, fried	1 thigh	11.3	180	0
w/skin, roasted	1 thigh	9.6	153	0
w/o skin, roasted	1 thigh	5.7	109	0
wing				
w/skin, fried	1 wing	9.1	121	0
w/skin, roasted	1 wing	6.6	99	0
duck,				
w/skin, roasted	3½ oz.	28.4	337	0
w/o skin, roasted	3½ oz.	11.2	201	0
pheasant, w/ or w/o skin, cooked	3½ oz.	9.3	181	0
quail, w/o skin, cooked	3½ oz.	9.3	213	0
turkey				
breast				
barbecued	3½ oz.	3.2	140	0
honey roasted	3½ oz.	2.8	112	0
oven roasted	3½ oz.	3.2	120	0
smoked	3½ oz.	3.5	112	0

Item	Serving	Total Fat (g)	Calories	Fiber (g)
dark meat				
w/skin, roasted	3½ oz.	11.5	221	0
w/o skin, roasted	3½ oz.	7.2	187	0
ground	3½ oz.	13.3	219	0
ham, cured	3½ oz.	5.1	128	0
light meat				
w/skin, roasted	3½ oz.	8.3	197	0
w/o skin, roasted	3½ oz.	3.2	157	0
loaf, breast meat	3½ oz.	1.6	110	0
patties, breaded/fried	1 patty	16.9	266	0
roll, light meat	3½ oz.	7.2	147	0
sausage, cooked	1 oz.	3.4	50	0
SALAD DRESSINGS				
blue cheese				
fat free	1 T	0	10	0
low cal	1 T	1.9	27	0
regular	1 T	8.0	77	0
buttermilk, from mix	1 T	5.8	58	0
Caesar	1 T	7.0	70	0
French				
creamy	1 T	6.9	70	0
fat free	1 T	0	18	0
low cal	1 T	0.9	22	0
regular	1 T	6.4	67	0
garlic, from mix	1 T	9.2	85	0
Green Goddess				
low cal	1 T	2.0	27	0
regular	1 T	7.0	68	0
honey mustard	1 T	6.6	89	0
Italian				
creamy	1 T	5.5	54	0
fat free	1 T	0	6	0
low cal	1 T	1.5	16	0

Item	Serving	Total Fat (g)	Calories	Fiber (g)
regular zesty, from mix	1 T	9.2	85	0
Kraft, free	1 T	0	20	0
Kraft, reduced cal	1 T	1.0	25	0
mayonnaise type				
low cal	1 T	1.8	19	0
regular	1 T	4.9	57	0
oil & vinegar	1 T	7.5	69	0
ranch style, prep. w/mayo	1 T	6.0	58	0
Russian				
low cal	1 T	0.7	24	0
regular	1 T	7.8	76	0
sesame seed	1 T	6.9	68	0
sweet & sour	1 T	0.9	29	0
Thousand Island				
fat free	1 T	0	20	0
low cal	1 T	1.6	24	0
regular	1 T	5.6	59	0
SNACK FOODS				
bagel chips or crisps	1 oz.	4.0	130	1
Cheese Puffs, Cheetos	1 oz.	10.0	160	0
cheese straws	4 pieces	7.2	109	1
Chex snack mix, traditional	1 oz.	4	130	1
corn chips, Frito's				
barbecue	1 oz.	9.0	150	1
regular	1 oz.	10.0	160	1
corn nuts, all flavors	1 oz.	4.0	130	2
Cracker Jack	1 oz.	2.2	115	2
party mix (cereal, pretzels, nuts)	1 cup	23.0	312	3
popcorn				
air popped	1 cup	0.3	31	1
caramel	1 cup	4.5	150	1
microwave, "lite"	1 cup	1.0	27	1
microwave, plain	1 cup	3.0	47	1

Item	Serving	Total Fat (g)	Calories	Fiber (g)
microwave, w/butter	1 cup	4.5	61	1
popped w/oil	1 cup	3.1	55	1
pork rinds, Frito-Lay	1 oz.	9.3	151	0
potato chips				
individually	10 chips	8.0	113	0
baked, Lays	1 oz.	1.5	110	2
by weight	1 oz.	11.2	159	1
barbecue flavor	1 oz.	9.5	149	1
potato sticks	1 oz.	10.2	152	0
pretzels	1 oz.	1.0	110	1
rice cakes	1	0	35	0
tortilla chips				
Doritos	1 oz.	6.6	139	1
no oil, baked	1 oz.	1.5	110	1
Tostitos	1 oz.	7.8	145	1
WOW chips, Frito-Lay	1 oz.	0	75	1
SOUPS				
asparagus				
cream of, w/milk	1 cup	8.2	161	1
cream of, w/water	1 cup	4.1	87	1
bean				
w/bacon	1 cup	5.9	173	4
w/franks	1 cup	7.0	187	3
w/ham	1 cup	8.5	231	3
w/o meat	1 cup	3.0	142	5
beef				
broth	1 cup	0.5	33	0
chunky	1 cup	5.1	171	2
beef barley	1 cup	1.1	72	1
beef noodle	1 cup	3.1	84	1
black bean	1 cup	1.5	116	2
broccoli, creamy w/water	1 cup	2.8	69	1

Item	Serving	Total Fat (g)	Calories	Fiber (g)
Campbell's Healthy Request				
chicken, cream of, w/water	1 cup	2.5	80	0
mushroom, cream of, w/water	1 cup	3.0	70	0
tomato, w/water	1 cup	2.0	90	0
canned vegetable type, w/o meat	1 cup	1.6	59	1
cheese w/milk	1 cup	14.6	230	0
chicken				
chunky	1 cup	6.6	178	2
cream of, w/milk	1 cup	11.5	191	0
cream of, w/water	1 cup	7.4	116	0
chicken & dumplings	1 cup	5.5	97	0
chicken & stars	1 cup	1.8	55	1
chicken & wild rice	1 cup	2.3	76	1
chicken/beef noodle or veg.	1 cup	3.1	83	1
chicken gumbo	1 cup	1.4	56	1
chicken mushroom	1 cup	9.2	132	1
chicken noodle				
chunky	1 cup	5.2	149	2
w/water	1 cup	2.5	75	0
chicken vegetable				
chunky	1 cup	4.8	167	2
w/water	1 cup	2.8	74	1
chicken w/noodles, chunky	1 cup	5.0	180	2
chicken w/rice				
chunky	1 cup	3.2	127	2
w/water	1 cup	1.9	60	1
clam chowder				
Manhattan chunky	1 cup	3.4	133	1
New England	1 cup	6.6	163	1
consommé w/ gelatin	1 cup	0	29	0
crab	1 cup	1.5	76	1
dehydrated				
bean w/bacon	1 cup	3.5	105	2

Item	Serving	Total Fat (g)	Calories	Fiber (g)
beef broth cube	1 cube	0.3	6	0
beef noodle	1 cup	0.8	41	0
chicken, cream of	1 cup	5.3	107	1
chicken broth cube	1 cube	0.2	9	0
chicken noodle	1 cup	1.2	53	0
chicken rice	1 cup	1.4	60	0
clam chowder				
Manhattan	1 cup	1.6	65	1
New England	1 cup	3.7	95	0
minestrone	1 cup	1.7	79	0
mushroom	1 cup	4.9	96	0
onion				
dry mix	1 pkg.	2.3	115	1
prepared	1 cup	0.6	28	0
tomato	1 cup	2.4	102	0
vegetable beef	1 cup	1.1	53	0
gazpacho	1 cup	0.2	40	2
hmde or restaurant style				
beer cheese	1 cup	23.1	308	1
cauliflower, cream of w/whole				
milk	1 cup	9.7	165	1
celery, cream of, w/whole milk	1 cup	10.6	165	1
chicken broth	1 cup	1.4	38	0
clam chowder				
Manhattan	1 cup	2.2	76	2
New England	1 cup	14.0	271	1
corn chowder, traditional	1 cup	12.0	251	3
fish chowder, w/whole milk	1 cup	13.5	285	1
gazpacho, traditional	1 cup	7.0	100	2
hot & sour	1 cup	7.1	134	1
mock turtle	1 cup	15.5	246	2
onion, French w/o cheese	1 cup	5.8	114	0
oyster stew, w/whole milk	1 cup	17.7	268	0
seafood gumbo	1 cup	3.9	155	3

Item	Serving	Total Fat (g)	Calories	Fiber (g)
lentil	1 cup	1.0	161	3
minestrone				
chunky	1 cup	2.8	127	2
w/water	1 cup	2.5	83	1
mushroom, cream of				
condensed	1 can	23.1	313	1
w/milk	1 cup	13.6	203	1
w/water	1 cup	9.0	129	1
mushroom barley	1 cup	2.3	76	1
mushroom w/beef stock	1 cup	4.0	85	1
onion	1 cup	1.7	57	1
oyster stew, w/water	1 cup	3.8	59	1
pea				
green, w/water	1 cup	2.9	164	2
split	1 cup	0.6	58	1
split w/ham	1 cup	4.4	189	1
potato, cream of				
w/milk	1 cup	7.4	157	2
shrimp, cream of, w/milk	1 cup	9.3	165	1
tomato				
w/milk	1 cup	6.0	160	1
w/water	1 cup	1.9	86	0.5
tomato beef w/noodle	1 cup	4.3	140	1
tomato bisque w/milk	1 cup	6.6	198	1
tomato rice	1 cup	2.7	120	1
turkey, chunky	1 cup	4.4	136	2
turkey noodle	1 cup	2.0	69	1
turkey vegetable	1 cup	3.0	74	1
vegetable, chunky	1 cup	3.7	122	2
vegetable w/beef, chunky	1 cup	3.0	134	2
vegetable w/beef broth	1 cup	1.9	80	1
vegetarian vegetable	1 cup	1.2	73	1
wonton	1 cup	1.0	40	1

Item	Serving	Total Fat (g)	Calories	Fiber (g)
VEGETABLES				
alfalfa sprouts, raw	½ cup	0.1	5	0
artichoke, boiled	1 medium	0.2	53	3
artichoke hearts, boiled	½ cup	0.1	37	3
asparagus, cooked	½ cup	0.3	22	2
avocado				
California	1 (6 oz.)	30.0	306	4
Florida	1 (11 oz.)	27.0	339	4
bamboo shoots, raw	½ cup	0.2	21	2
beans				
all types, cooked w/o fat	½ cup	0.4	143	9
baked, brown sugar & molasses	½ cup	1.5	132	4
baked, vegetarian	½ cup	0.6	118	5
baked w/pork & tomato sauce	½ cup	1.3	123	5
homestyle, canned	½ cup	1.6	132	5
beets, pickled	½ cup	0.1	75	4
black-eyed peas				
(cowpeas), cooked	½ cup	0.6	100	2
broccoli				
cooked	½ cup	0.3	22	7
frzn, chopped, cooked	½ cup	0.1	25	2
frzn in butter sauce	½ cup	1.5	50	2
frzn w/cheese sauce	½ cup	6.2	116	1
raw	½ cup	0.2	12	1
brussels sprouts, cooked	½ cup	0.4	30	2
butter beans, canned	½ cup	0.4	76	4
cabbage				
Chinese, raw	1 cup	0.2	10	2
green, cooked	½ cup	0.1	16	2
red, raw, shredded	½ cup	0.1	10	2
carrot				
cooked	½ cup	0.1	35	2
raw	1 large	0.1	31	2

Item	Serving	Total Fat (g)	Calories	Fiber (g)
cauliflower				
cooked	1 cup	0.2	30	3
frzn w/cheese sauce	½ cup	4.8	75	1
raw	1 cup	0.1	12	4
celery				
cooked	½ cup	0.1	13	1
raw	1 stalk	0.1	6	1
chard, cooked	½ cup	0.1	18	2
chilies, green	¼ cup	0	10	0
Chinese-style vegetables, frzn	½ cup	4.0	74	3
chives, raw, chopped	1 T	0	1	0
collard greens, cooked	½ cup	0.1	13	2
corn				
corn on the cob	1 medium	1.0	120	4
cream style, canned	½ cup	0.5	93	4
frzn, cooked	½ cup	0.1	67	4
frzn w/butter sauce	½ cup	2.2	110	3
whole kernel, cooked	½ cup	1.1	89	5
cucumber				
w/skin	½ medium	0.2	20	1
w/o skin, sliced	½ cup	0.1	7	0
dandelion greens, cooked	½ cup	0.3	17	2
eggplant, cooked	½ cup	0.1	13	2
endive lettuce	1 cup	0.2	8	1
garbanzo beans				
(chick peas), cooked	½ cup	2.1	135	5
green beans				
french style, cooked	½ cup	0.2	26	2
snap, cooked	½ cup	0.2	22	2
hominy, white or yellow, cooked	1 cup	0.7	138	3
Italian-style vegetables, frzn	½ cup	5.5	102	2
kale, cooked	½ cup	0.3	21	2
kidney beans, red, cooked	½ cup	0.5	112	8

Item	Serving	Total Fat (g)	Calories	Fiber (g)
leeks, chopped, raw	¼ cup	0.1	16	1
lentils, cooked	½ cup	0.4	116	8
lettuce, leaf	1 cup	0.2	10	1
lima beans, cooked	½ cup	0.4	108	5
miso				
(soybean product)	½ cup	8.4	284	4
mushrooms				
canned	½ cup	0.2	19	1
fried/sautéed	4 medium	7.4	90	1
raw	½ cup	0.2	9	1
mustard greens, cooked	½ cup	0.2	11	2
okra, cooked	½ cup	0.1	25	3
onions				
canned, french-fried	1 oz.	15.0	175	0
chopped, raw	½ cup	0.1	30	1
parsley, chopped, raw	¼ cup	0.1	5	0
parsnips, cooked	½ cup	0.2	63	3
peas, green, cooked	½ cup	0.2	67	4
pepper, bell, chopped, raw	½ cup	0.1	13	2
pimentos, canned	1 oz.	0	10	0
potato				
au gratin				
from mix	½ cup	6.0	140	2
hmde	½ cup	9.3	160	1
baked w/skin	1 medium	0.2	220	4
boiled w/o skin	½ cup	0.1	116	2
french fries				
frzn	10 pieces	4.4	111	2
hmde	10 pieces	8.3	158	1
hash browns	½ cup	10.9	163	2
knishes	1	3.2	73	1
mashed				
from flakes, w/milk & marg	½ cup	6.0	130	1
w/milk & marg.	½ cup	4.4	111	1

Item	Serving	Total Fat (g)	Calories	Fiber (g)
pan fried, O'Brien	½ cup	15.0	231	3
potato pancakes	1 cake	12.6	237	1
potato puffs, frzn, prep. w/oil	½ cup	11.6	183	3
scalloped				
from mix	1 serving	5.9	127	1
hmde	½ cup	4.8	105	1
w/cheese	½ cup	9.7	177	1
twice-baked potato, w/cheese	1 medium	11.8	370	4
pumpkin, canned	½ cup	0.3	41	4
radish, raw	10	0.2	7	1
rhubarb, raw	1 cup	0.2	29	2
sauerkraut, canned	½ cup	0.2	22	4
scallions, raw	5 medium	0.2	60	4
soybeans, mature, cooked	½ cup	7.7	149	4
spinach				
cooked	½ cup	0.2	21	3
creamed	½ cup	5.1	79	3
raw	1 cup	0.2	12	3
squash				
acorn				
baked	½ cup	0.1	57	4
mashed w/o fat	½ cup	0.1	41	3
butternut, cooked	½ cup	0.1	41	4
summer				
cooked	½ cup	0.3	18	2
raw, slice	½ cup	0.1	13	1
winter, cooked	½ cup	0.6	39	4
succotash, cooked	½ cup	0.8	111	3
sweet potato				
baked	1 small	0.1	118	7
candied	½ cup	3.4	144	5
mashed w/o fat	½ cup	0.5	172	5
tempeh (soybean product)	½ cup	6.4	165	1
tofu (soybean curd), raw	4 oz.	5.4	90	1

Item	Serving	Total Fat (g)	Calories	Fiber (g)
tomato				
boiled	½ cup	0.5	32	1
raw	1 medium	0.4	26	1
stewed	½ cup	0.2	34	1
tomato paste, canned	½ cup	1.2	110	4
turnip greens, cooked	½ cup	0.2	15	2
turnips, cooked	½ cup	0.1	14	2
water chestnuts, canned, sliced	½ cup	0	35	1
watercress, raw	½ cup	0	2	0
wax beans, canned	½ cup	0.2	25	2
yam, boiled/baked	½ cup	0.1	79	3
zucchini, cooked	½ cup	0.1	14	2
VEGETABLE SALADS				
Caesar salad w/o anchovies	1 cup	7.2	80	1
carrot-raisin salad	½ cup	5.8	153	4
chef salad w/o dressing	1 cup	4.2	65	1
coleslaw				
w/mayo-type dressing	½ cup	14.2	147	1
w/vinaigrette	½ cup	3.0	78	1
gelatin salad w/fruit & cheese	½ cup	4.6	74	0
macaroni salad w/mayo	½ cup	12.8	200	1
pasta primavera salad	1 cup	5.9	149	3
potato salad				
German style	½ cup	3.5	140	1
w/mayo dressing	½ cup	11.5	189	1
salad bar items				
alfalfa sprouts	2 T	0	2	0
bacon bits	1 T	1.0	21	0
beets, pickled	2 T	0	18	0
broccoli, raw	2 T	0	3	0
carrots, raw	2 T	0	6	0
cheese, shredded	2 T	4.6	56	0
chickpeas	2 T	0.3	36	1

Item	Serving	Total Fat (g)	Calories	Fiber (g)
cottage cheese	½ cup	5.1	116	0
croutons	½ oz.	2.6	62	0
cucumber	2 T	0	2	0
eggs, cooked, chopped	2 T	1.9	27	0
lettuce	½ cup	0	4	0
mushrooms, raw	2 T	0	2	0
onion, raw	2 T	0.1	7	0
pepper, green, raw	2 T	0	3	0
potato salad	½ cup	10.3	179	0
tomato, raw	2 slices	0	2	0
seven-layer salad	1 cup	17.8	226	2
tabbouli salad	½ cup	9.5	173	3
taco salad w/taco sauce	1 cup	14.0	202	2
three-bean salad	½ cup	8.2	145	3
three-bean salad, w/o oil	½ cup	0.2	90	3
Waldorf salad w/mayo	½ cup	12.7	157	2

Additional Items	Total Fat (g)	Calories	Fiber (g)

Index

Note: Page numbers in **boldface** refer to recipes

770701